Arthritis Sourcebook

Basic Information about Specific Forms of Arthritis and Related Rheumatic Disorders, Including Rheumatoid Arthritis, Osteoarthritis, Gout, Polymyalgia Rheumatica, Psoriatic Arthritis, Spondyloarthropathies, Juvenile Rheumatoid Arthritis, and Juvenile Ankylosing Spondylitis; Along with Information about Medical, Surgical, and Alternative Treatment Options and Including Strategies for Coping with Pain, Fatigue, and Stress

Edited by Allan R. Cook. 600 pages. 1998. 0-7808-0201-2. $78.

Back & Neck Disorders Sourcebook

Basic Information about Disorders and Injuries of the Spinal Cord and Vertebrae, Including Facts on Chiropractic Treatment, Surgical Interventions, Paralysis, and Rehabilitation, Along with Advice for Preventing Back Trouble

Edited by Karen Bellenir. 548 pages. 1997. 0-7808-0202-0. $78.

"The strength of this work is its basic, easy-to-read format. Recommended."
— *Reference and User Services Quarterly, Winter '97*

Blood & Circulatory Disorders Sourcebook

Basic Information about Blood and Its Components, Anemias, Leukemias, Bleeding Disorders, and Circulatory Disorders, Including Aplastic Anemia, Thalassemia, Sickle-Cell Disease, Hemochromatosis, Hemophilia, Von Willebrand Disease, and Vascular Diseases; Along with a Special Section on Blood Transfusions and Blood Supply Safety, a Glossary, and Source Listings for Further Help and Information

Edited by Karen Bellenir and Linda M. Shin. 575 pages. 1998. 0-7808-0203-9. $78.

Burns Sourcebook

Basic Information about Various Types of Burns and Scalds, Including Flame, Heat, Electrical, Chemical, and Sun; Along with Short- and Long-Term Treatments, Tissue Reconstruction, Plastic Surgery, Prevention Suggestions, and First Aid

Edited by Allan R. Cook. 600 pages. 1998. 0-7808-0204-7. $78.

Cancer Sourcebook, 1st Edition

Basic Information on Cancer Types, Symptoms, Diagnostic Methods, and Treatments, Including Statistics on Cancer Occurrences Worldwide and the Risks Associated with Known Carcinogens and Activities

Edited by Frank E. Bair. 932 pages. 1990. 1-55888-888-8. $78.

"Written in nontechnical language. Useful for patients, their families, medical professionals, and librarians."
— *Guide to Reference Books, '96*

"Designed with the non-medical professional in mind. Libraries and medical facilities interested in patient education should certainly consider adding the *Cancer Sourcebook* to their holdings. This compact collection of reliable information . . . is an invaluable tool for helping patients and patients' families and friends to take the first steps in coping with the many difficulties of cancer."
— *Medical Reference Services Quarterly, Winter '91*

"Specifically created for the nontechnical reader . . . an important resource for the general reader trying to understand the complexities of cancer."
— *American Reference Books Annual, '91*

"This publication's nontechnical nature and very comprehensive format make it useful for both the general public and undergraduate students." — *Choice, Oct '90*

New Cancer Sourcebook, 2nd Edition

Basic Information about Major Forms and Stages of Cancer, Featuring Facts about Primary and Secondary Tumors of the Respiratory, Nervous, Lymphatic, Circulatory, Skeletal, and Gastrointestinal Systems, and Specific Organs; Statistical and Demographic Data; Treatment Options; and Strategies for Coping

Edited by Allan R. Cook. 1,313 pages. 1996. 0-7808-0041-9. $78.

"This book is an excellent resource for patients with newly diagnosed cancer and their families. The dialogue is simple, direct, and comprehensive. Highly recommended for patients and families to aid in their understanding of cancer and its treatment"
— *Booklist Health Sciences Supplement, Oct '97*

"The amount of factual and useful information is extensive. The writing is very clear, geared to general readers. Recommended for all levels." — *Choice, Jan '97*

Cancer Sourcebook for Women

Basic Information about Specific Forms of Cancer That Affect Women, Featuring Facts about Breast Cancer, Cervical Cancer, Ovarian Cancer, Cancer of the Uterus and Uterine Sarcoma, Cancer of the Vagina, and Cancer of the Vulva; Statistical and Demographic Data; Treatments, Self-Help Management Suggestions, and Current Research Initiatives

Edited by Allan R. Cook and Peter D. Dresser. 524 pages. 1996. 0-7808-0076-1. $78.

". . . written in easily understandable, non-technical language. Recommended for public libraries or hospital and academic libraries that collect patient education or consumer health materials."
— *Medical Reference Services Quarterly, Spring '97*

Cancer Sourcebook for Women *(Continued)*

"Would be of value in a consumer health library. . . . written with the health care consumer in mind. Medical jargon is at a minimum, and medical terms are explained in clear, understandable sentences."
— *Bulletin of the MLA, Oct '96*

"The availability under one cover of all these pertinent publications, grouped under cohesive headings, makes this certainly a most useful sourcebook."
— *Choice, Jun '96*

"Presents a comprehensive knowledge base for general readers. Men and women both benefit from the gold mine of information nestled between the two covers of this book. Recommended."
— *Academic Library Book Review, Summer '96*

"This timely book is highly recommended for consumer health and patient education collections in all libraries."
— *Library Journal, Apr '96*

Cardiovascular Diseases & Disorders Sourcebook

Basic Information about Cardiovascular Diseases and Disorders, Featuring Facts about the Cardiovascular System, Demographic and Statistical Data, Descriptions of Pharmacological and Surgical Interventions, Lifestyle Modifications, and a Special Section Focusing on Heart Disorders in Children

Edited by Karen Bellenir and Peter D. Dresser. 683 pages. 1995. 0-7808-0032-X. $78.

". . . comprehensive format provides an extensive overview on this subject."
— *Choice, Jun '96*

". . . an easily understood, complete, up-to-date resource. This well executed public health tool will make valuable information available to those that need it most, patients and their families. The typeface, sturdy non-reflective paper, and library binding add a feel of quality found wanting in other publications. Highly recommended for academic and general libraries. "
— *Academic Library Book Review, Summer '96*

Communication Disorders Sourcebook

Basic Information about Deafness and Hearing Loss, Speech and Language Disorders, Voice Disorders, Balance and Vestibular Disorders, and Disorders of Smell, Taste, and Touch

Edited by Linda M. Ross. 533 pages. 1996. 0-7808-0077-X. $78.

"This is skillfully edited and is a welcome resource for the layperson. It should be found in every public and medical library."
— *Booklist Health Sciences Supplement, Oct '97*

Congenital Disorders Sourcebook

Basic Information about Disorders Acquired during Gestation, Including Spina Bifida, Hydrocephalus, Cerebral Palsy, Heart Defects, Craniofacial Abnormalities, Fetal Alcohol Syndrome, and More, Along with Current Treatment Options and Statistical Data

Edited by Karen Bellenir. 607 pages. 1997. 0-7808-0205-5. $78.

"Recommended reference source." — *Booklist, Oct '97*

Consumer Issues in Health Care Sourcebook

Basic Information about Health Care Fundamentals and Related Consumer Issues, Including Exams and Screening Tests, Physician Specialties, Choosing a Doctor, Using Prescription and Over-the-Counter Medications Safely, Avoiding Health Scams, Managing Common Health Risks in the Home, Care Options for Chronically or Terminally Ill Patients, and a List of Resources for Obtaining Help and Further Information

Edited by Karen Bellenir. 592 pages. 1998. 0-7808-0221-7. $78.

Contagious & Non-Contagious Infectious Diseases Sourcebook

Basic Information about Contagious Diseases like Measles, Polio, Hepatitis B, and Infectious Mononucleosis, and Non-Contagious Infectious Diseases like Tetanus and Toxic Shock Syndrome, and Diseases Occurring as Secondary Infections Such as Shingles and Reye Syndrome, Along with Vaccination, Prevention, and Treatment Information, and a Section Describing Emerging Infectious Disease Threats

Edited by Karen Bellenir and Peter D. Dresser. 566 pages. 1996. 0-7808-0075-3. $78.

Diabetes Sourcebook, 1st Edition

Basic Information about Insulin-Dependent and Noninsulin-Dependent Diabetes Mellitus, Gestational Diabetes, and Diabetic Complications, Symptoms, Treatment, and Research Results, Including Statistics on Prevalence, Morbidity, and Mortality, Along with Source Listings for Further Help and Information

Edited by Karen Bellenir and Peter D. Dresser. 827 pages. 1994. 1-55888-751-2. $78.

. . . very informative and understandable for the layperson without being simplistic. It provides a comprehensive overview for laypersons who want a general understanding of the disease or who want to focus on various aspects of the disease." — *Bulletin of the MLA, Jan '96*

Blood and Circulatory

DISORDERS SOURCEBOOK

Health Reference Series

AIDS Sourcebook, 1st Edition
AIDS Sourcebook, 2nd Edition
Allergies Sourcebook
Alternative Medicine Sourcebook
Alzheimer's, Stroke & 29 Other Neurological Disorders Sourcebook
Alzheimer's Disease Sourcebook, 2nd Edition
Arthritis Sourcebook
Back & Neck Disorders Sourcebook
Blood & Circulatory Disorders Sourcebook
Burns Sourcebook
Cancer Sourcebook, 1st Edition
New Cancer Sourcebook, 2nd Edition
Cancer Sourcebook for Women
Cardiovascular Diseases & Disorders Sourcebook
Communication Disorders Sourcebook
Congenital Disorders Sourcebook
Consumer Issues in Health Care Sourcebook
Contagious & Non-Contagious Infectious Diseases Sourcebook
Diabetes Sourcebook, 1st Edition
Diabetes Sourcebook, 2nd Edition
Diet & Nutrition Sourcebook, 1st Edition
Diet & Nutrition Sourcebook, 2nd Edition
Ear, Nose & Throat Disorders Sourcebook
Endocrine & Metabolic Disorders Sourcebook
Environmentally Induced Disorders Sourcebook
Fitness & Exercise Sourcebook
Food & Animal Borne Diseases Sourcebook
Gastrointestinal Diseases & Disorders Sourcebook
Genetic Disorders Sourcebook
Head Trauma Sourcebook
Health Insurance Sourcebook
Immune System Disorders Sourcebook
Kidney & Urinary Tract Diseases & Disorders Sourcebook
Learning Disabilities Sourcebook
Men's Health Concerns Sourcebook
Mental Health Disorders Sourcebook
Ophthalmic Disorders Sourcebook
Oral Health Sourcebook
Pain Sourcebook
Pregnancy & Birth Sourcebook
Public Health Sourcebook
Rehabilitation Sourcebook
Respiratory Diseases & Disorders Sourcebook
Sexually Transmitted Diseases Sourcebook
Skin Disorders Sourcebook
Sleep Disorders Sourcebook
Sports Injuries Sourcebook
Substance Abuse Sourcebook
Women's Health Concerns Sourcebook

Health Reference Series

First Edition

Blood and Circulatory
DISORDERS
SOURCEBOOK

*Basic Information about Blood and Its
Components, Anemias, Leukemias, Bleeding
Disorders, and Circulatory Disorders,
Including Aplastic Anemia, Thalassemia,
Sickle Cell Disease, Hemochromatosis,
Hemophilia, Von Willebrand Disease, and
Vascular Diseases; Along with a Special
Section on Blood Transfusions and Blood
Supply Safety, a Glossary, and Source
Listings for Further Help and Information*

Edited by
Linda M. Shin and Karen Bellenir

Omnigraphics, Inc.

Penobscot Building / Detroit, MI 48226

BIBLIOGRAPHIC NOTE

Because this page cannot legibly accommodate all the copyright notices, the Bibliographic Note portion of the Preface constitutes an extension of the copyright notice.

Beginning with books published in 1999, each new volume of the *Health Reference Series* will be individually titled and called a "First Edition." Subsequent updates will carry sequential edition numbers. To help avoid confusion and to provide maximum flexibility in our ability to respond to informational needs, the practice of consecutively numbering each volume will be discontinued.

Edited by Linda M. Shin and Karen Bellenir

Peter D. Dresser, Managing Editor, *Health Reference Series*
Karen Bellenir, Series Editor, *Health Reference Series*

Omnigraphics, Inc.

Matthew P. Barbour, *Manager, Production and Fulfillment*
Laurie Lanzen Harris, *Vice President, Editorial Director*
Peter E. Ruffner, *Vice President, Administration*
James A. Sellgren, *Vice President, Operations and Finance*
Jane J. Steele, *Marketing Consultant*

Frederick G. Ruffner, Jr., Publisher

©1999, Omnigraphics, Inc.

Library of Congress Cataloging-in-Publication Data

Blood and circulatory disorders sourcebook : basic information about blood and its components ... / edited by Linda M. Shin and Karen Bellenir. — 1st ed.
    p. cm. — (Health reference series : v. 39)
    Includes bibliographical references and index.
    ISBN 0-7808-0203-9 (lib. bdg. : alk. paper)
    1. Blood—Diseases—Popular works. I. Shin, Linda M. II. Bellenir, Karen. III. Series.
RC636.B556 1998
616.1'5—dc21   98-33704
                                                        CIP

∞
This book is printed on acid-free paper meeting the ANSI Z39.48 Standard. The infinity symbol that appears above indicates that the paper in this book meets that standard.

Printed in the United States

Table of Contents

Part III: Leukemias

Part IV: Bleeding Disorders

Part V: Circulatory Disorders

Preface

About This Book

Blood is a living tissue composed of many parts, each of which serves a vital function. The typical adult male has approximately 12 pints of blood in his body; on average an adult female has about nine pints. Disorders that affect the blood's ability to carry oxygen, nourishment, hormones, antibodies, and many other important compounds to other body tissues can have serious health consequences. Diseases of the veins and arteries may cause damage or blockage in blood vessels, which can lessen blood flow; diseases of the blood itself take many forms.

Anemias are the most common form of blood disorder. They occur when the amount of hemoglobin in the blood decreases. Hemoglobin, the red-colored substance in red blood cells, takes oxygen from the lungs and carries it through the bloodstream to all the body's tissues. Other blood and circulatory disorders include bleeding disorders, leukemias, and vascular diseases. Treatment for many blood disorders may include transfusion regimes or even bone marrow transplantation.

This *Sourcebook* provides information so that the layperson can identify early warning signs of blood and circulatory disorders such as aplastic anemia, thalassemia, sickle cell disease, hemochromatosis, leukemia, hemophilia, von Willebrand disease, vascular disease, aneurysms, and thrombosis. In addition to describing common blood and circulatory disorders, it provides answers to questions about blood donation and the safety of the U.S. blood supply. A glossary and a list of resources for further help and information are also provided.

How to Use This Book

This book is divided into parts and chapters. Parts focus on broad areas of interest. Chapters are devoted to single topics within a part.

Part I: Blood Components and Bone Marrow Transplantation provides basic information about whole blood and blood components including red blood cells, white blood cells, platelets, and plasma. It describes the important role played by bone marrow in blood development, lists diseases for which bone marrow transplantation is a treatment option, and gives data about the bone marrow transplantation process.

Part II: Anemias and Other Hemoglobin Diseases describes the different types of anemias and hemoglobin diseases that result from infections or other diseases, medication problems, poor nutrition, and genetic factors. These include iron-deficiency anemia, pernicious anemia, aplastic anemia, Cooley's anemia (also called Thalassemia), sickle cell anemia, hemochromatosis, and immune thrombocytopenic purpura.

Part III: Leukemias gives an overview of leukemia, a type of cancer that affects the blood cells. It also offers specific information to patients with adult acute lymphocytic leukemia, childhood acute lymphocytic leukemia, chronic lymphocytic leukemia, chronic myelogenous leukemia, adult acute myeloid leukemia, childhood acute myeloid leukemia, and hairy-cell leukemia. In addition to the information presented here, readers with further questions about general cancer treatment options and concerns may wish to consult Omnigrahics' *New Cancer Sourcebook*.

Part IV: Bleeding Disorders provides information about hemophilia, von Willebrand disease, other clotting factor deficiencies, and thrombocytopenia. Additional information about heritable bleeding disorders can be found in Omnigraphics' *Genetic Disorders Sourcebook*.

Part V: Circulatory Disorders describes conditions that disrupt the body's ability to circulate blood efficiently and disorders that result from impaired circulation. These include peripheral vascular disease, thrombophlebitis, Buerger's disease (also known as thromboangiitis obliterans), Raynaud's phenomenon, varicose veins, venous ulcers, aneurysms, strokes, syncope (fainting), low blood pressure (hypotension), high blood pressure (hypertension), and high blood cholesterol which leads to hardening of the arteries (atherosclerosis). Additional information about circulatory disorders with cardiovascular implications can be found in Omnigraphics' *Cardiovascular Disorders Sourcebook*.

Part VI: Blood Transfusions and Blood Supply Safety supplies answers to questions about blood donation and the safety of the blood supply. Topics covered include whole blood transfusion, blood component transfusion, and alternatives to regular blood transfusion such as autologous transfusion (donating your own blood for planned surgical procedures), recycling blood during surgery, red cell conservation, and directed blood donations.

Part VII: Additional Help and Information provides a glossary of blood-related terminology and a list of resources for patients with blood and circulatory disorders.

Bibliographic Note

This volume contains documents and excerpts from publications issued by the following U.S. government agencies: Agency for Health Care Policy and Research (AHCPR), Federal Trade Commission (FTC), Food and Drug Administration (FDA), General Accounting Office (GAO), Health Resources and Services Administration (HRSA), National Cancer Institute (NCI), National Center for Research Resources (NCRR), National Heart, Lung, and Blood Institute (NHLBI), National Institute on Alcohol Abuse and Alcoholism (NIAAA), National Institute of Arthritis and Musculoskeletal and Skin Diseases (NIAMS), National Institute of Neurological Disorders and Stroke (NINDS), and National Institutes of Health (NIH) Consensus Development Program.

In addition, this volume contains copyrighted documents from the following organizations: American Association of Blood Banks, Aplastic Anemia Foundation of America, Cooley's Anemia Foundation, Hemochromatosis Foundation, MedicineNet, and the National Hemophilia Foundation. Copyrighted articles from *Current Science* and *Mayo Clinic Health Letter* are also included.

Acknowledgements

In addition to the many organizations and agencies who contributed the material that is included in this book, thanks go to Margaret Mary Missar for her tireless efforts in tracking down documents, Jenifer Swanson for her researching and internet expertise, and Dawn Matthews for her verification assistance.

Note from the Editor

This book is part of Omnigraphics' *Health Reference Series*. The series provides basic information about a broad range of medical concerns. It is not intended to serve as a tool for diagnosing illness, in prescribing treatments, or as a substitute for the physician/patient relationship. All persons concerned about medical symptoms or the possibility of disease are encouraged to seek professional care from an appropriate health care provider.

Health Reference Series *Update Policy*

The inaugural book in the *Health Reference Series* was the first edition of *Cancer Sourcebook* published in 1992. Since then, the *Series* has been enthusiastically received by librarians and in the medical community. In order to maintain the standard of providing high-quality health information for the lay person, the editorial staff at Omnigraphics felt it was necessary to implement a policy of updating volumes when warranted.

Medical researchers have been making tremendous strides, and the challenge to stay current with the most recent advances is one our editors take seriously. Each decision to update a volume will be made on an individual basis. Some of the considerations will include how much new information is available and the feedback we receive from people who use the books. If there's a topic you would like to see added to the update list, or an area of medical concern you feel has not been adequately addressed, please write to:

Editor
Health Reference Series
Omnigraphics, Inc.
2500 Penobscot Bldg.
Detroit, MI 48226

The commitment to providing on-going coverage of important medical developments has also led to some technical changes in the *Health Reference Series*. Beginning with books published in 1999, each new volume will be individually titled and called a "First Edition." Subsequent updates will carry sequential edition numbers. To help avoid confusion and to provide maximum flexibility in our ability to respond to informational needs, the practice of consecutively numbering each volume will be discontinued.

Part One

Blood Components and
Bone Marrow Transplantation

Chapter 1

Blood Development and Composition

Blood vessels reach every organ and tissue in the body, indicating that the blood and the integrity of the blood vessels are essential to maintaining the body's health and functioning. The blood's most important functions include transporting substances, such as oxygen, nutrients, waste products to be excreted, and chemical messengers; defending the body against foreign organisms and substances, such as bacteria, viruses, and fungi; and repairing injured blood vessels.

Blood cells make up about 45 percent of the blood volume; the remaining 55 percent consists of a watery liquid called plasma. In addition to water, plasma contains minerals; nutrients; regulatory substances, such as hormones; gases, such as oxygen and carbon dioxide; and proteins. These proteins include those involved in blood clotting as well as immune proteins (i.e., antibodies or immunoglobulins).

Blood Cells

Blood cells fall into three major categories, each of which has specific functions, as follows:

- **Red blood cells (RBCs),** also called erythrocytes, transport oxygen from the lungs to all the cells in the body and carry carbon dioxide from the cells back to the lungs.

National Institute on Alcohol Abuse and Alcoholism, *Alcohol Health & Research World*, Winter 1997.

- **White blood cells (WBCs),** or leukocytes, engage in the body's defense against foreign microorganisms or toxic substances as well as mediate the immune response.

- **Platelets** help maintain the integrity of the blood vessels by stimulating blood clotting (i.e., coagulation) after an injury and thereby stopping the bleeding.

The WBCs are subdivided further into three groups—granulocytes, monocytes and macrophages, and lymphocytes—each with specific functions. Granulocytes recognize and eliminate microorganisms, especially bacteria, by ingesting them. Several types of granulocytes exist. Cells of the most common type are called neutrophils. Monocytes (which circulate in the blood) and macrophages (monocytes that have entered the tissues) also ingest and destroy foreign organisms and substances. In addition, these cells display foreign proteins and other molecules (i.e., antigens) on their surface and thereby help activate the body's immune response. Lymphocytes, which mediate and regulate the immune response, consist of two main groups: T cells and B cells. T cells secrete messenger substances (i.e., cytokines) that activate and regulate the immune response. T cells also kill cells displaying foreign antigens on their surface (e.g., virus-infected or transplanted cells). B cells produce and secrete antibodies that can bind to foreign antigens. This binding often is required to initiate the elimination of foreign microorganisms.

Hematopoiesis

Although the different blood cells have distinct structures and functions, they are all produced at the same site, the bone marrow, in a complex process called hematopoiesis. Hematopoiesis involves the multiplication (i.e., proliferation) of precursor cells, their specialization (i.e., differentiation) into cells with a specific function (e.g., oxygen transport or antibody secretion), and their maturation into functional cells that eventually circulate in the blood. The production of all types of blood cells begins with undifferentiated precursor cells— so-called, pluripotent stem cells—that can develop into whichever cell type is needed at that time. Through a series of tightly regulated intermediary stages, these stem cells multiply, differentiate, and mature into hundreds of thousands of functional RBCs, WBCs, or platelets, which then can be released into the bloodstream.

4

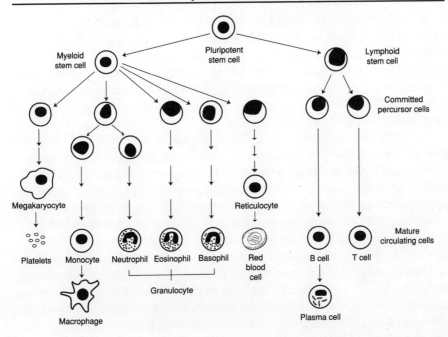

Figure 1.1. *Blood cell development. All types of circulating blood cells develop from a pluripotent stem cell. Under the influence of certain proteins (i.e., growth factors), this stem cell multiplies and differentiates into increasingly committed precursor cells. Through several intermediate states, these precursors differentiate further and develop into the mature cells circulating in the blood or residing in the tissues.*

Detection of Blood Disorders

To detect blood disorders, physicians frequently examine small blood samples (known as blood smears) under a microscope and assess the appearance, size, and number of the various blood cells. Each type of blood cell has a characteristic appearance that allows its identification in blood samples. Moreover, the proportion of the different cell types in the blood is relatively constant. Consequently, physicians can diagnose many blood disorders based on changes in the appearance or proportion of certain blood cells. For example, stomatocytosis (an RBC disorder associated with alcoholism) is characterized by abnormal, mouth-shaped RBCs.

Another way to identify blood disorders is to perform a complete blood count (CBC), in which a machine counts all the cells within a blood sample. In addition, these machines can determine several other parameters of blood cells, such as their average size, which may be diagnostic for certain disorders. For example, an increase in the average RBC volume (i.e., the mean corpuscular volume—MCV) is characteristic for a certain type of anemia.

Many blood disorders result from impaired or abnormal production of blood cells. These disorders can be diagnosed by microscopic analysis of bone marrow samples. (Bone marrow samples can be obtained by withdrawing tissue from the bone's interior with a needle or by removing a small "core" of marrow.) This type of diagnosis allows the physician to determine the overall number of cells in the bone marrow as well as the proportion of abnormal cells. Moreover, because each of the intermediary precursors of the various blood cell types has a characteristic appearance that can be discerned during microscopic examination, physicians can identify certain blood disorders based on the number and type of specific precursors in the marrow. For example, different types of leukemia are characterized by the accumulation in the bone marrow of WBC precursors at specific developmental stages.

—by Susanne Hiller-Sturmhöfel

Susanne Hiller-Sturmhöfel is a science editor of *Alcohol Health & Research World*.

Chapter 2

Facts about Blood

Whole Blood and Blood Components

Background

Whole blood is a living tissue that circulates through the heart, arteries, veins, and capillaries carrying nourishment, electrolytes, hormones, vitamins, antibodies, heat, and oxygen to the body's tissues. Whole blood contains red blood cells, white blood cells and platelets suspended in a watery fluid called plasma.

If blood is treated to prevent clotting and permitted to stand in a container, the red blood cells, weighing the most, will settle to the bottom; the plasma will stay on top; and the white blood cells and platelets will remain suspended between the plasma and the red blood cells. A centrifuge may be used to hasten this separation process. The platelet-rich plasma is then removed and placed into a sterile bag, and it can be used to prepare platelet concentrates and cryoprecipitated AHF. To make platelets, the platelet-rich plasma is centrifuged, causing the platelets to settle at the bottom of the bag. Plasma and platelets are then separated and made available for transfusion. The plasma may also be pooled with plasma from other donors and further processed, or fractionated, to provide purified plasma proteins such as albumin, immunoglobulin, and clotting factors.

Red blood cells are perhaps the most recognizable component of whole blood. Red blood cells contain hemoglobin, a complex iron-containing protein that carries oxygen throughout the body and gives blood its red color. The percentage of blood volume composed of red blood cells is called the "hematocrit." The average hematocrit in an adult male is 47 percent. There are about one billion red blood cells in two to three drops of blood, and, for every 600 red blood cells, there are about 40 platelets and one white cell. Manufactured in the bone marrow, red blood cells are continuously being produced and broken down. They live for approximately 120 days in the circulatory system and are eventually removed by the spleen. Red blood cells are prepared from whole blood by removing the plasma, or the liquid portion of the blood, and can raise the patient's hematocrit and hemoglobin levels while minimizing an increase in blood volume.

Patients who benefit most from transfusions of red blood cells include those with chronic anemia resulting from kidney failure, malignancies, or gastrointestinal bleeding and those with acute blood loss resulting from trauma. Since red blood cells have reduced amounts of plasma, they are well-suited for treating anemia patients who would not tolerate the increased volume provided by whole blood, such as patients with congestive heart failure or those who are elderly or debilitated.

Red blood cells may be treated and frozen for extended storage (up to 10 years).

Plasma is the liquid portion of the blood—a protein-salt solution in which red and white blood cells and platelets are suspended. Plasma, which is 90 percent water, constitutes 55 percent of blood volume. Plasma contains albumin (the chief protein constituent), fibrinogen (responsible, in part, for the clotting of blood), and globulins (including antibodies). Plasma serves a variety of functions, from maintaining a satisfactory blood pressure and volume to supplying critical proteins for blood clotting and immunity. It also serves as the medium of exchange for vital minerals such as sodium and potassium, thus helping maintain a proper balance in the body, which is critical to cell function. Plasma is obtained by separating the liquid portion of blood from the cells.

Fresh frozen plasma is frozen within hours after donation to preserve clotting factors, stored for up to one year, and thawed immediately before it is transfused. It is used to treat certain bleeding disorders for which no factor-specific concentrate is available.

Cryoprecipitated AHF is the portion of plasma that is rich in clotting factors, including Factor VIII. Cryoprecipitated AHF is removed from plasma by freezing and then slowly thawing the plasma. It is used to prevent or control bleeding in individuals with hemophilia and von Willebrand syndromes, which are the most common, inherited major coagulation abnormalities.

Platelets (or thrombocytes) are very small cellular components of blood that help the clotting process by sticking to the lining of blood vessels. Platelets are made in the bone marrow and survive in the circulatory system for an average of 9-10 days before being removed from the body by the spleen. The platelet is vital to life, because it helps prevent both massive blood loss resulting from trauma and blood vessel leakage that would otherwise occur. Units of platelets are prepared by using a centrifuge to separate the platelet-rich plasma from the donated unit of whole blood. The platelet-rich plasma is then centrifuged again to concentrate the platelets further.

Platelets may also be obtained from a donor by a process known as apheresis, or plateletpheresis. In this process, blood is drawn from the donor into an apheresis instrument, which, using centrifugation, separates the blood into its components, retains the platelets, and returns the remainder of the blood to the donor. The resulting component contains about six times as many platelets as a unit of platelets obtained from whole blood. Platelets are used to treat a condition called thrombocytopenia, in which there is a shortage of platelets, and platelet function abnormalities. Platelets are stored at room temperature for up to five days.

White blood cells are responsible for protecting the body from invasion by foreign substances such as bacteria and viruses. The majority of white blood cells are produced in the bone marrow, where they outnumber red blood cells by two to one. However, in the blood stream, there are about 600 red blood cells for every white blood cell. There are several types of white blood cells. Granulocytes and macrophages protect against infection by surrounding and destroying invading bacteria and viruses, and lymphocytes aid in the immune defense.

Granulocytes are prepared by apheresis or by centrifugation of whole blood. They are transfused within 24 hours after collection and are used for infections that are unresponsive to antibiotic therapy. The effectiveness of white blood cell transfusion is still being investigated.

Plasma derivatives are concentrates of specific plasma proteins that are prepared from pools (many units) of plasma. Plasma derivatives are obtained through a process, known as fractionation, developed during World War II, and are heat-treated and/or solvent detergent–treated to kill certain viruses, including those that cause AIDS and hepatitis B and C. Plasma derivatives include:

- Factor VIII Concentrate
- Factor IX Concentrate
- Anti-Inhibitor Coagulation Complex (AICC)
- Albumin
- Immune Globulins, including Rh Immune Globulin
- Anti-Thrombin III Concentrate
- Alpha 1-Proteinase Inhibitor Concentrate

Highlights of Transfusion Medicine History

1628   English physician William Harvey discovers the circulation of blood. Shortly afterward, the earliest known blood transfusion is attempted.

1665   The first recorded successful blood transfusion occurs in England: Physician Richard Lower keeps dogs alive by transfusion of blood from other dogs.

1667   Jean-Baptiste Denis in France and Richard Lower in England separately report successful transfusions from lambs to humans. The next year, transfusing the blood of animals to humans becomes prohibited by law, delaying transfusion advances for about 150 years.

1795   In Philadelphia an American physician, Philip Syng Physick, claims to perform the first human blood transfusion, although he does not publish this information.

1818   James Blundell, a British obstetrician, performs the first successful transfusion of human blood to a patient for the treatment of postpartum hemorrhage. Using the patient's husband as a donor, he extracts approximately four ounces of blood from the husband's arm and, using a syringe, successfully transfuses the wife. Between 1825 and 1830, he performs 10 transfusions, five of which prove beneficial to his patients, and publishes these results.

1840   At St. George's School in London, Samuel Armstrong Lane, aided by consultant Dr. Blundell, performs the first successful whole blood transfusion to treat hemophilia.

circa 1867	English surgeon Joseph Lister uses antiseptics to control infection during transfusions.
1900	Karl Landsteiner, an Austrian physician, discovers the first three human blood groups, A, B, and O. The fourth, AB, is added by his colleagues A. Decastello and A. Sturli in 1902. Landsteiner receives the Nobel Prize for Medicine for this discovery in 1930.
1907	Hektoen suggests that the safety of transfusion might be improved by crossmatching blood between donors and patients to exclude incompatible mixtures. Reuben Ottenberg performs the first blood transfusion using blood typing and crossmatching in New York.
1908	French surgeon Alexis Carrel devises a way to prevent clotting by sewing the vein of the recipient directly to the artery of the donor. This vein-to-vein or direct method, known as anastomosis, is practiced by a number of physicians, among them J.B. Murphy in Chicago and George Crile in Cleveland. The procedure, however, proves unfeasible.
1912	Roger Lee, a visiting physician at the Massachusetts General Hospital, along with Paul Dudley White, develops the Lee-White clotting time. Adding another important discovery to the growing body of knowledge of transfusion medicine, Lee demonstrates that it is safe to give group O blood to patients of any blood group, and that blood from all groups can be given to group AB patients. The terms "universal donor" and "universal recipient" are coined.
1914	Long-term anticoagulants, among them sodium citrate, are developed, allowing longer preservation of blood.
1915	At Mt. Sinai Hospital in New York, Richard Lewisohn uses sodium citrate as an anticoagulant to transform the transfusion procedure from direct to indirect. Although this is a great advance in transfusion medicine, it takes 10 years for sodium citrate use to be accepted.

1916   Francis Rous and J.R. Turner introduce a citrate-glucose solution that permits storage of blood for several days after collection. Allowing for blood to be stored in containers for later transfusion aids the transition from the vein-to-vein method to direct transfusion. This discovery also allows for the establishment of the first blood depot by the British during World War I. Oswald Robertson is credited as the creator of the blood depots.

1930   The first blood bank is established at a London hospital.

1937   Bernard Fantus, director of therapeutics at the Cook County Hospital in Chicago, establishes the first hospital blood bank. In creating a hospital laboratory that can preserve and store donor blood, Fantus originates the term "blood bank." Within a few years, hospital and community blood banks begin to be established across the United States. Some of the earliest are in San Francisco, Miami, and Cincinnati.

1939/40   The Rh blood group system is discovered by Karl Landsteiner, Alex Wiener, Philip Levine and R.E. Stetson and is soon recognized as the cause of the majority of transfusion reactions. Identification of the Rh factor takes its place next to ABO as one of the most important breakthroughs in the field of blood banking.

1940   Edwin Cohn, a professor of biological chemistry at Harvard Medical School, develops cold ethanol fractionation, the process of breaking down plasma into components and products. Albumin, a protein with powerful osmotic properties, is isolated.

1941   Isodor Ravdin, a prominent surgeon from Philadelphia, effectively treats victims of the Pearl Harbor attack with Cohn's albumin for shock. Injected into the blood stream, albumin absorbs liquid from surrounding tissues, preventing blood vessels from collapsing and thus causing shock. With the entry of the United States into World War II, the American National Red Cross establishes a nationwide blood program.

1943   The introduction by J.F. Loutit and Patrick L. Mollison of acid citrate dextrose (ACD) solution, which reduces the volume of anticoagulant, permits transfusions of greater volumes of blood.

1947   The American Association of Blood Banks (AABB) is formed to promote common goals among blood banking practitioners and the blood donating public.

1950   Audrey Smith reports the use of glycerol cryoprotectant for freezing red blood cells.

1951   The AABB Clearinghouse is established, providing a centralized system for exchanging blood among blood banks. Today the Clearinghouse is called the National Blood Exchange.

1952   In one of the single most influential technical developments in blood banking, Carl Walter introduces the plastic bag for blood collection. Replacing breakable glass bottles with durable plastic bags allows for the evolution of a collection system capable of safe and easy preparation of multiple blood components from a single unit of blood. Invention of the refrigerated centrifuge the following year further expedites blood component therapy.

Mid-1950s   In response to the heightened demand created by open heart surgery and advances in trauma care patients, blood use enters its most explosive growth period.

1957   The AABB forms its committee on Inspection and Accreditation to monitor the implementation of standards for blood banking.

1958   The AABB publishes its first edition of *Standards for a Blood Transfusion Service* (now titled *Standards for Blood Banks and Transfusion Services*).

1959   Max Perutz of Cambridge University deciphers the molecular structure of hemoglobin, the molecule that transports oxygen and gives red blood cells their color.

1960   The AABB begins publication of *Transfusion*, the first American journal wholly devoted to the science of blood banking and transfusion technology. In this same year, A. Solomon and J.L. Fahey report the first therapeutic plasmapheresis procedure.

1961	The role of platelet concentrates in treating cancer patients undergoing chemotherapy is recognized.
1962	The first antihemophilic factor (AHF) concentrate to treat coagulation disorders in hemophilia patients is developed through fractionation.
1964	Plasmapheresis is introduced as a means of collecting plasma for fractionation.
1965	Judith G. Pool and Angela E. Shannon report a method for producing Cryoprecipitated AHF.
1967	Rh immune globulin is commercially introduced to prevent Rh disease in the newborns of Rh-negative women.
1970s	Blood banks move toward an all-volunteer blood donor system.
1971	Hepatitis B testing of donated blood begins.
1972	Apheresis is used to extract one cellular component, returning the rest of the blood to the donor.
1979	A new anticoagulant preservative, CPDA-1, extends the shelf life of whole blood and red blood cells to 35 days, increasing the blood supply and facilitating resource sharing among blood banks.
Early 1980s	With the growth of component therapy, products for coagulation disorders, and plasma exchange for the treatment of autoimmune disorders, hospital and community blood banks enter the era of transfusion medicine, in which doctors trained specifically in blood transfusion actively participate in patient care.
1983	Additive solutions extend the shelf life of red blood cells to 42 days.
1985	to the present. The first blood screening test to detect HIV is licensed and quickly implemented by blood banks to protect the blood supply. The development and implementation of five more tests for other infectious diseases (tests for hepatitis B and syphilis were already in place) and donor questioning and deferral procedures add more layers of safety to the American blood supply.

Facts about Blood Donation and Transfusion

Blood may be transfused as whole blood or as one of its components. Because patients seldom require all of the components of whole blood, it makes sense to transfuse only that portion needed by the patient for a specific condition or disease. This treatment, referred to as "blood component therapy," allows several patients to benefit from one unit of donated whole blood. Blood components include red blood cells, plasma, platelets, and cryoprecipitated antihemophilic factor (AHF). Up to four components may be derived from one unit of blood. Improvements in cell preservative solutions over the last 15 years have increased the shelf-life of red blood cells from 21 to 42 days.

How much blood is donated each year? How much blood is transfused each year?

About 14 million units (including approximately one million autologous donations) of blood are donated each year by approximately eight million volunteer blood donors. These units are transfused to as many as four million patients per year. A unit of whole blood is roughly equivalent to a pint. Adult males have about 12 pints of blood in their circulatory systems, and adult females have approximately nine pints. Each unit is usually separated into multiple components, which may be transfused to a number of different individuals. Up to four components can be derived from one unit of blood.

The need for blood is great—on any given day, approximately 40,000 units of red blood cells are needed. Accident victims, people undergoing surgery, and patients receiving treatment for leukemia, cancer or other diseases, such as sickle cell disease and thalassemia, all utilize blood. More than 23 million units of blood components are transfused every year.

Who donates blood?

Less than 5 percent of healthy Americans eligible to donate blood actually donate each year. According to studies, the average donor is a college-educated white male, between the ages of 30 and 50, who is married and has an above-average income. However, these statistics are changing, and women and minority groups are volunteering to donate in increasing numbers. While persons 65 years and older compose 13 percent of the population, they use 25 percent of all blood units transfused. Using current screening and donation procedures, a growing number of blood banks have found blood donation by the elderly to be safe and practical.

Where is blood donated?

There are many places where blood donations can be made. Bloodmobiles travel to high schools, colleges, churches, and community organizations. People can also donate at community blood centers and hospital-based donor centers. Many people donate at blood drives at their place of work. Community blood centers collect approximately 88 percent of the nation's blood, and hospital-based donor centers account for the other 12 percent. Consult the yellow pages to locate a nearby blood center or hospital to donate.

What are the criteria for blood donation?

To be eligible to donate blood, a person must generally be at least 17 years of age (although some states permit younger people to donate with parental consent); be in good health; and weigh at least 110 pounds. Most blood banks have no upper age limit. All donors must pass the physical and health history examinations given prior to donation.

Nearly all blood used for transfusion in the United States is drawn from volunteer donors. The donor's body replenishes the fluid lost from donation in 24 hours. It may take up to two months to replace the lost red blood cells. Whole blood can be donated every eight weeks.

An increasingly common procedure is apheresis, or the process of removing a specific component of the blood and returning the red blood cells to the donor. This process allows more of a particular component—platelets, for instance—to be drawn in one sitting than could be separated from a unit of whole blood. Apheresis is also performed to collect plasma and granulocytes.

What is the most common blood type?

The approximate distribution of blood types in the US population is as follows. Distribution may be different for specific racial and ethnic groups:

- O   Rh-positive   38 percent
- O   Rh-negative   7 percent
- A   Rh-positive   34 percent
- A   Rh-negative   6 percent
- B   Rh-positive   9 percent

- B   Rh-negative   2 percent
- AB Rh-positive   3 percent
- AB Rh-negative   1 percent

In an emergency, anyone can receive type O red blood cells, and type AB individuals can receive red blood cells of any ABO group. Therefore, people with type O blood are known as "universal donors" and those with AB blood as "universal recipients."

What tests are performed on donated blood?

After blood is drawn, it is tested for ABO group and Rh type, as well as for any unexpected antibodies that may cause problems in the recipient. Screening tests are also performed for hepatitis B surface antigen (HbsAg), the hepatitis B core antibody (anti-HBc), antibody to hepatitis C virus (anti-HCV), and for antibodies to the human immunodeficiency virus (anti-HIV-1 and HIV-2), the human immunodeficiency virus-1 (HIV) p24 antigen, the human T lymphotropic virus type 1 (HTLV-1), and syphilis.

How is blood stored and used?

Each unit of blood is normally separated into several components. Red blood cells may be stored under refrigeration for a maximum of 42 days, or they may be frozen for up to 10 years. Red cells carry oxygen and are commonly used to treat anemia.

Platelets are important in the control of bleeding and are used in patients with leukemia and other forms of cancer. Platelets may be kept for a maximum of five days. Granulocytes (white cells) are sometimes used to fight infections, although their efficacy is not well established. They must be transfused within 24 hours of donation. Plasma, used to control bleeding, is usually kept in the frozen state for up to one year. Cryoprecipitated AHF, which contains clotting factors, is made from fresh-frozen plasma and may be stored frozen for one year.

Other products manufactured from blood include albumin, immune globulin, specific immune globulins and clotting factor concentrates. These blood products are commonly made by commercial manufacturers.

How much does blood cost?

While donated blood is free, and most blood collecting organizations (blood centers as well as collecting hospitals) are not-for-profit, there are significant costs associated with collecting, storing, testing, and transfusing blood. As a result, processing fees are charged to recover costs. Processing fees for red blood cells vary and may be more than $100 per unit in certain parts of the country. The national average is between $65 and $75. Other components may be more expensive.

Chapter 3

How Blood Clots Are Formed

How poor are they that have not patience! What sound did ever heal but by degrees?

—Iago, in Shakespeare's *Othello*

The mending of any wound takes time. Although the lines from *Othello* refer to the mysterious and gradual healing of a broken heart or wounded pride, they also apply to the repair of physical injury, which is nearly as complex and inscrutable. Even with today's sensitive instruments and technologies, scientists are only beginning to understand the atomic-scale activities and molecular machinations that cause blood to clot and tissues to mend.

By putting the spotlight on the protein fibrinogen, a key player in the formation of blood clots, structural biologists are beginning to uncover the intricacies of clot assembly at the molecular and atomic levels. Assisted by the NCRR-supported synchrotron resource at Stanford University and instruments purchased through NCRR Shared Instrumentation Grants (SIG), Dr. Russell Doolittle and his colleagues at the University of California, San Diego (UCSD), used X-ray crystallography to acquire the most detailed three-dimensional (3-D) image yet of a critical portion of human fibrinogen.

"We also showed, for the first time at the atomic level, how two molecules of fibrinogen butt up against each other, as they do when

National Center for Research Resources (NCRR), *NCRR Reporter*, January-March 1998.

a clot has stabilized," says Dr. Doolittle, professor of chemistry and biology, who solved the structures along with postdoctoral researchers Drs. Glen Spraggon and Stephen J. Everse. Knowledge of fibrinogen's 3-D form might facilitate drug discovery and lead to improved therapies for heart disease, stroke, and many disorders caused by abnormal blood clotting.

First discovered nearly a century and a half ago, fibrinogen has since been the subject of intense scientific scrutiny. "There have probably been 10,000 or more papers written about fibrinogen in the last 10 years," says Dr. Doolittle, who has studied the molecule nearly that long. Scientists now know that this large, rod-like protein is manufactured in the liver and can stack together to build a double-stranded water-resistant protein known as fibrin. Fibrin strands are then woven into a stable, 3-D scaffolding for a blood clot.

Fibrinogen is so critical to clot formation that individuals who lack the normal protein may bleed excessively when injured or develop potentially dangerous internal blood clots—a condition known as thrombosis. Fibrinogen can also be hazardous in excess. Elevated plasma fibrinogen is an independent risk factor for cardiovascular disorders and stroke and can increase health risks for patients with diabetes and certain inflammatory diseases.

Most studies of fibrinogen's structure and function have depended on advanced microscopy of biochemical techniques such as amino acid sequencing. Using these methods, researchers discovered more than 20 years ago that fibrinogen is a three-segmented protein, akin to a bowtie with a knot in the middle and identical loops on either end. To create fibrin, the "loops" of two fibrinogen molecules abut end-to-end, each also attaching to the center "knot" of a third fibrinogen. So linked, this molecular trio is now a fibrin building block, a dozen or more of which spontaneously stack to construct a double-stranded filament of fibrin.

Despite a wealth of information pieced together over the years, scientists have been unable to pinpoint the precise locations of atoms and amino acids within fibrinogen's 3-D structure, nor could they be certain how fibrinogen molecules manage to combine to create fibrin. Such details can be inferred from biochemical and microscopic analyses, says Dr. Doolittle, "but there are no real assurances that such conclusions are correct."

In the case of fibrinogen, the details of atomic-scale structure are not trivial. Fibrinogen's intricate contours are so critical to fibrin formation, says Dr. John Weisel, professor of cell and developmental biology at the University of Pennsylvania in Philadelphia, that "even a slight alteration—such as changing a single amino acid—can deform the molecule and dramatically affect its ability to polymerize and form a clot."

One technique that can provide atomic-scale information is X-ray crystallography, which involves shinning an X-ray beam through a crystallized sample of the molecule and then measuring how the X-rays are diffracted. Computers can then analyze the diffraction pattern to determine the molecule's atomic-scale architecture precisely.

Unfortunately, fibrinogen is so large and complex that even today it defies crystallization. In the early 1970s one team of investigators, led by Dr. Carolyn Cohen at Brandeis University in Waltham, Massachusetts, managed to crystallize a large portion of bovine fibrinogen containing most of the protein's "bowtie" structure. "However, the crystals proved so difficult to work with that 20 years later Dr. Cohen and her colleagues had obtained only a low-resolution, 18-angstrom structure," notes Dr. Doolittle.

To avoid the complications of working with the entire molecule, Dr. Doolittle focused only on a portion of fibrinogen—one of the bowtie "loops," technically known as fragment D. Because fragment D is only one-quarter size of the entire fibrinogen molecule, it is a more feasible target for crystallization efforts. And because each molecule of fibrinogen contains two D fragments, solving the crystal structure of fragment D amounts to determining half of fibrinogen's molecular structure.

By 1993, after nearly two decades of painstaking effort, Dr. Doolittle and his colleagues had produced pure crystals of fragment D and had collected preliminary diffraction data at UCSD. But it soon became apparent that a more brilliant radiation source—a synchrotron—would be needed to solve the fragment's structure at high resolution.

Synchrotrons are huge, ring-shaped facilities, nearly a mile in circumference, that produce X-ray beams thousands times brighter than those from conventional sources. "We could not have solved the structures without the synchrotron data," says Dr. Doolittle. "It's really a marvelous resource."

Synchrotron analyses revealed the precise twists and turns of fragment D's 3-D shape at a resolution of 2.9 angstroms. The scientists were also able to crystallize "double-D," which shows how bowtie "loops" from two fibrinogen molecules align end-to-end, each also linking to the "knot" on a third fibrinogen molecule. "It shows for the first time at atomic resolution how this molecule is packed together in a clot," says Dr. Doolittle. "It means that all the inferences built up over a half-century can now be checked."

The new atomic-scale findings largely agree with earlier studies of fibrinogen, including Dr. Cohen's 18-angstrom structure. However, crystallography has its drawbacks, notes Dr. Michael W. Mosesson, professor of medicine at the University of Wisconsin Medical School in Madison. "Crystals are formed under very specific and rigid conditions that may not reflect how molecules actually engage one another in a more physiological setting," says Dr. Mosesson, who has used the NCRR-supported Electron Microscope Facility at Brookhaven National Laboratory in Upton, New York, to study fibrinogen and fibrin formation for more than 20 years. Dr. Mosesson appreciates the structural details provided by Dr. Doolittle's work, but has reached different conclusions about the location of chemical crosslinks that bind fibrinogen molecules to one another.

With half of fibrinogen's 3-D organization now understood, Dr. Doolittle's team is competing with several other laboratories to crystallize and solve 3-D structures of additional portions of fibrinogen, including the central "knot" known as fragment E.

Meanwhile, at the University of Pennsylvania, Dr. Weisel is using an NCRR-supported electron microscopy resource and SIG-purchased instruments to determine how mutant versions of fibrinogen contribute to clotting disorders. By studying a French family susceptible to thrombosis, Dr. Weisel and colleagues in France have found that an inherited fibrinogen mutation—caused by a single amino acid modification—results in fibrin strands that are too thick to form a normal clot. Therefore, family members are at increased risk for heart attack and stroke. "These studies could have significance not only for people with rare genetic mutations, but also for larger populations at risk for heart attack or stroke," says Dr. Weisel.

Dr. Doolittle's crystal structures may also have clinical implications, since they revealed the atomic minutiae of a tiny indentation on fragment D that fastens to small knobs on other fibrinogen molecules. These indentations might be targeted in drug discovery efforts, thus setting the state for improved treatment of clotting disorders.

More Information

This research is supported by the Biomedical Technology area of the National Center for Research Resources; the National Heart, Lung, and Blood Institute; and the American Heart Association.

For information about NCRR-supported synchrotron research and other molecular X-ray technologies, visit http://www.ncrr.nih.gov/ncrrprog/btxray.htm.

For information about Shared Instrumentation Grants, see http://www.ncrr.nih.gov/biotech/btshrgr.htm.

Additional Reading

Spraggon G, Everse SJ, and Doolittle RF. Crystal structures of fragment D from human fibrinogen and its crosslinked counterpart from fibrin. *Nature* 389:4550462, 1997.

Chapter 4

Facts about Bone Marrow Transplantation

What Is Bone Marrow?

Bone marrow is a spongy tissue found inside bones. Blood cells are produced in the bone marrow by in a complex process called hematopoiesis. Bone marrow transplantation is sometimes used in the treatment of several different types of blood diseases, cancers, and immune disorders.

Diseases Treatable by Bone Marrow Transplant

- Acute lymphoblastic leukemia
- Acute myelogenous leukemia
- Chronic myelogenous leukemia
- Histiocytic disorders
- Hodgkin's lymphoma
- Inherited erythrocyte abnormalities
- Inherited immune system disorders
- Myelodysplastic disorders
- Non-Hodgkin lymphoma
- Other leukemias

Information in this chapter is adapted from material posted in 1996 by the Health Resources and Services Administration (HRSA) at http://www.hrsa.dhhs.gov and a report on current NIH-sponsored clinical research studies underway at the Clinical Center in Bethesda, Maryland.

- Other malignancy
- Other non-malignant diseases
- Plasma cell disorder
- Severe aplastic anemia

Facts and Figures from the National Marrow Donation Program (NMDP)

Number of Donors on Registry: 1,982,499

Number of Patients Searching: At any given time, there are an average of 2,000 active searches of the NMDP Registry.

Number of NMDP Transplants: 4,135

Current NMDP Transplants Monthly: 81 per month

Likelihood of Finding a Match: Approximately 30 percent of patients have a family member, generally a sibling, who is suitably matched and able to donate marrow.

The chances of any two unrelated individuals matching vary widely depending on how frequently the individual's antigens are found in the population. Currently, almost 65 percent of patients searching the NMDP Registry have at least one identical matched donor.

The level of match for bone marrow must be closer than that for heart, liver and other solid organ transplants, since the marrow contains the cells responsible for the immune system. In organ or marrow transplantation, the patient's body may reject the organ. In marrow transplantation the donated marrow may attack the recipient's body (graft-versus-host disease).

Survival Rates: The success rate of marrow transplants depends on the disease of the patient being treated, stage of the disease, age and condition of the patient and level of match between the patient and the donor. Overall, survival rates are generally in the 30 percent to 60 percent range for diseases that would be fatal without marrow transplants.

Unrelated donor transplants represent a therapeutic option for selected pediatric and adult patients with leukemia, aplastic anemia and certain congenital blood disorders. In some situations, unrelated marrow transplant is initial therapy while in others it represents a treatment strategy used following the failure of other treatments.

The Donation and Transplantation Process

The Donation Process

- A small amount of blood is taken from the volunteer donor at an NMDP-approved donor center or recruitment drive site.

- The sample is typed for markers on the surface of white blood cells (called HLA-A and B antigens) and the results are entered on the computerized NMDP Registry.

- If the donor's A and B antigens (two of each) match the patient's, the donor is asked to give another small sample of blood. The donor's HLA-DR antigens are typed and compared to the patient's.

- If all six antigens match, the donor is counseled about the donation process and given a physical examination after a thorough information session. The donor makes the decision to donate and signs an "intent to donate" form.

- Donated marrow is extracted in a simple surgical procedure under general or spinal anesthesia at an NMDP-approved Collection Center (hospital). Two to five percent of the donor's liquid marrow is extracted from the back of the pelvis through a special needle and syringe.

- The donor usually is kept in the hospital overnight for observation.

- After the marrow collection procedure, the donor may experience slight discomfort for a week or so in the lower back. The donor's marrow replenishes itself within a few weeks.

The Transplantation Process

- A patient's physician begins a preliminary search of the NMDP Registry.

- A list of potential matches (donors whose HLA-A and B antigens match the patient) are sent to the physician, who requests further testing of the donor's blood.

- From these results, the physician determines whether there is a match.

- If a match is found, the patient undergoes pre-transplant conditioning, consisting of radiation and/or chemotherapy, for seven to ten days.

- The donated marrow is transfused directly into the patient's blood stream, much like a blood transfusion. Healthy marrow cells travel to bone cavities, where they begin to grow and replace the old marrow.

- The patient must be isolated in a protected environment until the new marrow produces enough white blood cells to fight off disease.

- An increased white blood count, a sign that the new marrow is beginning to function, generally appears about three to four weeks after the procedure.

- The patient may be removed from protective isolation three to six weeks after transplant, as long as the new marrow continues to produce white blood cells and there are no serious complications.

Health History Guidelines for Bone Marrow Donors

Before being tested as a volunteer donor you will answer a series of questions that screen out volunteers who may have health problems barring them from becoming a marrow donor. If you are unsure of your eligibility please contact your donor center. All donors must be between the ages of 18-60 and in good health. It is the purpose of the following information is to be an informative tool, not a policy document. **Difficult questions are ideally handled by a medical director or donor center staff with medical training.** There may be exceptions to the recommendations on the medical conditions chart. Good judgement and sound medical advice should overrule these guidelines.

Health History Guidelines

AIDS: If you have or are at risk for HIV (AIDS), you cannot become a marrow donor.

Asthma: Active asthma is not acceptable. If a donor has not had an episode in five years and is not on medication, he or she is acceptable. Exercise-induced asthma is acceptable.

Back Problems: Back problems (sprains, strains and aches) are common and may not interfere with a marrow donation. Serious back problems, particularly those requiring surgery, may be a cause for deferral. If you have significant back problems, consult your donor center.

Blood Pressure: Elevated blood pressure (hypertension) is acceptable if controlled by medication. High blood pressure is acceptable provided it is not associated with a heart condition.

Cancer: Cured local skin cancer (only simple basal cell or squamous cell) is acceptable. Cervical cancer in situ is acceptable. All other forms of cancer are unacceptable.

Diabetes: Medication-dependent diabetes is not acceptable. Diabetes controlled by a diet is acceptable.

Epilepsy: More than one seizure in the past year or multiple seizures are not acceptable. Epilepsy controlled with medication, when there has been no more than one seizure in the past year, is acceptable.

Heart Disease: Prior heart attack, bypass surgery or other heart disease is not acceptable. Mitral valve prolapse that does not require medication or restrictions is acceptable. Irregular heartbeat not requiring medication is acceptable.

Hepatitis: History of hepatitis A is acceptable. Antibody to hepatitis B core antigen is acceptable. Hepatitis B surface antigen is not acceptable. Hepatitis C antibody is not acceptable. Hepatitis vaccine is acceptable.

Hospitalization: If hospitalized within the last six months, consult your donor center coordinator.

Lyme Disease: Asymptomatic Lyme disease is acceptable if the donor has been treated successfully with antibiotics. Chronic Lyme disease is unacceptable.

Malaria: Malaria more than three years ago is acceptable. If the volunteer finished a full course of antimalarial drugs more than six months ago, he or she is acceptable.

Obesity: Greater than 25 percent more than medical standards for weight is unacceptable.

Organ or Tissue Transplant: Heart, lung, kidney, bone or other organ or tissue transplant recipients are deferred.

Pregnancy: Marrow cannot be collected at any time during pregnancy. Women who are pregnant are temporarily deferred.

Sexually Transmitted Diseases: Genital herpes will be evaluated at time of physical exam, but is usually acceptable. Gonorrhea is acceptable if it has been treated prior to the past 12 months. Syphilis is acceptable if it was treated prior to the past 12 months.

Tuberculosis: Pulmonary active tuberculosis within the last two years is not acceptable.

Vaccinations: Vaccinations are acceptable, excluding HBIG and investigational.

Current NIH-Sponsored Bone Marrow Transplantation Studies

The Hematology Branch at the National Institutes of Health in Bethesda, Maryland conducts clinical research studies on a number of hematologic diseases. For patients to be admitted to the Clinical Center, they must be referred by a physician and meet protocol requirements. There is no charge for medical care at the Clinical Center because patients are participating in research studies. In most instances, patients will be expected to pay the costs of their travel and local lodging.

The Hematology Branch has an active experimental bone marrow transplantation unit. Patients with acute myelogenous leukemia, chronic myelogenous leukemia in stable phase or in transformation, and a variety of other hematologic malignancies may satisfy protocol requirements.

Patients can contact Wanda Zamani by e-mail (zamaniw@ gwgate.nhlbi.nih.gov) or by phone at 301-402-0764 or telefax at 301-402-3088 for more information.

Physicians are welcome to call Dr. Neal Young, Chief of the Hematology Branch or Dr. John Barrett, Chief of the Bone Marrow Transplant Unit at 301-496-5093 or telefax at 301-496-8396.

Part Two

Anemias and
Other Hemoglobin Diseases

Chapter 5

Understanding Anemia

Anemia is the most common form of blood disorder. It occurs when the amount of hemoglobin in the blood decreases. Hemoglobin, the red-colored substance in red blood cells, takes oxygen from the lungs and carries it through the bloodstream to all the body's tissues.

Anemia also occurs when there is a drop in the hematocrit, which is the fraction of red blood cells found in whole blood. The drops in hemoglobin and hematocrit can happen for several reasons: red blood cells are being destroyed faster than is normal; there is bleeding; or the bone marrow is not making enough red blood cells.

There are many types of anemia, and they have various causes. Some anemias are caused by infections or certain diseases. Others result from medication problems or poor nutrition.

General Symptoms

The first symptoms of anemia are usually mild and may go unnoticed. These symptoms include being more tired or pale than usual. The symptoms worsen as the condition progresses. The underside of the eyelids, nails, and lips may become very pale. Also, creases in the palms may lighten and appear be the same color as the surrounding skin.

An undated fact sheet produced by the National Heart, Lung, and Blood Institute, distributed in 1997.

Diagnosis

Because early symptoms are mild, anemia often is not discovered until routine blood tests are done as part of a yearly physical or medical exam for another problem. Once anemia is detected, the doctor will try to find its cause. This includes taking a thorough medical history, performing a physical examination, performing various blood tests, and evaluating symptoms.

Types of Anemia

There are many types of anemia, including iron-deficiency anemia, pernicious anemia, anemia from folic acid deficiency, hemolytic anemia, aplastic anemia, sickle cell disease, and Cooley's anemia (thalassemia).

Iron-Deficiency Anemia

Iron-deficiency anemia is the most common anemia. The body needs iron to make hemoglobin; thus, too little iron leads to a lack of hemoglobin, which causes anemia.

An iron deficiency can result from blood loss, poor diet, an increased need for iron, or an underlying condition. By far, the most serious cause of iron deficiency is blood loss. Women of childbearing age may lose too much iron because of menstruation. Otherwise, blood loss usually occurs in the digestive tract, mostly due to problems such as ulcers.

A dietary deficiency, although rare, can result from not eating enough iron-rich foods. Such foods include eggs, green leafy vegetables, meats (especially liver), fish, and poultry.

Iron deficiency from an increased need for iron has various causes. For example, children and adolescents occasionally become anemic during their growth spurts. Pregnancy and breastfeeding also increase the need for iron. Both conditions can increase iron requirements by 1 to 4 mg daily. An iron supplement can help meet this added need. Supplements usually come in pill form and are taken until the hemoglobin returns to normal and the body has stored a supply of iron. Iron pills can cause side effects, such as nausea, constipation, and black stools. A doctor should be told if side effects occur.

When iron deficiency occurs because of some other disease, the other disorder must be treated before the anemia, which usually then disappears.

Pernicious Anemia

Pernicious anemia, which is fairly rare, results when the body does not absorb enough vitamin B_{12} from the digestive tract to make red blood cells. Its symptoms can include fatigue, a fast pulse, a sore tongue, and weight loss. These symptoms may be very mild in the anemia's early stages but worsen as the disease progresses.

If not diagnosed and treated properly, pernicious anemia can become severe and cause permanent damage to the nervous system and digestive tract. Pernicious anemia is easily treated with injections of vitamin B_{12}. These injections are given first every few days and then monthly. With them, patients can live a normal life.

Anemia from Folic Acid Deficiency

Anemia from folic acid deficiency also is caused by the lack of a substance needed to make red blood cells in this case, folic acid. Normally, folic acid is absorbed from foods, such as meat and dairy products. A poor diet may lead to folic acid deficiency. Sometimes, however, medications or other diseases prevent its absorption.

Symptoms include weight loss and diarrhea. A blood test is used to help make a diagnosis.

Treatment calls for correcting the underlying problem or improving the diet. Sometimes, folic acid supplements are given.

Hemolytic Anemia

Hemolytic anemia occurs when red blood cells get destroyed too soon. This type of anemia has various causes, including medications, infections, congenital (present at birth) abnormalities, or an autoimmune response, in which the body mistakenly tries to kill its own red blood cells.

Symptoms of hemolytic anemia include fatigue, paleness, increased heart rate, breathlessness, yellow-tinged skin (jaundice), dark-tea-colored urine, and an enlarged spleen.

To diagnose the condition and identify its cause, the doctor will take a medical history and do a physical exam and various blood tests. The doctor will check particularly for an enlarged spleen or liver.

Hemolytic anemia can be hard to treat but is rarely fatal. Patients usually resume a normal life after treatment. The treatment depends on the cause. If caused by a medication, the anemia will go away after the medication is stopped. For an immune-related hemolytic anemia, drugs known as corticosteroids (such as prednisone) are given. In some cases, the spleen must be removed.

Aplastic Anemia

Aplastic anemia occurs when the bone marrow makes too few of all types of blood cells—red cells, white cells, and platelets. The lack of enough red blood cells creates a shortage of hemoglobin. The drop in white cells, which fight invading organisms, leaves the patient susceptible to infections. The decrease in platelets, which help blood to clot, means that the patient bruises and bleeds easily.

Causes of aplastic anemia include radiation, chemotherapy, and toxic products, such as insecticides and solvents, as well as immune system problems. For example, certain medicines and cancer chemotherapy may injure blood-forming cells in the bone marrow, and this may lead to aplastic anemia.

Symptoms of aplastic anemia include headache, dizziness, nausea, shortness of breath, and bruising.

Diagnosis requires a complete blood cell count and removal of a bone marrow sample.

Treatment begins by eliminating the cause, if known. For example, a drug causing the anemia will be stopped. Then, the anemia is treated. In mild cases, transfusions of red blood cells and platelets will replenish the supply of blood cells. Antibiotics also are used to protect the patient against infection until the immune system has been restored.

Severe aplastic anemia is sometimes treated with a bone marrow transplantation. Marrow is taken from a donor and injected into the patient's vein. It then travels through the bloodstream to the bone marrow, where it begins producing new blood cells.

Bone marrow transplantation poses problems and risks. First, it can be hard to find a suitable donor. A donor must be a "match"—or have the same mix of immune proteins as the recipient; otherwise, the donor marrow is rejected. Donors may be family members. The odds of finding a match among two siblings (brothers or sisters) are about 25 percent; among six siblings, about 75 percent.

Still, a match with a family member occurs in only about 30 to 40 percent of cases. Using bone marrow from unrelated persons has become a standard practice. Even so, the odds of finding a suitable unrelated donor are small, estimated to be anywhere from 1 in 100 to only about 1 in 1 million. The National Marrow Donor Program was established to help patients find an unrelated match. The program has a registry of potential donors. A patient's doctor can contact the program to ask about finding a donor.

The chances of a transplantation curing the anemia depends on more than just the donor-recipient match. Other key factors are the severity of the disease and the patient's age.

The procedure also poses risks. The major risk from a transplantation is a complication called graft-versus-host disease. This can affect the skin, liver, digestive tract, and lungs and may cause death. Only bone marrow transplantations between identical twins do not carry this risk.

Families should discuss the benefits and risks of transplantation with their doctors.

Sickle Cell Disease

Sickle cell disease (SCD) is an inherited disease that alters the shape of red blood cells. Normally, red blood cells are flexible and shaped like a disk. But SCD red cells have an abnormal hemoglobin, called hemoglobin S, that causes them to become rigid and crescent- or sickle-shaped, especially during periods of exertion, when the body's need for oxygen increases. The cells' distorted shape makes it hard for them to flow easily through blood vessels, and they can get stuck and clog the vessels, causing severe pain.

Hemoglobin S also makes the red cells fragile, and they tend to break down too soon. This produces anemia. In addition, SCD makes the body more vulnerable to infection, possibly by hindering the production of immune system cells in the spleen.

SCD mostly affects persons of African ancestry. In the United States, about 80,000 African Americans have the disease.

The disease is caused by a defect in a gene, the basic unit of heredity. Genes tell the body how to produce proteins, such as hemoglobin, and occur in pairs within cells. Every person has two genes for hemoglobin, one inherited from each parent. Each parent also has two genes, and each can be either normal or defective. If two hemoglobin S genes are inherited, then the child will have SCD. However, if at least one normal hemoglobin gene is inherited, then the child can produce normal hemoglobin.

A person who has only one gene for hemoglobin S is said to have the trait or is called a "carrier" of SCD. About 1 in 12 African Americans are carriers of the disease but do not have SCD. Carriers can be detected through a special test. Persons who may have the trait and who want to have children should take the test; at the same time, they should consult with a genetic counselor, an expert who can discuss the test results and the options available.

Treatment for SCD remains limited. Antibiotics are prescribed for infections, and certain medicines can relieve the pain. A medicine called hydroxyurea may help to reduce the frequency of painful episodes in some patients. In addition, bone marrow transplantation may be an option for others.

Cooley's Anemia (Thalassemia)

Cooley's anemia, or thalassemia, also is an inherited hemoglobin disease. It causes chronic anemia, poor growth, an enlarged spleen, and sometimes heart failure. Without treatment, death usually occurs in early childhood.

There are two treatments for this type of anemia: blood transfusions combined with drug therapy and bone marrow transplantation. As noted, bone marrow transplantation may pose serious risks but, if successful, can cure the thalassemia. The patient and his or her family should discuss the risks and benefits with the doctor.

Blood transfusions must be given throughout the patient's life. Because blood contains a lot of iron, the repeated transfusions cause excess iron to build up in the body. The excess iron is poisonous to the body, especially to key glands and organs, including the heart and liver. The excess iron must be removed with a special medicine.

Rare Hemoglobin Diseases

Rare hemoglobin diseases are uncommon types of hemoglobinopathy, disease that results from a genetically abnormal hemoglobin. Sickle cell disease is a common hemoglobinopathy. In fact, there are more than 400 known varieties of abnormal hemoglobin.

These abnormal hemoglobins do not carry oxygen as well as normal hemoglobin. The lack of enough normal hemoglobin produces mild to moderate anemia.

The rare hemoglobinopathies can cause attacks of pain similar to those in sickle cell disease.

Finding a Doctor

Internists, family doctors, and pediatricians can treat some types of anemia. However, a patient may need to consult a hematologist, a doctor with special training in blood diseases. Hematologists can be found in most cities and at large hospitals. Patients can get a referral to a hematologist from their primary care doctor or other health care professional.

Research

Various components of the National Institutes of Health are conducting research on anemia. The National Heart, Lung, and Blood Institute has clinical trials under way on aplastic anemia and sickle cell anemia; the National Institute of Diabetes and Digestive and Kidney Diseases is studying iron deficiency and pernicious anemias; and the National Institute of Allergy and Infectious Diseases conducts research on hemolytic and autoimmune anemias.

For More Information

More information on anemia is available from the following organizations. Full contact information, including addresses, phone numbers, e-mail addresses, and web sites, can be found in the chapter titled "Resources for Patients with Blood and Circulatory Disorders" in end section "Additional Help and Information".

- Aplastic Anemia Foundation of America
- Cancer Information Service
- Cooley's Anemia Foundation
- National Institute of Allergy and Infectious Diseases
- National Institute of Diabetes and Digestive and Kidney Diseases
- National Organization for Rare Disorders (NORD)

Chapter 6

Aplastic Anemia

Aplastic Anemia—The Disease

Aplastic anemia is a rare but extremely serious disorder that results from the unexplained failure of the bone marrow to produce blood cells. In all probability you had never heard of this disease until the time of diagnosis. We hope that this chapter helps you deal with your situation by providing basic information about aplastic anemia and the various treatment options. This chapter is not intended as a substitute for the advice of a physician. It is important that you ask questions and learn as much as you can about this disease. By contacting the Aplastic Anemia Foundation of America, you can be connected with others in your same situation and receive information free of charge. There are AAFA chapters around the country. You do not need to be alone in dealing with aplastic anemia.

Normal Bone Marrow Function

The central portion of bones is filled with a spongy red tissue called bone marrow. The bone marrow is essentially a factory producing the cells of the blood: red cells that carry oxygen from the lungs to all areas of the body, white cells that fight infection by attacking and destroying

Aplastic Anemia Answer Book ©1995 Aplastic Anemia Foundation of America, Inc., P.O. Box 613, Annapolis, MD 21404, (800) 747-2820; reprinted with permission.

41

germs, and platelets that control bleeding by forming blood clots in areas of injury.

Continuous production of blood cells is necessary all through life because each cell has a finite life span once it leaves the bone marrow and enters the blood: red cells—120 days; platelets—6 days; and, white cells—1 day or less!

Fortunately, the bone marrow is a superb blood cell factory and ordinarily supplies as many cells as needed, increasing production of red cells and platelets when bleeding occurs and of white cells when infection threatens.

Bone Marrow Stem Cells and Environment

The bone marrow contains a small number of precious stem cells. Just as plant seeds give rise to both mature plants and new seeds for the next generation of plants, so do the bone marrow stem cells produce blood cells and new stem cells in a lifelong cycle of production and self-renewal. Bone marrow stem cells require a proper environment for normal function. Just as a seed cannot grow in poor soil, bone marrow stem cells cannot survive and multiply in a poor environment.

Failure of the bone marrow cell production can result from damage to the stem cells or to the environment. The result is aplastic anemia.

Bone Marrow Failure

When the bone marrow cell production fails, normal blood levels of red cells, white cells, and platelets begin to fall. Symptoms of anemia, bleeding, and infection develop when blood cell levels fall to dangerously low levels.

The Diagnosis

The diagnosis of aplastic anemia begins with a blood test. Blood cell levels are normally maintained within certain ranges. The diagnosis of aplastic anemia is suspected when all three blood cell levels are very low. Confirmation of the diagnosis requires examination of a small sample of bone marrow under the microscope. Aspiration and biopsy of the bone marrow is easily carried out in the examining room or hospital bed by inserting a sturdy needle into the large pelvic bone just beneath the belt line on either side of the spine. This procedure is made more tolerable by the use of Novocain-like drugs to "numb up" the skin and bone. In aplastic anemia, the bone marrow biopsy shows a great reduction in the number of cells in the bone marrow, with a normal appearance of the few remaining cells. The diagnosis of aplastic anemia is usually made or confirmed by a hematologist— a specialist in blood disorders.

Initial Treatment

Aplastic anemia is a medical emergency. Patients with severe aplastic anemia require immediate hospital treatment.

Blood transfusion: Aplastic anemia patients are often given transfusions. Anemia is corrected by red cell transfusions. Since anemia in itself is not an emergency, red cell transfusions are usually given only when symptoms are not relieved by restriction of activity. By contrast, bleeding due to low platelets is an acute medical emergency, which should be treated with platelet transfusions to prevent fatal hemorrhage. You may be asked to provide platelet donors. Do not ask close family members to donate platelets until after a bone marrow transplant has been done or ruled out, since this may interfere with the effectiveness of a bone marrow transplant if a family member donor is found.

Platelets are collected from donors through a process called hemapheresis. Donating usually takes three hours. Platelets are collected from a vein in the donor's arm, passed through a blood-separating machine, and returned to the donor. The platelets that are removed are then given to the aplastic anemia patient. The donor's body replaces the platelets within a day or two.

Antibiotics: Because of their extremely short life span, white cells cannot be effectively replaced by a transfusion. Therefore, control of infection depends on prompt, appropriate intravenous antibiotic therapy as soon as fever or other signs of infection appear.

Isolation: To prevent transfer of infection to aplastic anemia patients, they must often be isolated from even healthy people ("reverse quarantine"). Necessary visitors may have to wear masks and gowns and must always thoroughly wash their hands before touching the patient.

Activity: Activity must be restricted to reduce symptoms of anemia. Avoid falls or accidents that could provoke bleeding and reduce contact with other people.

What You Can Do:

1. Take charge of your illness!

2. Research all you can about aplastic anemia and treatment options.

3. Gather information from as many people as possible: health professionals and other patients.

4. Don't be afraid to ask questions from different sources until you fully understand the answers.

5. Record information in a notebook. Take a tape recorder to appointments and meetings.

6. Encourage friends and family to become platelet and bone marrow donors.

7. Join a support group and read about ways to cope.

8. Check with the doctor about what things to avoid.

Bone Marrow Transplantation

Bone marrow transplantation is now being used more and more frequently for aplastic anemia patients who are good candidates and who have a matched donor. Identical twins or perfectly matched siblings are the best choices for bone marrow donors for patients. If a patient does not have a perfect match within the family, a search of existing bone marrow registries may be undertaken to find a matched, unrelated donor.

When a suitable donor is identified, he or she will be "harvested"— having between ½ to 1½ quarts of marrow drawn out through a large needle. The filtered bone marrow cells are then transfused by IV into the patient. Production of new blood cells should be seen in 2-4 weeks as the patient's counts begin to recover.

Immunosuppressive drugs, such as cyclosporin, play an important role in suppressing the transplanted donor white cells from fighting against those of the patient. Graft-versus-host disease (GVHD) is a reaction of the donor marrow against the body of the patient; donor white cells cause skin thickening, rashes, liver disease, jaundice, drying out of the eyes and mouth, weight loss, and diarrhea. Graft-versus-host disease, while it can be quite serious, can be successfully treated in most patients.

For young patients in relatively good health prior to transplant, and who have a matched donor, more than 75% are successfully cured by bone marrow transplantation. For patients who do not have a matched donor, who are over 50 years of age, or who are not good candidates for bone marrow transplantation, other forms of therapy are being used.

Drug Therapies

Doctors may recommend that the patient start on drug therapy while searching for a donor, or drug therapy may be the best choice for treatment for that patient. New therapies are being developed all the time. Be sure to talk with the doctor about what is available.

Immunosuppressive therapies work with a patient's immune system. One theory about aplastic anemia is that the patient's immune system is fighting against itself, thereby interfering with production of blood cells. These drugs are believed to work by stimulating the bone marrow to produce cells or by reducing the patient's immune response and thereby allowing the bone marrow to work. ATG, antithymocyte globulin, or ALG, antilymphocyte globulin, are two types of immunosuppressive therapies that have been used for treating aplastic anemia.

Another immunosuppressive drug is cyclosporin, which may be given alone or in combination with androgens, antilymphocyte globulin, or serum. It is thought that cyclosporin plus androgens may stimulate blood cell production.

Hematopoetic growth factors are products of the new genetic engineering. These are copies of substances that occur naturally in the human body, but are produced in larger quantities in the laboratory. Colony stimulating factors (CSFs) act to stimulate colonies of cells, such as red cells. Erythropoietin (EPO) stimulates production of red cells. Interleukin-3 (IL-3) stimulates production of other cells. It is thought that a combination of the growth factors might work in treating aplastic anemia.

Other drug therapies are being developed; your doctor will be able to help you explore these options.

Frequently Asked Questions

Who gets aplastic anemia?

Aplastic anemia can strike down literally anyone: men and women, children as well as adults, any race or socioeconomic status.

Don't blood transfusions replace the cells needed by aplastic anemia patients?

Unfortunately, blood transfusions are only a temporary solution to some of the problems of aplastic anemia patients. Consider each type of cell in turn:

1. **Red Cells.** Red cells are the easiest to replace by transfusion. There are only 4 major blood types, so "matching" is usually easy, and transfused cells may remain in the body for a month or longer. However, after years of regular red cell transfusions, patients begin to accumulate toxic amounts of iron (carried inside the red cells) in critical body organs, such as the liver or heart. Iron overload from transfusions is eventually fatal.

2. **Platelets.** Successful, long-term platelet transfusion therapy is a challenge. Since the normal life span of a platelet is so short, transfused platelets may only survive a few days; thus regular platelet transfusions several times a week may be needed. In addition, platelets carry tissue-type "markers" that are almost unique for each person. Patients "learn" to recognize foreign platelets and produce antibodies that destroy the transfused platelets instantly. Thus, aplastic anemia patients rapidly develop a need for "matched" platelets, that is platelets from donors whose tissue-type markers resemble the patient's own markers. To support one small child with matched platelets for a year, 20 matched donors may be needed.

3. **White Cells.** White cells cannot be effectively supplied by transfusion. The life span of the number of white cells obtained from donors is so short (a few hours) that routine white cell transfusion is technically impossible.

What are the causes of aplastic anemia?

Aplastic anemia has been clearly linked to radiation, environmental toxins, insecticides, and drugs in much the same fashion that cancer has been linked to these agents. Benzene-based compounds, airplane glue, and drugs such as chloramphenicol have been linked to aplastic anemia. In some individuals, aplastic anemia is believed to be caused by a virus. To date, the exact cause of the disease in over half the cases is unknown, or idiopathic.

Are there any experimental treatments available for those who do not respond to ATG and do not have a bone marrow transplant match?

Yes. There are several alternative therapies that can be tried and some are successful to some extent. These include the use of cytokines (growth factors) or granulocyte monocyte colony stimulating factor (GM-CSF) or erythropoietin (EPO). These are approved and commercially available cytokines that are available to all physicians. In addition, several experimental cytokines are being evaluated and could potentially be useful in some aplastic anemia patients. These include interleukin-3, monocyte colony stimulating factor, stem cell factor (SCF or C-kit ligand), and IL-6. Several newer cytokines are being developed and will be available for study in the near future.

How do I find out where there is experimental research going on in my area?

In the United States of America, nearly all experimental therapy for aplastic anemia is being carried out at hospitals associated with either one of the medical schools, or one of the NIH designated cancer centers. In addition, experimental therapies are being carried out at the National Institutes of Health in Bethesda, Maryland. A letter or call to the Hematology Division (either pediatric or adult) of the nearest medical school or designated cancer center should result in information concerning the availability of experimental therapy.

What activities should I avoid?

Patients with low red cell counts should avoid excessive exercise; going to high altitudes; or any activity that brings on a fast heart rate, any chest pain, or severe shortness of breath. Patients with low white counts may be more susceptible to infection with bacteria, not viruses. These are usually acquired from cuts in the skin or lining of the mouth or throat, which might result from dental work, burns from hot food, etc. Patients with low platelets should avoid activities that result in trauma, especially head trauma.

Glossary

Aplastic anemia: bone marrow failure; for unknown reasons, production of blood cells slows or stops.

Antibody: a complex molecule produced by lymph tissue in response to the presence of an antigen; antibodies neutralize the effect of the antigen.

Antigen: foreign substance, which is not usually part of the body's makeup, that stimulates antibody production; this antibody reacts specifically with a particular antigen to destroy or weaken it.

Bacteria: organism that can cause infection.

Bone marrow: soft tissue within the bones where blood cells are manufactured.

Bone marrow aspiration: test in which a sample of bone marrow cells is removed with a needle and examined under a microscope.

Bone marrow biopsy: procedure in which a small piece of bone marrow tissue is removed with a needle; sample is processed by softening the bone and examining thin slices of the softened bone under a microscope.

Bone marrow transplant: procedure in which bone marrow filled with disease is destroyed by radiation or chemotherapy and then replaced with healthy cells from a donor.

Chromosome: a rod-like structure that appears in the nucleus of a cell during division; contains the genes responsible for heredity.

Complete blood count: CBC; the amount or level of blood cells present: white cells, red cells, and platelets.

Cross match: type and cross; test in which the blood cells of a donor and a recipient are mixed together to determine if they are compatible.

Culture: procedure used to identify the source of infection; specimen of blood, urine, sputum or stool is taken and tested to determine the type of infection and the appropriate antibiotic.

Differential: percentage of different types of blood cells in the blood.

Erythroblast: an immature red blood cell.

Erythrocyte: a mature red blood cell that carries oxygen.

Granulocyte: a white blood cell produced in the bone marrow that engulfs and destroys invading organisms.

Hematocrit: the percentage of blood that is made up of cells. Normal values for men range from 42-52%, and for females 38-48%.

Hemoglobin: Hg; iron-containing coloring in the red cells that combines with oxygen from the lungs and carries it to the body's cells. Normal values for men are 13-16 gms/100 ml and 12-14 gms/100 ml for women.

Histocompatibility antigens: HLA; a group of DNA substances in chromosomes that determine whether certain tissues can be transplanted; also can be used to determine the most compatible platelet donors.

Human leukocyte antigen: HLA; the tissue typing test done on white cells to determine if a donor and recipient are compatible.

Immunoglobulins: kill microbes directly or make it easier for white cells to kill them.

Immunosuppression: decrease in the ability of the body's normal immune response to the invasion of foreign material.

Leukocyte: a white blood cell.

Leukopenia: a low number of white blood cells.

Lymphocyte: a type of white cell that fights infection by producing antibodies and other defense substances; occurs in 2 forms: B cells that recognize specific antigens and produce antibodies against them, and T cells that are agents of the immune system.

Megakaryocyte: a cell in the bone marrow that produces platelets.

Neutropenia: low neutrophil (poly) count.

Pancytopenia: low number of blood cells.

Petechiae: tiny red dots on the skin due to bleeding under the skin caused by low platelet counts.

Peripheral blood: blood in the bloodstream.

Phagocytosis: "cell eating"; the engulfment and destruction of dangerous microorganisms or cells by certain white blood cells

Platelet: blood cell that prevents bleeding and bruising.

Red blood cell: oxygen carrying cell in the blood, which contains the pigment hemoglobin, produced in the bone marrow; erythrocyte.

Refractory (to platelets): the immune system's response to platelet transfusions; platelets are recognized as foreign and destroyed.

Reticulocyte: an immature red blood cell.

Stem cell: cell from which platelets, red blood cells, and white blood cells grow in the marrow.

Thrombocytopenia: a low number of platelets in the blood. When the platelet level falls below 5 (or 5,000/cu.mm) it is considered a life-threatening emergency and may be corrected by a platelet transfusion.

Thymocytes (T cells): white blood cells that have traveled through the thymus.

White blood cells: blood cells that fight infection.

Blood counts: Adult normal value ranges

White blood cells 3.5-10.6 (1000/cu.mm)
Red blood cells 4.27-5.69 (million/cu.mm)
Platelets 150.0-450.0 (1000/cu.mm)
Hemoglobin 13.3-17.1 (grams/100 ml.)
Hematocrit 38.9-49.7%

Original text was written by Dr. Robert K. Stuart, updates and edits by Linda B. Kaufman and Dr. Lyle L. Sensenbrenner.

About the Aplastic Anemia Foundation of America

The Aplastic Anemia Foundation of America, Inc. (AAFA) is solely supported through individual contributions and is a tax-exempt organization as described under the Internal Revenue Code, section 50l(c)(3).

The AAFA offers free educational materials on aplastic anemia and myelodysplastic syndromes. The AAFA serves as a resource directory for patient assistance and emotional support through the volunteer efforts of patients, family members, and health care professionals throughout the world. Major research studies to find effective prevention and a cure for aplastic anemia and myelodysplastic syndromes are also financially supported by the AAFA. Patients can participate in the AAFA National Registry, which collects data for statistical analysis.

Contact the AAFA to receive a free information packet and to learn more about aplastic anemia, myelodysplastic syndromes, and the AAFA National Registry.

Chapter 7

Cooley's Anemia (Thalassemia)

What Is Thalassemia? How Is It Inherited?

The thalassemias are blood disorders, so we have to describe blood and its functions before we can talk about thalassemia.

What is blood?

Blood is a part of your body. It is pumped round by your heart, and circulates in the blood vessels that spread it through your whole body. Blood vessels are arteries, capillaries and veins. When your heart pumps blood out, it flows first into the big arteries, and then into smaller arteries to reach the capillaries. Capillaries are so small that you can only see them with a microscope, but they are very important because while the blood is flowing through them, it gives out the air and food it is carrying to the tissues of the body, and picks up wastes to take away. After this the blood flows into the veins which finally carries it back to your heart.

What is blood made of?

Blood is made up of a light yellow liquid, called plasma, and of three types of "cells." In fact, your whole body is made up of tiny building

Excerpted from *What Is Cooley's Anemia*, second edition, by Rino Vullo MD, Bernadette Modell, MD and Eugenia Georganda, PhD, with help from Beatrix Wonke, MD and Alan Cohen, MD © 1995 Cooley's Anemia Foundation, Inc. 129-26st Street, Flushing, New York, 11354, (718) 321- CURE, (800) 522-7222, (718) 321-3340 fax; reprinted with permission.

blocks called cells, far too small to see. In most tissues they are stuck together, but in the blood they float round freely in the plasma. There are 3 types of blood cells: red cells, white cells and platelets.

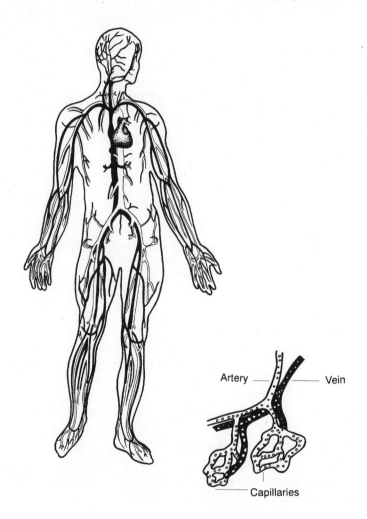

Figure 7.1. *The main part of the picture shows how the blood vessels are arranged in your body. The smaller picture shows some capillaries, as they look through a microscope. You can see that blood passes from arteries through capillaries that are far too small to be seen, into your veins. Then it goes back to your heart to be pumped round again.*

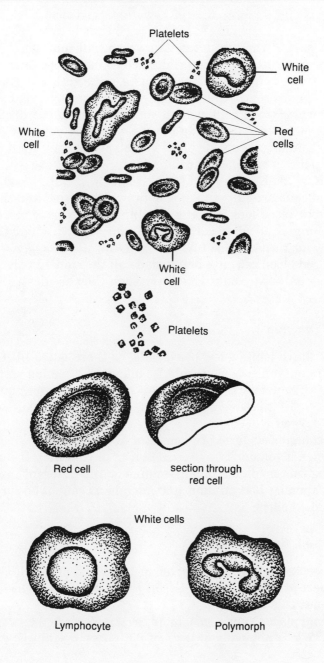

Figure 7.2. Drawing of what blood cells look like through a microscope. Blood contains red cells, white cells, and platelets.

What does blood do?

Each part of the blood has its own special function. The plasma carries water, salts, and materials such as food, hormones, and drugs to your tissues, and carries away waste, to be got rid of through your lungs (in your breath) and through your kidneys, in your urine.

Your white blood cells defend your body against infections. Your platelets stop you from losing blood if you hurt yourself. They stick together and block up your blood vessels when they get damaged, so they stop any more blood escaping.

You have many more red blood cells than white blood cells. The red blood cells are full of hemoglobin, which is red, and this is what makes your blood look red. Hemoglobin picks up oxygen from the air in your lungs, and carries it round to your tissues, where it lets it go. To live, your tissues need to breath, so they need oxygen.

New red blood cells are being made all the time in your bone marrow. They only live about 120 days. Then they are destroyed in your spleen.

What is "anemia"?

If you have too few red blood cells, or there is too little hemoglobin in them, you have "anemia." This simply means a shortage of blood. If the anemia is mild, it does no harm and you may not even notice it: but if it is severe, you are ill, because your tissues don't have enough oxygen.

The commonest form of anemia is "iron deficiency anemia." This can happen if you don't have enough iron in your diet. It can be cured by taking iron medicine. Thalassemia is quite different from iron deficiency anemia. It is an inherited anemia. It cannot be cured by taking any medicines.

How do you measure anemia?

By measuring the amount of hemoglobin in your blood. This is quite easy. There are two ways to describe the result, and we use both ways throughout this chapter.

In some places your hemoglobin level is described as a "percent of normal," e.g. a hemoglobin level of 63%. Hemoglobin is written Hb, for short.

Described this way, the usual Hb level for men is about 90–110%, for women and children it is about 77–100%.

Moderate anemia means an Hb level of about 55–70%.

Severe anemia means an Hb level of less than 55%.

In other places your Hb level is described as grams (g) of hemo-globin (Hb) per deciliter (1/10th of a liter) of blood. One gram is the same as 7% of hemoglobin. So, for example, a hemoglobin level of 63% = 9g/dl (nine grams per deciliter).

Described this way, the usual Hb level for men is about 13–16 g/dl, for women and children it is about 11–14 g/dl.

Moderate anemia means an Hb level of about 8–11 g/dl.

Severe anemia means an Hb level of less than 8 g/dl.

Of course, in thalassemia major your hemoglobin level changes all the time, because of the transfusions you receive.

Thalassemias

Thalassemia is an inherited characteristic of the blood. It reduces the amount of hemoglobin your body can make, so it can cause ane-mia.

How is thalassemia passed on from parents to their children?

Every characteristic of your body is controlled by "genes," which control your growth from an embryo, and all your physical functions. Genes are present in every cell of your body. You have two of every kind of gene, one passed on from your mother, the other passed on from your father. Among many other genes, you have two genes that control how hemoglobin is made in each of your red blood cells.

"Normal" people are normal because they have two normal genes for hemoglobin.

Healthy carriers of ß-thalassemia trait have one normal gene for hemoglobin and one altered one. They are healthy because one gene is working well. Since one gene is inherited from each parent, at least one of their parents must be a carrier.

People with ß-thalassemia major have two altered genes for he-moglobin, one inherited from each parent, so both their parents must be carriers.

Children are conceived when a sperm from the father meets an egg from the mother. Eggs and sperms are made so that they carry only one of each gene from the parent. When the sperm and egg meet and become one, the material the baby will be made from has two genes for every characteristic again, one from the mother and one from the father.

The eggs or sperms from normal people always carry normal genes for hemoglobin, and so cannot transmit thalassemia. When healthy carriers of thalassemia produce eggs or sperms, each egg or sperm carries either a normal gene or a thalassemia gene, but not both—so half the eggs are thalassemic and half are normal; and half the sperms are thalassemic and half are normal.

Now let us consider three sorts of married couples:

1. Both parents are "normal."

They cannot possibly pass on thalassemia trait or thalassemia major to their children.

2. One parent has a thalassemia trait and one is "normal."

All the children must inherit a normal gene from the "normal" parent. However, they may inherit a normal or a thalassemia gene from the carrier parent. For each child there is a one in two (50%) chance of inheriting the thalassemia gene from the carrier parent: if this happens the child will have thalassemia trait. There is also a one in two (50%) chance of inheriting the normal gene from the carrier parent: if this happens the child will be completely normal. None of this couple's children can have thalassemia major.

3. Both the parents are β-thalassemia carriers: i.e., they are a "couple at risk."

When the mother produces an egg (once a month) the egg is either completely normal or completely thalassemic. There is no way of telling in which order they will come. And when the father produces sperm, half are completely normal and half are thalassemic.

When the mother produces a normal egg, it does not matter what kind of sperm meets it. If the normal egg meets a normal sperm, the child will be completely normal. If the normal egg meets a thalassemic sperm, the child will be a healthy carrier.

But if the mother produces a thalassemic egg, it matters very much what kind of sperm meets it. If the sperm is normal, the child will be a healthy carrier of thalassemia. But if the thalassemic egg meets a thalassemic sperm, the child will have thalassemia major.

This is why couples of carriers have a one in four (25%) chance in each pregnancy of having a child with thalassemia major: a one in two (50%) chance of having a child with thalassemia trait: and a one in four (25%) chance that the child will inherit a normal gene from both parent, and so will be completely normal.

These chances are the same in each pregnancy.

It is possible to test the fetus during pregnancy, to see if it has thalassemia major. Then the parents can decide whether or not to keep the pregnancy. This is called prenatal diagnosis. To do this test, it is necessary to study blood from both parents, to find out exactly which type of thalassemia gene they carry.

Thalassemia Major

Usually thalassemia is severe, and people who have it need regular blood transfusions in order to live. This is called thalassemia major. In some cases the disorder is milder, or even very mild, and the person can live quite well without blood transfusions. This is called thalassemia intermedia. We discuss thalassemia intermedia in a separate section below.

This section is about thalassemia major. Other names for thalassemia major are:

- Cooley's anemia
- ß-thalassemia major
- Homozygous ß-thalassemia
- Homozygous thalassemia
- Mediterranean anemia

How does thalassemia major first show itself?

During pregnancy, thalassemia major does not affect the fetus. This is because the fetus has a special sort of hemoglobin, called "fetal hemoglobin" (HbF for short). Children and adults have a different hemoglobin called "adult hemoglobin" (HbA for short). When a baby is born, most of its hemoglobin is still the fetal kind, but during the first 6 months of life it is gradually replaced with adult hemoglobin. The problem with thalassemia, is that the child cannot make enough adult hemoglobin. Therefore children with thalassemia major are well at birth, but usually become ill before they are 2 years old. They usually become quite anemic (their hemoglobin level is usually less than 55% (8 g/dl). So they become pale, do not grow as well as they should, and often have a big spleen. The number of months that can pass before a thalassemic child becomes ill can differ quite a lot from case to case. This is because thalassemia can be caused by several different defects in the hemoglobin genes. However, nearly all children with severe ß-thalassemia become ill by 4 years of age, and need blood transfusions.

How do the tissues of a child with thalassemia manage to breathe, if there is no adult hemoglobin?

The child's body reacts to the shortage of adult hemoglobin by making some fetal hemoglobin, so most of the hemoglobin in a thalassemic's own blood is HbF. But our bodies are programmed to make fetal hemoglobin only in the fetus. Our body can only make a very small amount later on—not nearly enough to keep a child alive for long.

What happens if thalassemia major is not treated?

The anemia gets worse, the child stops growing altogether, and the spleen goes on getting bigger, so the stomach gets very big. The bone marrow, the tissue that forms the red blood cells, expands inside the bones because of this. But its efforts to make more and more red blood cells are useless. The red cells it makes do not contain enough hemoglobin, and most simply die without ever getting out of the bone marrow. However, the marrow's efforts to expand makes the bones weak and alters their shape. The cheekbones and the bones of the forehead begin to bulge and the child's face gets a characteristic look, so that people can see from a distance that something is wrong. The spleen's normal job is to destroy old red blood cells in the circulation, but as time passes it begins to destroy young red blood cells as well. Finally it also kills white blood cells and platelets. This is called "hypersplenism." So in the end, the spleen makes the child's illness worse.

How do we treat thalassemia major?

Two different treatments are now possible, traditional treatment, and bone-marrow transplantation. We describe bone marrow transplantation a later section. Here we describe the traditional treatment. This consists of (1) blood transfusion, sometimes (2) removing the spleen (splenectomy), and (3) Desferal treatment.

Blood transfusion. To be precise, the treatment is not blood transfusion, but transfusion of red blood cells. Thalassemics are only short of red blood cells: they make the other parts of the blood quite normally.

Blood transfusions should be arranged to keep the child's hemoglobin in the normal range. The child is sick because the hemoglobin is low. So obviously, for the child to be well the hemoglobin should be about normal. The normal hemoglobin level for women and children is 77 -100% (11-14 g/dl). So thalassemics should be transfused when the hemoglobin is around 70%, and the hemoglobin should be raised to around 100%. (Or, in grams, they should be transfused at about 10g/dl, and the hemoglobin should be raised to about 14g/dl). To do this it is initially necessary to give a transfusion about every 4 weeks.

Until recently, some doctors recommended transfusion at about 42% (6 g/dl) and raised the hemoglobin only to about 70% (10 g/dl). This is called a "low transfusion regimen" because the patient's hemoglobin is never in the normal range. However, this therapy does not keep the children strong. They don't grow as well as other children, they usually get a big spleen and liver, and they can have other problems such as bone deformities, or fragile bones that break easily. Few children on a low transfusion regimen live long enough to grow up. The "high transfusion regimen" recommended here avoids most of these problems. It has been used for many years in Western countries. There are three reasons for high transfusion.

- It corrects your anemia, and makes sure that your tissues get a normal amount of oxygen. This allows you to live and grow normally.

- It lets your bone marrow rest, so that your bones can develop normally and will be strong, and your face looks normal.

- It slows down, or prevents, any increase in the size of your spleen, so it prevents hypersplenism.

Splenectomy. When the spleen becomes too active and starts to destroy red blood cells, transfusions become less and less effective. Then it may become necessary for a surgeon to take the spleen out. This operation is called splenectomy. (Splenectomy is discussed in a later section.)

Desferal treatment. Every 400ml of blood transfused contains about 200 milligrams of iron. (One milligram is a 1000th of a gram. Since one gram is a thousandth of a kilogram, you can see that one milligram is a millionth of a kilogram. It is not much, but it can add up with time!) Packed red cells in the U.S. have 200 mg of iron per 200–250 ml of blood. This iron can't be taken out of the blood because it is part of the hemoglobin, which your body needs. On its own, your body can only get rid of a tiny amount of iron, so if you have transfusions regularly, iron gradually accumulates in your body. It is stored in certain organs, especially the liver, the heart, and the "endocrine" glands (see Figure 7.3). Your body can store a lot of iron safely, but in

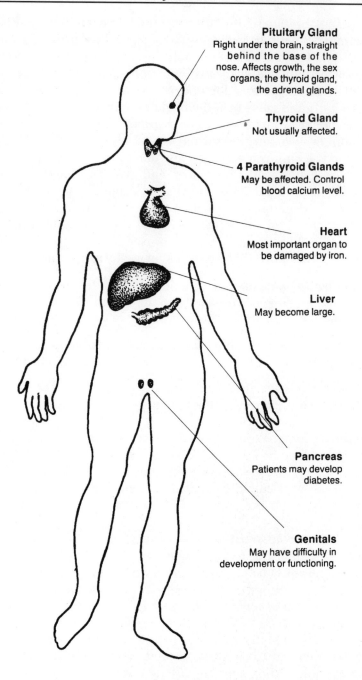

Pituitary Gland
Right under the brain, straight behind the base of the nose. Affects growth, the sex organs, the thyroid gland, the adrenal glands.

Thyroid Gland
Not usually affected.

4 Parathyroid Glands
May be affected. Control blood calcium level.

Heart
Most important organ to be damaged by iron.

Liver
May become large.

Pancreas
Patients may develop diabetes.

Genitals
May have difficulty in development or functioning.

Figure 7.3. *Parts of the body that can be damaged if iron overload is not controlled by Desferal.*

the end it can damage the organs where it is stored. Fortunately, there are drugs that can pick up the iron, and carry it out of your body in your urine and feces. The only one that is used regularly at present is desferrioxamine, which is also called "Desferal." If you use Desferal regularly, you can keep the amount of iron in your body down to a safe level.

What happens when thalassemia is treated correctly?

For a well-treated patient thalassemia is quite different from the untreated disorder. There is no anemia, growth is normal, and the face and the bones look normal. Figures 7.4 and 7.5 show the same child, aged 4 on low transfusion and aged 10 on high transfusion. However, there can be complications because of stored iron, or because of infections passed on in transfused blood. It is possible for viruses to get into your body with the blood and to make you ill. In particular, it is possible to get hepatitis, which is an infection of the liver, this way. It is also possible for the virus that causes AIDS (HIV), to be transmitted by the transfusion, but this is a very remote possibility,

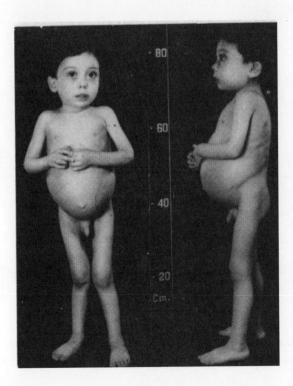

Figure 7.4. *A four and a half year old boy, on a low transfusion regimen.*

because all blood donors are first tested for this virus. People who are found to be carriers, or who have been infected with the HIV virus are not allowed to give blood.

What should you do now?

Remember that thalassemia will be life-long. Therefore it is necessary to look ahead and plan your treatment carefully, so as to get the best results in the long-term. With modern treatment there is real hope for thalassemics of leading a long and useful life. And there will be time for a lot of improvements in treatment. So keep a careful record of your treatment.

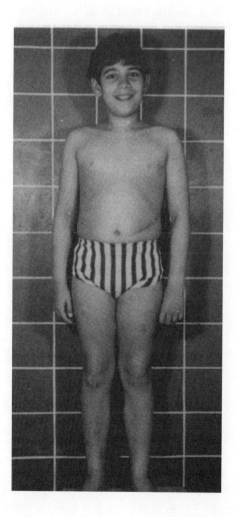

Figure 7.5. The same boy, now older, on a high transfusion regimen.

So You Want to Know More?

Some people will feel that they have enough information now, but perhaps you want to go into some things more deeply? In the following sections we answer questions that thalassemics and their families often ask. In this section we talk about some general questions. There are separate sections on important topics like blood transfusion, Desferal, splenectomy, etc.

Questions about Life-Expectancy and "Quality of Life" for Thalassemics on Regular Transfusion

How long can a person with thalassemia major live?

People sometimes don't like to ask this question directly, but thalassemics and their parents must often ask themselves.

The fact is that people with thalassemia are living longer and longer. Children who have good modern treatment are just like normal children, and can grow up, complete their education, work, and perhaps have a family. In countries where modern treatment has been available for a long time, there are now many patients in their thirties, who have had transfusion all their lives. They all work, and some have children.

On the other hand, it is true that thalassemics live with more risks than others, because of the amount of medical treatment they need. All medical treatments include some risk. But even so, a well-treated thalassemic at the present day can have an excellent life-expectancy.

What is the "quality of life" for a thalassemic?

A chronic disorder always causes some limitation of quality of life, especially when it requires frequent and complex treatment, as thalassemia does.

All the same, the treatment should not be allowed to have a profound effect on a thalassemic's life. In particular doctors and hospitals should make the effort to arrange out-patient visits and visits for transfusions so that they interfere as little as possible with normal life. One should try not to let treatment interrupt schooling or work. To manage this, some centers arrange transfusions for weekends, others in the late afternoon or at night.

In fact, most thalassemics do lead an essentially normal existence. They go to school, take part in social activities and work, get engaged, and get married like everyone else. We are certain that, as time passes, the quality of life will steadily improve.

Do thalassemics necessarily have thalassemic children?

No. Usually their children will be healthy, but it does depend on who they may marry.

If a thalassemic marries a "normal," all the children will be healthy carriers. They must inherit a thalassemia gene from their thalassemic parent, but they must inherit a normal one from the normal parent, so none of them can possibly have thalassemia major.

If a thalassemic marries a thalassemia carrier, in each pregnancy there is a 50% chance that the child will be thalassemic, and a 50% chance that it will be a healthy carrier. This is quite a common situation, since some thalassemia carriers have a special understanding for people with thalassemia major. Then they have the choice whether to use prenatal diagnosis or not.

If one thalassemic marries another, all their children will be thalassemics. This situation arises sometimes too, because thalassemics have so much in common, that they often feel particularly close to each other. When it does happen, they usually decide not to have any children, or to try to have children with medical help, for example, by artificial insemination (using semen from a man who is not a carrier). But in the future, if it becomes possible to correct thalassemia by gene therapy, even for such couples might have their own, healthy children.

These days, some thalassemic patients are cured, by bone marrow transplantation.

Can transplanted thalassemics still pass thalassemia onto their children?

Bone marrow transplantation may cure you, but it does not change your genes. You will still pass one thalassemia gene on to all your children. So make sure your partner has a thalassemia test before you have children!

Do thalassemics have to have a special diet?

In general, no, but we do recommend avoiding animal foods that are rich in iron, such as liver. And also some foods such as prunes, raisins and spinach contain iron. Breakfast cereals sometimes contain added iron.

It is also wise to avoid alcoholic drinks, or to drink them only moderately. This is because the liver is specially vulnerable in thalassemia, because of the iron stored in it, and the possibility that you were exposed to hepatitis in the past.

These are only recommendations, not absolute rules.

Can thalassemics take vitamin supplements?

Yes, in general they can. But if you do take vitamin preparations, avoid any with added iron. You should also avoid taking extra vitamin C tablets, except when you take Desferal. You should also avoid extra Vitamin D, unless it has been shown that you really need it.

Can thalassemics join in sports?

The answer is the same as for non-thalassemics—it depends on whether or not you have any heart problems. You can discuss it with your doctor. However, as a general rule, most thalassemics can take part in most sports, up to their own capacity. Your body itself will tell you when to stop, because if you "overdo" it you will get tired.

Can thalassemics take any kind of vacation they want?

Visits to high mountain areas need acclimatization, and a normal hemoglobin level. It might be wise for thalassemics to avoid altitudes above 11,480 feet, or to make sure they have a transfusion immediately before going to high mountains. Otherwise, there are no restrictions. Also the Cooley's Anemia Foundation (CAF) provides a travel directory containing the names, addresses and telephone numbers of hospitals and doctors who treat thalassemia worldwide. Call or write to the CAF National office (1-800-522-7222).

Questions about Blood Transfusion

Most thalassemics alive today will need regular transfusion for many years—perhaps for their whole life—so it is worth taking time and thought to organize the treatment in the best possible way.

How can you tell when you need to start a child on regular blood transfusion?

It can sometimes be very difficult to decide when to start transfusions. The following must all be taken into account:

1. *The hemoglobin level.* If the child cannot keep a steady hemoglobin level of more than 50% (7 g/dl) he or she will almost certainly need regular transfusions.

2. *The HbA level.* Many thalassemic patients have no adult hemoglobin (hemoglobin A). These will certainly need transfusion if

they cannot keep their hemoglobin above 50% (7g/dl). Some patients have from 30%–70% of hemoglobin A. Some of these patients can do well with a hemoglobin level around 50% (7g/dl).

3. *The child's growth.* A growth chart should be used for every thalassemic patient. If the child's growth does not follow steadily along the right line, but falls off, the child probably needs transfusion.

4. *Bone change.* Very obvious facial changes (especially if there is deafness, which can be due to bone marrow expanding into the ear), or broken bones, indicate the need for starting blood transfusion.

5. *Age of the patient and spleen size.* A patient who starts to need transfusion above 5 or 6 years of age, and has a large spleen may in fact have a mild form of thalassemia. If the spleen is taken out, some of these patients may not need transfusion.

It is important not to leave the start of transfusion too late, or some changes may be irreversible.

At what hemoglobin level should blood be given? (i.e., What is the best "pretransfusion hemoglobin " level?)

Everyone agrees that we should aim for a normal hemoglobin level, that is to say, the mean Hb level should be between 85 and 90% (12 and 13 g/dl). This is called a "high transfusion regimen"—though in fact it would be more correct to call it a normal transfusion regimen.

You can see from Table 7.6 that to keep a mean hemoglobin level of 12 g/dl (85%), you need to be transfused at different pre-transfusion hemoglobin levels, depending on the number of weeks between transfusions.

If you have had your spleen taken out, these calculations are almost always correct. If you have your spleen in, you may need transfusion a little more often to keep a high hemoglobin level.

What is the right number of weeks between transfusions?

There are several possible "regimens" for transfusion. Your own regimen can depend on things like whether you have to travel a long distance and stay overnight for your transfusion; or whether you live

Table 7.6. This table shows how the average Hb level may be the same, but Hb level before and after transfusion will be different, depending on the number of weeks between transfusions.

Weeks between Transfusions	Before transfusion	Hb level (g/dl) After transfusion	Mean
2	11.0	13.0	12.0
3	10.5	13.5	12.0
4	10.0	14.0	12.0
5	9.5	14.5	12.0
6	9.0	15.0	12.0

Or, if you measure the hemoglobin level in "per cent"

Weeks between Transfusions	Before transfusion	Hb level, % After transfusion	Mean
2	77	90	85
3	74	95	85
4	70	98	85
5	66	100	85
6	64	106	85

nearby and your center is able to provide "day transfusion," and on the number of units of blood you need. In Cyprus they give small transfusions every 2 weeks, in Italy they give moderate transfusions every 3 weeks, and in the UK they usually give larger transfusions every 4 or 5 weeks. In the United States, transfusions of one to three units are given as often as necessary to keep the hemoglobin level above 9–10 g/gl.

How much blood must you have at each transfusion?

This depends on the interval between transfusions. Here we show how to work out how much blood to give in two ways, depending on whether you describe the hemoglobin level in grams per deciliter (g/dl) or as a per cent.

In gd/l. Between transfusions, your hemoglobin level falls at about 1g/dl per week. So if you are transfused every 4 weeks, your hemoglobin level will fall about 4 g/dl. Therefore at each transfusion you need enough blood to raise your hemoglobin level by about 4g/dl.

To raise your Hb 1g/dl, you need 3 ml of packed red cells per kg = 5ml of donor blood. So to raise your Hb 4g/dl, you need 12 ml of packed red cells per kg = 20ml of donor blood.

For example, if you weigh 20 kg, you need 240 ml of packed cells (equivalent to 400 ml of donor blood) to raise your hemoglobin level by 4g/dl.

In per cent. Between transfusions, your hemoglobin level falls at about 7% per week. So if you are transfused every 4 weeks, your hemoglobin level will fall about 28%.

Therefore at each transfusion you need enough blood to raise your hemoglobin level by about 28% (or 4g/dl). To raise your Hb 7% you need 3ml of packed red cells per kg = 5ml of donor blood. So to raise your Hb 28% you need 12ml of packed red cells per kg = 20ml of donor blood.

For example, if you weigh 20 kg, you need 240 ml of packed cells (equivalent to 400 ml of donor blood) to raise your hemoglobin level by 28%.

Is it safe to give every patient 12ml of packed cells / kg at a single transfusion?

It is safe to give this amount to patients who are on a high transfusion regimen, because in general their heart is healthy.

However, if patients are on a low transfusion regimen their heart is often weak and their circulation is not healthy. Therefore it is wise to give less red cells at a time. This can be arranged by giving two smaller transfusions one or two days apart, or giving transfusions every 2 weeks.

As the child grows, obviously you need to give more blood at each transfusion. How does the blood requirement increase?

You do have to gradually increase the amount of blood you give at each transfusion. Figure 7.7 is a chart that shows how the amount of blood you need to give at each transfusion increases with body weight.

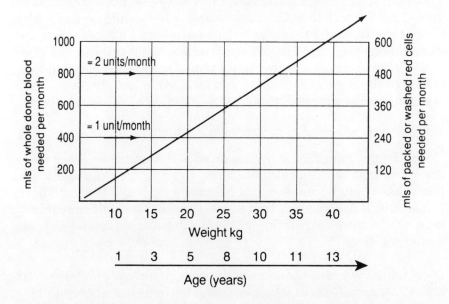

Figure 7.7. The amount of blood that must be given at each transfusion increases as the child grows. The chart shows how much blood is needed per monthly transfusion, in relation to a child's weight (and approximate age). If the person has a big spleen that is destroying blood too fast, they will need more blood than indicated here. If they have had their spleen removed, they may need slightly less.

But blood comes in "units. " How do you work out how many "units" you need?

Usually about 450ml of blood are taken from each blood donor. This is a unit of blood. Before it is given to patients, the plasma and most of the white cells are removed, so only about 250 ml of "packed red cells" are left in the blood pack. One "unit" of blood therefore means about 400 ml of donor blood, or about 250ml of packed red cells.

From the chart you can see that you need one unit of blood a month when you are 3–4 years old, but you usually need 2 units a month by the time you are 10 years old.

Blood is very precious, and should not be thrown away. As a child grows, you can increase the amount of blood you give, from one to two whole units, by changing the number of weeks between transfusions. Table 7.6 helps with this plan. For example, when a child needs 1.5 units every 4 weeks, he or she can be given 1 unit every 3 weeks for a year or so, and then changed to 2 units every 5 weeks. As the child goes on growing, you can change to 2 units every 4 weeks again. The important thing is to keep the same mean hemoglobin level. So in fact, the "transfusion regimen" can be arranged to suit the needs of each individual family.

How often do you need to measure the hemoglobin level?

The hemoglobin should be measured before and after every transfusion, so that you can calculate when to bring the child again. The hemoglobin before transfusion should not drop below 70%, and never below 60%. It is very important to measure the hemoglobin regularly, because if you are not careful you can slip down again to a lower transfusion regimen.

Does it matter if you do not measure the hemoglobin level after each transfusion? Many patients and doctors find it too complicated to do this.

No, though it is desirable to measure the hemoglobin again after each transfusion, it is not essential. In fact, it is usually possible to calculate the hemoglobin level after a transfusion. We know that the hemoglobin usually falls by about 1g/dl per week (7% per week). Therefore, you can work out how high your hemoglobin was after the last transfusion, when you measure your hemoglobin before your next transfusion. For example:

- If your pre-transfusion hemoglobin is 10g/dl, and it is four weeks since your last transfusion, your post-transfusion hemoglobin was probably about 14 g/dl.

- If your pre-transfusion hemoglobin is 10g/dl, and it is three weeks since your last transfusion, your post-hemoglobin was probably about 13g/dl.

Do patients differ in the amount of blood they need per month?

Yes, they can differ quite a lot. Most patients who have had their spleen out need the same amount of blood, as shown in the chart.

Patients with a normal spleen usually need about 20–30% more blood than patients who have had their spleen out.

Patients whose spleen is over-active can need 2 or 3 times as much as other patients. In this case, the spleen should be removed.

Why High Transfusion Is Better Than Low Transfusion

You are talking all the time about high transfusion. Can you explain why it is better than low transfusion?

Yes. It is easier to do this if we use a chart. Figure 7.8 summarizes the effects that thalassemia has on the body. We explained that the problem with thalassemia is that the bone marrow cannot make normal red blood cells. Most of the cells it makes die inside the bone marrow, and never come out. This explains the anemia.

But the bone marrow keeps trying harder and harder to make red blood cells, and the result is that it increases in size, up to 20 or even 30 times normal. In spite of all this effort, it still can't make enough red blood cells. But the effort that it makes leads to other problems:

1. Figure 7.8 shows that the bone marrow can distort the bones, especially the bones of the face, because it expands inside them. It also makes the bones fragile. As a result, they may break easily.

2. The huge bone marrow needs a big blood supply of its own. The result is that the total volume of blood in the body is increased, often to as much as twice normal. (You can often see enlarged veins pulsating in a thalassemic child's neck, and blue veins on their temples). This makes the anemia worse, and puts a big strain on the heart. It also means that when you give blood, the hemoglobin does not rise as much as you expect. It is as if you are trying to fill a bucket, and the bucket is bigger than normal.

3. Because a thalassemic is anemic, the body makes a mistake and thinks that they are short of iron. So it absorbs more iron from the food, in an attempt to correct the anemia. Of course this does not help. On the contrary, it makes the situation worse, by increasing the amount of iron in the body.

4. Many of the red cells that the bone marrow does manage to make become trapped in the spleen, because they are abnormal. This makes the spleen swell up. Then it traps more cells and begins to destroy them. Of course this makes the anemia, and all its consequences, worse.

5. Finally, because of all these strains on the system, thalassemics can not grow as well as normal children. Though their stomach

71

and face may be big, their arms and legs tend to get thin and weak, and they fall behind other children in height.

6.   Because the bone marrow cannot correct the anemia, you still need regular transfusions. And as a result, your body accumulates iron. But if you are low transfused you are still anemic all the time. Your bone marrow continues to try to make red cells, and you still have all these problems. In general, patients kept on a low transfusion regimen get gradually weaker, and the disease becomes more difficult to treat as they get older. Very few survive to adult life.

Well, how does high transfusion change things?

When your hemoglobin is kept in the normal range by blood transfusions, your bone marrow does not have to try to make blood any more. It gives up all its useless efforts and shrinks down to a normal size. This abolishes all the changes we have just described.

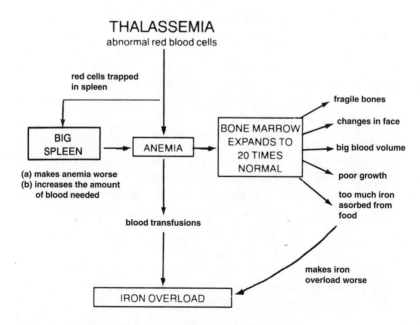

Figure 7.8. *This diagram shows the complex sequence of events in a child with thalassemia, who is on a low transfusion regimen.*

With high transfusion, your bones are strong and your face looks normal. You grow normally. Your heart is strong and your circulation is normal. When you are given blood, your hemoglobin rises as expected. You do not absorb too much iron from your food. The spleen usually may stay small and do no harm.

The main problem now is the problem of the iron overload from the blood that you receive.

You make high transfusion sound very good, but doesn't it need much more blood than a low transfusion regimen?

It does need about 30% (a third) more blood, to start with. But surprisingly, in the end, you may need less blood than on a low transfusion regimen. This is because some of the changes that can happen in low transfused patients increase the amount of blood they need.

Firstly, the total amount of blood in their body increases, because their bone marrow expands. So when you give blood, the hemoglobin does not rise as high as it should, and you have to give more blood. This does not happen in high transfused thalassemics.

Secondly, a big spleen increases the amount of blood a thalassemic needs, because it destroys red cells. In patients on a low transfusion regimen, the spleen nearly always enlarges and starts destroying transfused blood. This usually will not occur in patients who start on high transfusion from the beginning.

But if you need more blood, doesn't that make the problem of iron overload worse?

No, oddly enough, it doesn't. We explained above that when you are low transfused, you absorb too much iron from your food. When you are high transfused, this stops. So the total rate at which iron enters your body actually falls on high transfusion.

In addition, your body can resist any harmful effect of iron better when your hemoglobin level is normal, than when it is low.

How can you change from low transfusion to high transfusion?

It is quite simple. You only need one or two extra transfusions. Hemoglobin falls and rises on a low transfusion regimen. If a second transfusion is given 2 to 5 days after a transfusion is finished (instead of a month later), the hemoglobin will rise to nearly 14 g/dl (100%) (See Figure 7.9). Then you can go back to having transfusions about every 4 weeks, as before. At first you may need rather more blood than before, but this will only last 6 months or so. After that, your blood requirement will be only very little higher than it was before.

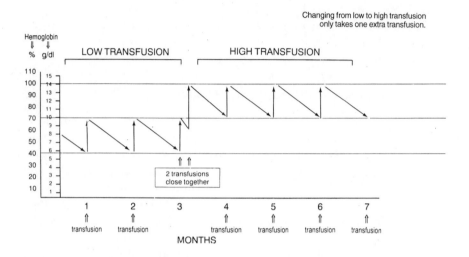

Figure 7.9. *It only takes one (or two) extra transfusions to switch a thalassemic from a low transfusion regimen to a high transfusion regimen.*

When you change to high transfusion, how quickly will you see the good effects?

You feel much more energetic, and start to eat and grow better almost at once, but the other benefits take longer. It takes 6 months to a year for the blood volume to decrease to normal. It also takes about 6 months for the bones to become stronger. So you have to be patient and persevere. But you will be encouraged because you feel so much more lively.

Does high transfusion always work?

Not always. If a patient already has a big spleen that is destroying much of the blood you receive, it may not be possible to keep to a high transfusion regimen. If this happens, it is necessary to take the spleen out before the high transfusion regimen can work.

Problems with Blood Transfusion

Don't you get a lot of problems with high transfusion as well as with low transfusion regimens?

Yes, you can get quite a lot of problems, but they can almost all be solved.

Does the hemoglobin always rise as the chart predicts after transfusion?

No, it does not always rise as high as expected. If it does not the reason should be found and corrected. Common reasons are:

1. The person has been on very low transfusion, so the blood volume is greatly increased. It is as if the bucket to be filled with blood is bigger than usual. In this case you have to give up to twice as much blood as you expect to get the desired rise in hemoglobin level. However, if the hemoglobin is kept at a high level, the blood volume shrinks down in time, as if the bucket you are trying to fill gets smaller. So if you persevere for 6 months or a year the hemoglobin should rise as predicted.

2. The spleen may be destroying the transfused blood. We discuss how you know whether the spleen is doing harm, and when to take it out, in the next section.

Does the hemoglobin level always fall at 1g/dl (7%) per week?

No, sometimes the hemoglobin level can fall more rapidly after a transfusion. If this happens only once there is no need to worry. But if it happens regularly you need to find the explanation. There are two possible reasons: (a) the spleen is destroying the red blood cells, (b) the patient has developed an antibody which tends to destroy the red blood cells.

Is something wrong if the interval between transfusions gets shorter and shorter?

Sometimes the interval gets shorter because your doctor has decided to change your transfusion regimen, but then you would know the reason.

If the interval between transfusions keeps getting shorter, without having been planned, an explanation is needed. It should not be difficult for your doctor to find the cause.

The commonest reason is growth. As a child grows, more blood is needed. If the same amount of blood is always given at each transfusion, obviously with time, it becomes necessary to give transfusions more often.

Another possibility is that the spleen is becoming over-active and destroying some of the transfused red cells.

What complications can be caused by blood transfusion?

Very important problems can arise from mistakes in preparing the blood, or mistakes when blood bags are changed during a transfusion. Such mistakes are very rare. It is always helpful if you look at the label on the blood bag, to check that it shows your name and blood group.

The commonest problems arise from sensitization (allergy) to white blood cells or plasma from other people, and from infections.

What are the signs of sensitization to white blood cells?

If you have become sensitive to white blood cells from other people, you can get a fever during transfusion. This means you have "antibodies" in your own blood, that react with white cells and platelets in the transfused blood. This sort of reaction, with a fever, feeling sick or even vomiting is called a "febrile transfusion reaction."

What are the signs of sensitization to a component of the plasma?

The most usual sign is "urticaria," which means an itchy blotchy skin rash, that can come up either during or after the transfusion. A much rarer, but more serious problem is "anaphylactic shock" when the blood-pressure falls and some tissues may become puffy. If the tissues round the mouth and throat puff up, there could be some difficulty in breathing. On the rare occasions when this happens, it can be treated with cortisone and adrenaline.

How can you prevent transfusion reactions?

They can be prevented in several ways.

For patients who only have occasional reactions, it may be enough to give paracetamol and an anti-histamine before the transfusion.

For patients who often have reactions, the white cells and plasma can be "washed" away from the red cells with salt solutions before the transfusion, so that only pure red cells are transfused.

Another method for preventing "febrile reactions" to white blood cells is to "filter" the white cells out of the blood. The filter is attached to the tubing from the blood bag. This is now routine in many Western clinics. However, filters are expensive, and one filter is needed for every 2 units of blood transfused.

In many places where thalassemia is common, filters are not available and there is no equipment for washing the blood. In these places it is possible to prevent transfusion reactions for patients who suffer from them regularly, by giving a single dose of cortisone immediately before the transfusion. (Given in this way once a month, cortisone is harmless.)

Can a patient become allergic to red cells?

25% of all thalassemics develop some type of "red cell antibodies." This means that they become sensitive to and destroy red cells in some of the units of blood they receive. The result is that their hemoglobin falls faster than it should, after transfusions. Patients who start regular transfusion after the age of 5 are more likely to make many antibodies to red blood cells. The solution is usually to find "fully compatible donors"—this means testing all units blood very carefully to be sure that it will not react with the patient's particular red cell antibodies. It is usually possible to find a set of compatible blood donors whose red cells are not destroyed by the patient's antibodies. Rarely it is not possible to find compatible donors. In this case, another solution is to give a low dose of cortisone or prednisone every day.

What infections can be passed on in transfusions?

Some infectious organisms can be transmitted through blood. For instance, malaria parasites, syphilis, and most recently the AIDS (Acquired Immune Deficiency Syndrome) virus have been shown to be transmitted by blood. However, transmission of these diseases is very rare indeed, because all blood donors are tested, and those who could pass on infections are identified and avoided.

It is more difficult to avoid a common virus called cytomegalovirus, but in people with normal immune defenses, it causes relatively little problem. However, it can sometimes cause problems after bone marrow transplantation. Therefore newly diagnosed patients who are likely to have a marrow transplant should be given "cytomegalovirus negative" blood, if this is possible.

What about hepatitis?

Hepatitis needs separate discussion. It means infection of the liver, and it can be caused by a number of different viruses that can be passed on in blood. Hepatitis is the commonest infection caused by transfusion.

One of the viruses that causes hepatitis, hepatitis B virus, is known. It is possible to identify carriers of hepatitis B virus, and they are no longer accepted as blood donors, so hepatitis B infections are now very rarely caused by transfusion. Also, it is possible to immunize people against hepatitis B with a course of hepatitis B vaccine. This involves three injections, two one month apart, and one six months later. All thalassemic patients should be immunized against hepatitis B.

However, there is another type of hepatitis, hepatitis C, caused by another type of virus. Hepatitis C virus is the most important cause of acute or chronic hepatitis caused by transfusion. Its frequency differs very much in different countries, and may differ from one region to another within the same country. This is because the proportion of healthy carriers of hepatitis C differs in different parts of the world. Blood donors are now tested for hepatitis C virus in most Western countries. There is no vaccine against the virus as yet.

Questions about the Spleen and Splenectomy

We have already said that if the spleen gets big, it may destroy too many red cells, and then it should be taken out.

Why does the spleen become big in thalassemia?

Normally, the spleen is a filter for the blood. It removes abnormal particles. For example it removes germs from the blood stream and kills them, and so helps to protect against infections. Normally, it also removes old used up red blood cells, and abnormal red cells.

Most of the red cells a thalassemic patient makes are abnormal. They often become stuck in the spleen, and this is why the spleen enlarges. Gradually more red cells become stuck, and the spleen starts to destroy them. The spleen just goes on getting bigger and bigger and destroying more and more red cells, until almost all the blood you transfuse just goes directly to the spleen and is destroyed. This process is called hypersplenism. It is irreversible. Once the spleen is doing harm, the only solution is to take it out.

High transfusion works so well because the patient's own bone marrow does not try to make any red cells. Therefore it does not make abnormal cells. They do not get stuck in the spleen, and the spleen usually stays small.

How can you tell when the spleen is doing harm?

The most important thing is to feel the size of the spleen. You can do this yourself, e.g. when a child is sitting comfortably on your knee, or sleeping. You cannot feel the spleen if a child is crying.

A normal spleen is small and is hidden under the ribs on your left side. You cannot feel it. In thalassemia you can usually, but not always, feel the spleen. You can measure it too, in centimeters from the edge of the ribs to the most distant part of the spleen.

In low-transfused thalassemic patients the spleen usually increases steadily in size. Figure 7.10 shows different stages of enlargement of the spleen, and the stage at which it is usually doing harm by destroying red blood cells. Usually there is no reason to remove the spleen if it is smaller than 4 cms. Between 4 and 6 cms it is hard to know what to do. If the spleen is bigger than 6 cms it is usually best to take it out.

However, the decision should not be hasty. In very small children, the spleen may shrink down again when high transfusion is started. It is also unwise to remove the spleen in children under 5 years old, because it increases the risk of a serious infection.

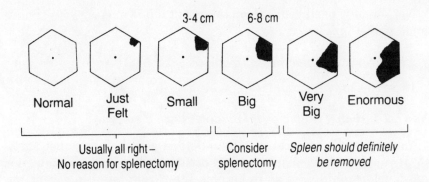

Figure 7.10. Stages in the enlargement of the spleen. In general, a small spleen does not cause problems, a spleen bigger than 6–8cm may cause problems, and a spleen larger than this should be removed.

Can taking the spleen out ever cure thalassemia?

No. Taking your spleen out never cures thalassemia. If you have thalassemia major you have a severe anemia, and a big spleen makes it worse. Taking the spleen out only removes this additional effect. Splenectomy only returns you to the situation you were in before the spleen made your thalassemia worse.

Then why do we sometimes hear of people being "cured" after splenectomy?

As you know, some people with thalassemia are born with a milder form called thalassemia intermedia which is described in a separate section below. These people can manage without regular blood transfusions. However, they can also get a big spleen. This can make their thalassemia so much worse that they need to start on regular transfusions. Of course, when the spleen is taken out, these people go back to having thalassemia intermedia again. Since they don't need transfusions any more, it is almost as if they had been cured. But their fundamental form of thalassemia has not been changed.

Patients who are well for the first 7 or 8 years of life, and then have to start on regular blood transfusions, and who have a big spleen, may in fact have thalassemia intermedia that has been made worse by the spleen. It is worth thinking about taking their spleen out.

Should everyone with thalassemia major or thalassemia intermedia have their spleen taken out?

No. You only need your spleen taken out if it is making your thalassemia worse.

Is splenectomy a dangerous operation?

It carries only a small risk.

Does it cause any problems if you don't have a spleen?

Your spleen is important to help defend your body against bacteria. If you don't have a spleen, very occasionally a bacterial infection can develop rapidly, so as to become life-threatening in a very few hours. Therefore, everyone who has had their spleen out should consider every infection as potentially serious. It is important to discuss this problem with your doctor, and decide precisely what to do if you get an illness with a fever.

What can we do to avoid serious infections after splenectomy?

There are some things you can do. One is to have "antipneumo-coccal vaccine" before your spleen is taken out.

Some doctors advise thalassemics whose spleen has been removed to take daily doses of penicillin to prevent some bacterial infections. This treatment may be recommended for a few years only, or for life.

Other doctors recognize that people often forget to take penicillin capsules regularly, and they only prevent some infections anyway. There are two ways to deal with this. Some doctors prescribe an injection of a long-acting penicillin once a month, but these injections are painful. Other doctors rely on a collaboration with the family. They tell them that if the patient has a fever that is not obviously just due to a cold, they must go immediately to the treatment center, or to the family doctor, for an examination and further advice. (In places where it is not easy to contact or reach the center very quickly, they sometimes give the family antibiotics to keep at home. These should be taken at once if there is a fever with no obvious explanation, and then the patient should be taken to the center.) This system seems to work very well. As with many other things, if you understand a risk, you can usually avoid it.

Does splenectomy cause any other problems?

No. Blood tests show that the number of platelets in the blood usually increases, sometimes to a really high level, following splenectomy. However, there is no evidence that the increased number of platelets causes any problems.

Questions about Bone-Marrow Transplantation

Why can transplanting bone marrow help?

A thalassemic's bone marrow is not able to make a normal amount of red blood cells. If the malfunctioning bone marrow can be replaced with normal bone marrow, that problem is solved.

Who can give bone marrow for a thalassemic?

It is necessary to have a "fully compatible donor," with tissues that match the thalassemic patient exactly, so that the thalassemic's body will not reject them. You can find out if someone is a fully compatible donor or not, by special blood tests. The most likely donors are a brother or a sister of the thalassemic patient. On average, one in four of a thalassemic's brothers or sisters is a suitable donor. Even quite small children (of about 2 years old) can be donors. Parents are very rarely a close enough match, unless they are first cousins. Unrelated people are never (as yet) a close enough match for a safe marrow transplant and are not recommended as donors.

Is it dangerous for the donor to give bone marrow?

Marrow is sucked out by a special needle from the hip-bone, and the sternum (the flat bone in front of the chest). The donor is given a general anesthetic and does not feel pain. It is not harmful to give marrow, and does not take longer than 30 minutes. If the donor is very young, a blood transfusion may be given after the procedure. The donor usually stays in the hospital 24 hours. The risk to the donor of bone marrow transplantation is the same as the risk of a general anesthetic: that is, it is very small.

How is a bone-marrow transplant done in practice?

To transplant bone-marrow, the first step is to make space in the thalassemic child's bones, for the new bone-marrow. To do this, the patient is treated with drugs (called cyclophosphamide and busulphan) to kill the thalassemic patient's own bone-marrow. The drugs are given by mouth, and can make the patient feel quite ill. Suppressing the bone marrow takes about 6 days. Once space has been made, marrow is taken from the donor, and "transplanted" into the recipient. This is done by putting it into a blood bag and running it into a vein, just like a blood transfusion.

Is bone-marrow transplantation dangerous?

Yes, it is. As we said, the patient has to be "prepared" by getting rid of their own bone-marrow. As white blood cells and platelets are also made in the marrow, they are lost too. But the white blood cells are an important part of our defense against infections, so if a patient who has been prepared for bone-marrow transplantation catches an infection, they can die from it. When the new marrow has become settled, it makes new white blood cells as well as normal red blood cells, so the danger of infection fades away.

Sometimes the patient's body reacts against the transplanted marrow and kills it. When this happens the graft fails, the thalassemia comes back and the patient needs regular transfusions again.

Sometimes the new marrow can react against the patient's body. This can lead to "graft-versus-host" disease, which is usually relatively mild, but sometimes is very severe.

Because of all the drugs that are used, the immune system cannot work as well as usual for at least 6 months after bone marrow transplantation. It is recommended for children to take at least 6 months off school after the procedure, to reduce their exposure to infections.

Can you summarize the risks, and the results, of bone-marrow transplantation?

Yes. Firstly, it is important to realize that the risk of bone-marrow transplantation is different in different countries, and also changes with time, as we become more experienced. The risk of marrow transplantation depends less on the age of the patient, than on how well he or she has been treated. The results are most likely to be favorable if the patient has been on regular treatment with Desferal (and so is not iron loaded), and if there is no liver problem. There is a good chance of success even in older patients providing the liver is healthy. Cirrhosis of the liver is a serious problem, and bone marrow transplantation is not recommended for such patients. In well-treated patients there is a 90% cure rate. However, there are many more problems in less well-treated patients.

How can you decide whether to have a bone-marrow transplant or not?

Firstly, it is necessary to have a fully compatible donor. So the thalassemic patient must have at least one healthy brother or sister. Special blood tests (called tissue-typing) will show whether they match the patient fully. If the patient has no brothers or sisters, and neither of the parents matches either, at present there is really no possibility of a bone-marrow transplant.

Secondly, you need to have considered the points for and against a transplant very carefully, in discussion with your own doctor, and also with the transplant specialist. Bone-marrow transplantation is a serious procedure, and both parents and patient need to consider all the possibilities before making up their minds.

Thirdly, bone-marrow transplantation is expensive. At most centers a transplant costs at least $60,000. In the U.S.A. it's over $100,000.

Questions about Iron Overload and Desferal

How much iron is there a normal person's body?

In most normal adults there are about 4 grams of iron. Three grams are in their red blood cells, and one gram is kept in a store in the liver, in case they need it. People get their iron by absorbing a small amount from the food they eat. Usually people absorb only about one tenth of the iron in their food.

There is no natural way of getting rid of iron once it is in your body, but a small amount gets lost every day in cells that rub off the surface of your skin or from the lining of your gut.

How does regular transfusion lead to iron overload?

Every unit of blood contains about one fifth of a gram of iron, so a thalassemic person who receives 20 units of blood a year, also receives about 4 grams of iron a year. There is no natural way of getting rid of this iron, so it has to be stored.

At first the extra iron is stored in the liver. The liver seems able to store away about 20 grams of iron without much difficulty. Most thalassemic children are able to store all the iron they receive safely, up to about 11 years of age. Your liver may enlarge a little to fit it all in, so it may be a bit easier to feel the liver edge in thalassemics than in other people. There is no harm in this. However, after about 11 years of age, the stores are full, and the iron begins to accumulate in places like the heart, where it can do damage. Figure 7.3 shows the parts of the body that can be damaged when iron is allowed to build up.

How does the iron that accumulates in the body do damage?

The right amount of iron is important for your body to be able to work normally. There is a small amount of iron in every cell. But if there is too much iron in a cell, parts of the cell may be damaged, and even die. Once this starts to happen it creates more problems, because the iron that was stored in that cell is freed, and has to be put into other cells.

How does Desferal help?

Desferal's only function is to prevent problems due to iron overload. It helps in two ways. Firstly, it picks up iron from your cells and brings it out in your urine and stool, and this keeps down the total amount of iron in your body. Secondly, it prevents the iron that is stored in your body from interfering with its normal functions.

When should you start Desferal treatment?

The iron that is given in blood causes visible damage only after about 10 years of age, and can cause death after about 16 years of age. Thalassemic patients who are on a low transfusion regimen usually die around the age of 12 years, for other reasons. Desferal treatment will not prevent this. It is therefore useless to give Desferal to patients who are on low transfusion.

Desferal does not solve any of the problems that are due to low transfusion. It does not help with anemia, bone changes, big liver, big spleen, or big blood volume. It should not be given to low-transfused thalassemics unless they are more than 10 years old, or their skin is slatey gray. Otherwise it is a waste of money for the parents, and uncomfortable for the child.

Problems must be solved one at a time. First and most important is to make sure that the patient is on high transfusion. Next, is to make sure that the spleen is not destroying the blood transfused. It is only worth worrying about iron overload when these two problems are under control.

How do you know when to start Desferal treatment and the amount of Desferal you need?

In principle, new patients should start after they have received about 20 units of blood. Older patients should start as soon as possible after they are settled on a high transfusion regimen. The best guide to your iron overload, and your need for Desferal, is your "serum ferritin" level. Ferritin is the substance that holds iron in the stores in your liver and other tissues. A small amount of ferritin gets out into the blood, and the amount in the blood reflects the amount of your iron stores. We can use it as a guide to tell us when you need Desferal, and how much. Figure 7.11 shows what different levels mean. Even if your ferritin is very high when you start treatment, Desferal treatment can bring it down to the recommended level with time.

What serum ferritin level should we aim for?

We do not think that thalassemics should aim for as low a serum ferritin level as other "normal" people. At present we think the best balance is reached when the serum ferritin is about 1,000 to 1,500 ng/ml.

WHAT DOES YOUR SERUM FERRITIN MEAN?

Ferritin, ng/ml	What it Means
Less than 1,000	Perhaps you are having *too much* Desferal!
1,000 – 2,000	Probably you are having ideal treatment.
2,000 – 4,000	Not low enough but not alarming. Work on it!
4,000 – 7,000	Much too high. It could lead to problems at puberty.
Over 7,000	This is getting dangerous!
Over 10,000	This needs *urgent* action.

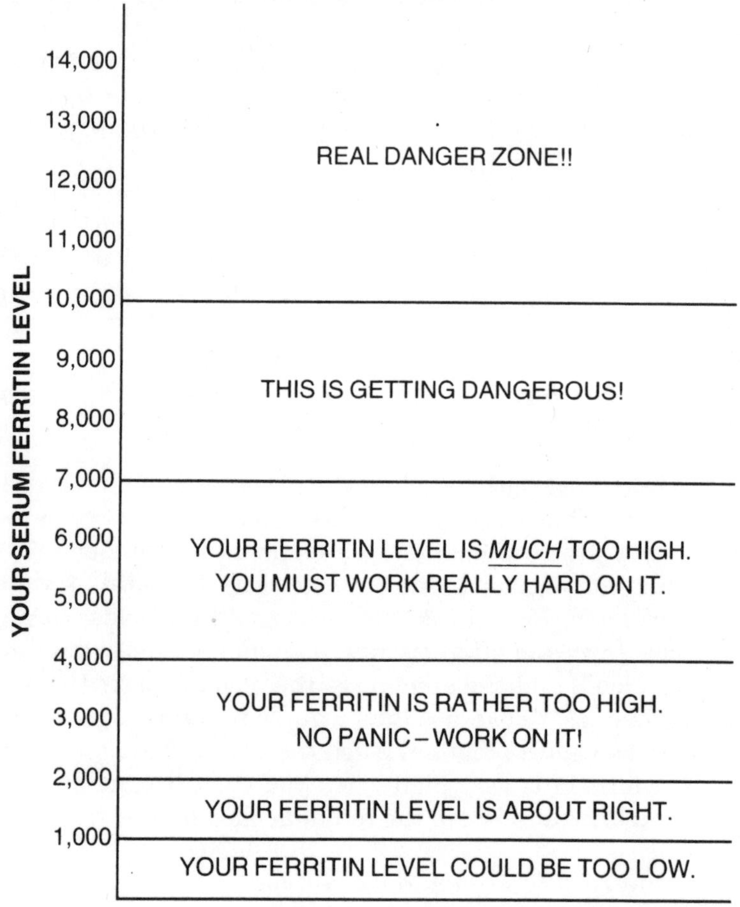

YOUR SERUM FERRITIN LEVEL

14,000
13,000
12,000
REAL DANGER ZONE!!
11,000
10,000
9,000
THIS IS GETTING DANGEROUS!
8,000
7,000
6,000
YOUR FERRITIN LEVEL IS *MUCH* TOO HIGH.
YOU MUST WORK REALLY HARD ON IT.
5,000
4,000
3,000
YOUR FERRITIN IS RATHER TOO HIGH.
NO PANIC – WORK ON IT!
2,000
YOUR FERRITIN LEVEL IS ABOUT RIGHT.
1,000
YOUR FERRITIN LEVEL COULD BE TOO LOW.

Figure 7.11. Your serum ferritin level.

What is the ideal dose of Desferal?

We are still not quite sure about this. In areas where Desferal is freely available, we recommend at least 25mg/kg/day (and not more than 50mg/kg/day except in exceptional circumstances). For most patients this means one to four vials (of 500mg) of Desferal most days. However, Desferal is very expensive. In many countries only a little, or even none at all, is available for most thalassemics.

Thalassemia Intermedia

"Thalassemia intermedia" simply means thalassemia of a milder kind, in which the patient can if necessary survive without regular transfusions. This includes a very wide range of people. A few are completely healthy, most are rather "delicate," while a few are chronic invalids. In the same person, the disease is fairly constant and should not change from time to time.

Thalassemia intermedia is usually caused by inheriting one of the common severe thalassemia genes and one milder thalassemia gene. (There is quite a large number of mild ß-thalassemia genes, but they are all rare, except Hb E, which is described in a separate section below).

How do you know if you have thalassemia intermedia, and not thalassemia major?

Children with thalassemia intermedia start to develop problems a bit later in life than those with thalassemia major. Most are reasonably well until after 2 years of age, and some with mild thalassemia intermedia may not have the diagnosis made until they are about 7 years old, or sometimes even older. Very occasionally, someone with a very mild thalassemia intermedia finds out only in adult life, for example when they become pregnant, or have a routine medical examination for some other reason.

There is not really a very clear distinction between thalassemia major and thalassemia intermedia. There are many borderline patients, who may have many of the problems mentioned below, but still manage just to survive without transfusion. Naturally enough, in countries where it is hard to find blood and Desferal, most borderline patients are not transfused, while in Mediterranean and European countries, most finally start on regular transfusions.

Can people with Thalassemia intermedia lead a normal life?

We can give a very general answer: yes, people with thalassemia intermedia should be able to lead a normal life.

What happens to people with thalassemia intermedia?

The very big differences between individual patients makes it hard to describe thalassemia intermedia as clearly as we can describe thalassemia major. Here we give only a very general description, which may not exactly fit your case.

How severe is the anemia?

Children with thalassemia intermedia usually become pale and ill only after their second year of life. They are moderately anemic, i.e., their hemoglobin level is usually between 8 and 9 g/dl. However, in some special cases it may be as low as 7 g/dl, and in a few others, as high as 10 or 11g/dl. In any case, you cannot really judge how severe your thalassemia is from your hemoglobin level alone. What really counts is how you feel in yourself: how strong you are, how well you grow, and whether you have any other problems.

Do people with thalassemia intermedia ever need blood transfusions?

Most people with thalassemia intermedia have occasional times when their anemia gets rather suddenly worse. This is usually a result of an infection, though sometimes it is hard to see a cause. If this makes you feel ill and stops you leading a normal life, your doctor will suggest that you should have a "top-up" transfusion, or even a course of transfusions. It is sensible to accept a transfusion when you need it, to give your bone-marrow a short rest, and help both you and it to recover. Having a few top-up transfusions will not make your thalassemia worse, and will not make you go on needing transfusions in the future.

What happens to the spleen?

In thalassemia intermedia, the spleen usually enlarges only rather slowly, and hypersplenism develops late, if at all. But finally, many people with thalassemia intermedia need to have their spleen taken out.

Are there any bone changes in thalassemia intermedia?

Most people with thalassemia intermedia have some changes in their bones and their face. The changes resemble those in children with thalassemia major who are not adequately transfused. But in thalassemia intermedia, the changes are usually quite mild, and do not spoil your looks.

Is there any problem with growth and puberty?

Children with thalassemia intermedia usually grow nearly normally in height, though they are often a bit thin. They go through a normal puberty, though often two to three years later than their "normal" friends.

Can people with thalassemia intermedia have children?

Yes, they can. Usually a woman will need regular transfusions during pregnancy, not so much for herself, but to help the baby to grow normally. Desferal treatment should be stopped during pregnancy, and probably so should other drugs. But pregnant women should take folic acid regularly.

Why do people with thalassemia intermedia sometimes need Desferal treatment?

People with thalassemia intermedia quite often have too much iron in their body, even if they are never transfused. This is because they usually absorb more iron from their food than the rest of us do. It is part of the body's attempt to cope with the anemia: it thinks that because you are anemic, you must be short of iron. So iron usually does build up slowly in your body, but it takes a long time (usually more than 10 years) for it to reach an undesirable level. To be honest, we are not certain what an undesirable level really is. To be absolutely safe, we usually say you should have some Desferal if your serum ferritin is more than 1000 mg/ml. When it does reach this level, it can usually be brought down again by a relatively short course of Desferal. About 6 weeks of subcutaneous infusions from a pump, or a course of intramuscular injections, twice a year (or an infusion once or twice a week) is usually adequate. It is important for you to have your serum ferritin measured at least once a year, to keep an eye on the iron build-up in your body, and to decide when to control it.

Particular Problems in Thalassemia Intermedia

A wide range of problems can arise in thalassemia intermedia, but they can all be dealt with. When these problems are severe, they may make it necessary to start on regular transfusion, even relatively late in life.

Most of the problems that can occur in thalassemia intermedia, happen because the thalassemia is not being controlled by regular blood transfusions. It can affect almost every part of the body. People with thalassemia major would have the same problems in a worse form, if they were not transfused. In fact, some older people with thalassemia major who were kept on low transfusion regimen in the past, when we did not know better, will remember having had some of these problems themselves.

The Spleen

Sometimes the spleen gets gradually bigger and the anemia gets gradually worse as the years pass. Finally some patients with thalassemia intermedia start to need transfusions. When that happens, removing the spleen often brings the situation back to what it was earlier in life. The anemia gets better, so some people can stop transfusions again after splenectomy.

Sometimes a mild thalassemia intermedia causes very little trouble in the first few years of life, so that no one notices that there is anything wrong with the child. But then the spleen may get bigger and make the thalassemia worse, and the diagnosis is made rather late. By this time the thalassemia intermedia may look like thalassemia major, because the spleen is making it worse, and the child may be started on regular transfusions. This is why we always wonder whether it is thalassemia major or thalassemia intermedia when a child with a big spleen starts to need transfusions for the first time after 4 years of age.

Occasionally, someone who really has thalassemia intermedia with a big spleen, who has been on regular transfusions for years, has their spleen taken out. After the operation, they may find they can manage without transfusions. This does not happen often. You may have heard stories of people who were "cured" by having their spleen taken out. This is the explanation of such cases. Splenectomy on its own does not improve thalassemia. It is helpful only if the spleen is making the thalassemia worse than it would be otherwise.

How do you know if your spleen is causing trouble and needs to come out?

The best way to follow what the spleen is doing in thalassemia intermedia, is to keep a regular record of your hemoglobin level and growth over the years.

In thalassemia intermedia, your hemoglobin level falls gradually below normal in the first 3 to 5 years of life. After that, in most cases, it remains more or less constant.

At this point it is important to explain exactly what a hemoglobin level means. Very many things can affect the measurement, such as the temperature of the room when the sample is taken, details of the method of taking the sample, and whether it is comes from a finger-prick or from a vein. These variations alone can make a difference of as much as a gram in the result. Also, your real hemoglobin level can vary by up to a gram either way, from week to week. And if you get an infection, even a relatively mild one, your hemoglobin level usually falls about a gram. Therefore, when you talk about your real hemoglobin level, it must be the average of several measurements taken some weeks apart. This is why we say people with thalassemia intermedia must have their hemoglobin measured at least 4 times a year. Then, if you keep a careful record of the measurements, you can see if your average hemoglobin level is changing from one year to the next.

The commonest cause for a steady fall in your hemoglobin level over the years is gradually developing hypersplenism. However, we do not recommend removing the spleen simply because your hemoglobin level is a bit lower than it used to be. It is only worth having the operation if you feel unwell, or there are other problems. For instance, an over-active spleen can slow down your growth-rate. This is one reason why it is important to keep a growth-chart.

The Bones

Some people with thalassemia intermedia can have severe bone problems. This is because their bone-marrow tries to work too hard to overcome the anemia, so that it expands inside the bones, and can weaken or even deform them. Some bones can be too fragile, and get fairly easily broken in the course of normal life. The growth of some bones can be disturbed, so that for instance, your upper arm may be shorter than other people's. Sometimes one leg bone may be shorter than the other, so that you develop a limp. This can usually be corrected by surgery after you have finished growing. Sometimes changes in the bones of the face can be severe, and some adults with thalassemia intermedia can get unpleasant, nagging pains in their bones and joints. If you have real problems of this type with your bones, you have a more severe form of thalassemia intermedia, verging on thalassemia major. Most bone problems can be controlled or cured by starting on regular transfusions.

The Bone Marrow and Folic Acid

In thalassemia intermedia, the bone marrow has to work very hard to make enough red blood cells to go round. One of the things it needs to make red cells is a vitamin called folic acid.

This vitamin is present in meat and in green vegetables. Usually people get as much folic acid as they need from their diet, but this is not always true for people with thalassemia intermedia, since they need considerably more than usual. This is why your doctor advises you to take a folic acid tablet every day.

What happens if you run short of folic acid?

Your anemia gets much worse, and people may think you have thalassemia major and start you on transfusions.

Are any particular people likely to get short of folic acid?

Yes. People who have a strict vegetarian diet can get short of folic acid. For instance, in England, some groups of people of Indian origin both have a high frequency of thalassemia and a strict vegetarian diet. People with thalassemia intermedia on this type of diet can get very ill without additional folic acid and may be thought to have thalassemia major. When they start on extra folic acid, they get better very quickly.

Can expansion of the bone-marrow cause any other problems?

Very occasionally, the bone marrow expands altogether too much, and makes the bones too thin and fragile, so that they break very easily. Sometimes it may even get into places where it should not be, and can interfere with the smooth working of other organs; for instance by putting pressure on nerves. Such important problems may indicate that, in this case, the thalassemia intermedia is too severe, and the patient should start on regular blood transfusions.

The Heart

In thalassemia intermedia, your heart has to work extra hard, because it helps to compensate for your anemia by pumping your blood round faster than usual. This does not, as a rule, do it any harm; the heart is a rather tough organ! But it does mean that when you have a chest X-ray your heart looks a little larger than usual. In itself, this is normal for you, and should not worry you.

But can't you have problems with your heart in thalassemia intermedia?

Yes, of course you can, but only under special circumstances. Firstly, if your thalassemia intermedia really is too severe, or if you get hyper-splenic, or short of folic acid, you become more anemic than you should be. When anemia is really severe, it does put too much strain on your heart. Then it really is not able to cope, and you can have problems. These things do not happen suddenly: the main thing is that you start to feel unwell and short of breath. If you really have heart problems, they can usually be "cured" by starting on regular blood transfusions.

Secondly, if you become iron overloaded, some of the iron may eventually find its way to your heart. Then, as in thalassemia major, you may have heart problems: but in thalassemia intermedia, this sort of problem rarely happens before about 30 years of age. It can be prevented by taking courses of Desferal treatment as your doctor advises, earlier in life.

The Kidneys

Thalassemia can sometimes affect your kidneys, because, as your bone marrow is so overactive, they make an unusual amount of wastes to be excreted in your urine. (The most important of these is uric acid.) As a rule this does not do your kidneys any harm, but they are often a bit larger than normal.

There may be an increased level of uric acid in your blood, and there certainly is in your urine. If the level is very high, the excess of uric acid can damage the kidneys. So it may be necessary to take a drug (Allopurinol) that prevents your body making so much uric acid.

Why do people with thalassemia intermedia often have to get up at night to pass water?

Quite often, people with thalassemia intermedia cannot make such concentrated urine as other people do. This means that you may lose more water than other people, and so may need more to drink. So many people with thalassemia intermedia need to get up once (or even twice) at night to pass water and to have a drink. This does no harm, but it is important always to have enough to drink, especially if you are ill and have a temperature.

Body Heat

Why do some people with thalassemia intermedia sweat a lot, and suffer from the heat in summer or at night?

This is because of the hard work your bone-marrow does all the time to make enough good red blood cells for you. For every good red blood cell, it has to make many that are no good and die in the bone-marrow without getting out into your blood. When they are broken down in the bone-marrow, each cell releases some heat, so altogether the body of a person with thalassemia intermedia generates more heat than other people. People with thalassemia intermedia have their own "central heating" that they can't switch off at night or in summer. So it is more comfortable for them not to have too many bed-clothes at night and to keep cool in warm weather.

The Liver

Your liver may be a bit big, so that the doctor can feel it, but this is harmless and a normal part of thalassemia intermedia.

Is it true that people with thalassemia intermedia are particularly likely to develop gallstones?

Yes, it is quite common for older people with thalassemia intermedia to get gallstones. The stones are made of a material called bile-pigments, that comes from your red cells that are made and broken down faster than normal. It collects in your gall-bladder; that is attached to your liver.

You can have an ultrasound examination from time to time, to see if you have any gallstones. If you get attacks of pain in the stomach, you should certainly have an ultrasound examination.

In fact, gallstones usually cause no trouble at all. But if they do cause uncomfortable stomach pains, the best thing is to have your gall-bladder removed, with the stones in it. You can manage very well without a gall-bladder.

Other Problems

What other problems can occur in thalassemia intermedia?

Ankle ulcers are a frequent and troublesome problem. They often arise just above the inside or outside of your ankle. They often start from a bruise or bang that takes a long time to heal. Once an ulcer has started, it can take a very long time to go, or simply refuse to go away at all. These ulcers are important, because they can interfere with your ability to work.

Ankle ulcers tend to occur in older patients (usually after puberty), especially if they are tall. They are caused partly by the fact that the blood supply to the skin over your ankles is rather poor. Your anemia also contributes because when blood does flow to this part of the skin, it may not be able to give it enough oxygen. And finally, when you stand or sit, the circulation in your legs is slower than when you are lying down because gravity keeps too much of the blood in your legs. There may be other reasons as well, why these ulcers happen.

What can you do to avoid ankle ulcers?

There are several things you can do to prevent ulcers from starting, but you only need to think about this after you have passed through puberty and if the skin on your ankles looks unusually thin and shiny or has brown marks on it.

Firstly, try to make sure that you do not bang your ankles. Most people bang their ankles accidentally from time to time, even with the heel of the opposite shoe. Try wearing a sock with a turned-down top (e.g. a toweling sock) to protect your shins or one of those toweling bands that tennis stars use on their wrists.

Secondly, make sure that the circulation is as free as possible in your ankles for at least several hours a day. To do this you need to raise your feet above the level of your heart. The easiest way to do this is to try sleeping with your feet slightly raised by putting a brick under the foot of your bed. It is even easier to raise your feet in a comfortable chair or on a sofa when you are resting, e.g. watching television. You should try to arrange to sit like this for about 2 hours every day if possible.

Thirdly, some people who have had ankle ulcers say that they can be prevented by taking zinc sulphate tablets daily by mouth. This has not been proved scientifically, but it is worth a try!

If you do actually get an ankle ulcer, discuss the best way to treat it with your own doctor.

Is it really better to have thalassemia intermedia than thalassemia major?

Usually it is better because you remain well enough to lead a reasonably normal life without having regular blood transfusions and daily tedious treatment with the pump.

However, there are some real disadvantages to having thalassemia intermedia. For instance, many people with thalassemia intermedia never feel completely well. In addition, you may hear a lot of things about thalassemia, but most of what people say, applies only to thalassemia major. Unless you understand that thalassemia intermedia really is different, and why, you may always feel uncertain about your health, and worried about your future. So sometimes people with thalassemia intermedia, and their families, worry more than families of people with thalassemia major.

One of the most worrying times is when the doctors think a small child of one or two years old may have thalassemia intermedia and not thalassemia major. Only time will give the answer. As time passes, if the child's hemoglobin level stays high, you get more and more hopeful that your child will have only a mild disease. But at the same time you get more and more anxious in case he or she finally turns out to have thalassemia major. We do understand that this can be a very trying time for parents.

Even after you know that you definitely have thalassemia intermedia, you may feel anxious in case something happens to make your thalassemia worse. We hope our explanation has reassured you that if it does get worse, we can usually find out why, and can correct the problem. It is rare for any sudden change to happen, so you always have time to notice it and bring it to the attention of your doctor. It is true that some people with severe thalassemia intermedia can develop quite serious problems and may have to change over to having regular transfusions. But really you should not be afraid of this. On the contrary, it is reassuring to know that if you do have a problem that cannot be solved in any other way, you can start on regular transfusions. This should make you feel secure and ready to try any form of treatment that your doctor proposes—because you know, if it does not work, you always have transfusion to fall back on.

And, though regular transfusions and daily Desferal are a bore, there is the advantage that you should feel fitter than ever before in your life, and you enjoy your food more!

Thalassemia Associated with an "Abnormal Hemoglobin"

Abnormal hemoglobins have an altered structure and sometimes an altered behavior. Occasionally a person inherits beta thalassemia from one parent and an abnormal hemoglobin from the other parent. Sometimes this causes problems, and sometimes not.

The important abnormal hemoglobin are:

- Hemoglobin S (Hb S)
- Hemoglobin C (Hb C)
- Hemoglobin E (Hb E)
- Hemoglobin D (Hb D)

They are carried in the same way as thalassemia, by healthy people who have one gene for normal hemoglobin, and one for the abnormal hemoglobin. Carriers of Hb S, for instance, are said to have sickle cell trait, and carriers of Hb E are said to have Hb E trait. Carriers of abnormal hemoglobin can be detected by blood tests, like thalassemia carriers can.

People who inherit Hb S from both parents have sickle-cell anemia, but people who inherit Hb C or Hb D or Hb E from both parents are perfectly well. People who inherit beta thalassemia from one parent and Hb S or Hb E from the other may have a severe anemia. But people who inherit beta thalassemia from one parent and Hb C or Hb D from the other, are perfectly healthy—just like healthy carriers of beta thalassemia trait.

Sickle Cell/Beta Thalassemia (HB S/β-Thalassemia)

Worldwide, Hb S is the commonest abnormal hemoglobin. So the commonest combination is Hb S/beta thalassemia. It is rather more like sickle-cell disease than like thalassemia.

Hemoglobin E/Beta Thalassemia (HB E/β-Thalassemia)

Hemoglobin E (HbE) is very common indeed in parts of India and South-East Asia and also in part of South Turkey and Eastern Saudi Arabia. So HbE/beta thalassemia is another "combined" form of thalassemia that is common among people from these areas.

It is usually, but not always, milder than beta thalassemia major. In fact, it is usually like thalassemia intermedia. A few people with Hb E/beta thalassemia need regular blood transfusions, some need transfusions occasionally, some need to have their spleen removed, and a few are very well with no treatment at all.

So if you have Hb E/beta thalassemia, read the section above on Thalassemia intermedia. But there is one thing you should remember as you read it. With Hb E/beta thalassemia, your blood carries oxygen rather better than in thalassemia intermedia, so you can stay well at a rather lower hemoglobin level. If your average hemoglobin level is above 7g/dl, you will probably lead a reasonably normal life without regular transfusions. If it is above 8g/dl, you should expect to be very well indeed. However, if it is less than 6.5g/dl, you will probably need blood transfusions, or you may need to have your spleen removed if it is very big.

The fact is, we do not know as much about Hb E/beta thalassemia as about other forms of thalassemia. However, we are learning, and we hope we will be able to write more about it in the future.

Psychological Aspects of Thalassemia

I have understood how thalassemia affects my body, but I don't yet understand how it affects me as a person and the effect it has had on my body.

Well, every person and every family is unique and is affected by thalassemia, reacts to it, and deals with it in unique ways. However, we do know a few things about individual and family development that could help you understand matters a little better. We must start by talking a little about what possibly happened to you and your family when your thalassemia was diagnosed.

When two people decide to get married, they start out with the idea that they want to be with each other through good times and bad times. Of course, no one knows beforehand what these good times and bad times are going to be, but both partners believe that together they can work things through. The last thing they imagine is that when they decide to have a child, their child will be born with a chronic illness because they are carriers.

In the beginning of their marriage the partners try to settle their ways of being with each other. They negotiate their differences and establish common ways of being together. Some couples have difficulty in resolving disagreements and conflicts from the start. Sooner or later most couples decide to have children. They hope that this will help strengthen their mutual commitment, but of course most people do not know how the presence of children in their life will change them or their relationship with their partner. When a child is born, it usually takes the couple some time to renegotiate their relationship and to fully adjust to the presence of a new family member.

The diagnosis of thalassemia usually comes at an early and crucial time in the life of both the child and the couple.

Usually the parents do not even know what thalassemia is. The result is normal and to be expected: the parents are shocked, disheartened and disappointed. They are in a state of despair because they do not know how to cope with such an unforeseeable and tragic event in their life and the life of their child. Often the presence of the illness brings the parents closer together to help each other deal with the common misfortune in their life. However, it can push them apart if the mother becomes completely preoccupied with the ill child and leaves her partner and any other children further out from her consideration. No matter how each family, each mother, father, brother and sister deal with this unexpected event, it is obviously not an easy task. Parents need to be informed and understand what thalassemia is. They need a lot of support and encouragement to learn how to deal with it in the most effective way, and in a way which will cause the least problems to their child. That is why help from a psychologist could be very useful at this time of crisis.

But how does thalassemia affect my psychological development?

It can have a profound effect in your psychological development both in childhood and in adult life. Erik Erikson, a prominent psychologist, has described how all human beings go through eight stages in life. Each stage has a positive, or desirable outcome, and a negative, or undesirable outcome. Whether the outcome of each stage will be positive and growth enhancing or not depends on thousands of factors. The presence of thalassemia can have an effect at every one of these stages

What effect do you think thalassemia has on childhood development?

There are four big steps in psychological development in childhood. Developing trust, autonomy, initiative, and industry. Let us look at each of these in turn, and the way thalassemia can affect it.

Year 1. The first thing we are called upon to learn in this life is how to trust. As infants we cannot survive on our own. We are completely dependent on the person who takes care of us. We hope and wish that this person (usually our mother) has the best possible intentions, but we can learn to trust her only by experiencing her consistent caring and affection. Her willingness and eagerness to be there for us is of utmost importance, especially during the first year of life.

The diagnosis of thalassemia during this first year of life makes things more complicated both for the child and the parents. Parents are passing through a time of grieving and shock, and often they do not know how to deal with their infant. They feel guilty, and they feel responsible. Often they also resent this sudden misfortune. This change in the parents, and in their behavior towards the child, combined with the beginning of painful treatments can make it very difficult for the young child to develop trust in other people. The child has no way of understanding what has suddenly happened, what it is that has changed its life so dramatically. The child feels the difference but has no way of explaining or understanding it. Although the child is far too young to understand the idea of a chronic hereditary disease, he/she is exceptionally capable of sensing when they are being really loved and treated with honesty.

Year 2. In order to become a mature, competent and independent adult a person needs to start developing a basic sense of autonomy from the time when they enter toddlerhood. The so called "terrible two's" is a difficult time for the parents (less of course than adolescence) because the child begins to say "no" and to have its own opinion. In addition, the child begins to move around on its own. It can now move away and towards its mother and other people and start exploring the world. If this newly developed autonomy and curiosity is thwarted by overprotective and fearful parents, the child develops shame and doubt in its desires and abilities. Very often other people, as well as parents and medical professionals, believe that a child who is ill is weak, vulnerable, and in more need of protection and constant surveillance. However, this attitude communicates the idea to the child that it is an inferior and less capable being. The fear that something may happen to the child or that the child will not be capable of making it on its own interferes with the development of autonomy. The autonomy of the child with thalassemia is thwarted not only by the parents, but also by the medical treatments which increase dependence on the presence of adults and helplessness in their absence. This includes parents and doctors as well as blood donors. Thus, issues of autonomy, dependence/independence, and trust in oneself and others are more complex, and more difficult to resolve than they are for children without thalassemia.

Year 3 to 5–6. In the next stage the child begins to initiate its own activities, like playing with other children, communicating with adults, etc. The development of initiative is important in order for the child to be prepared for school.

Fear, over-protectiveness, and the limiting factors of medical treatments (including Desferal treatment which usually begins about this time) may make the young child with thalassemia feel doubtful of its abilities and guilty for attempting to do its own thing. It is very important for parents and health care providers to allow thalassemic children to express themselves, and to participate in all activities appropriate for their age. Their physical disability must not be extended into an emotional or mental handicap, which does not exist.

Years 6–7 to 12–13. When the child enters school the parents must deal with another important concern; presenting their child to the world. All parents are concerned about how their child will do at school. Whether the child is bright enough, competent enough, admirable enough, etc.

How will the teachers and the other children accept and judge the child?

These concerns are even more prominent for the parents of a thalassemic child. The child has to develop industriousness and must be encouraged to be competent both academically and socially, and not be made to feel inferior to and less competent than other children. It is of course true that many adults can be very prejudiced against an ill child, partly because of ignorance and partly because of their own fears of what it means to be ill. However, the most important thing is how the parents feel and the message they transmit to the child and to the school system.

These four developmental stages can be resolved positively (i.e., the child develops trust, autonomy, initiative and industry) or negatively (i.e., the child develops mistrust, shame and doubt, guilt and inferiority). This is crucial for how well prepared the child will be for entering adolescence. Of course no one ever has such a perfect childhood that everything will be positive. But it is important to recognize the extent to which, for example, we are distrustful or guilt-ridden, and fearful of being our own person.

But why is adolescence always thought to be such a difficult time?

Adolescence is basically a preparatory stage for entering adulthood. Adulthood means leaving home, establishing intimate relationships outside the family, finishing one's education and entering the working world. The adolescent is becoming increasingly more aware of these tasks and has to start preparing her or himself. In order to do this, teenagers have to start forming their own identity. A number of

101

things make adolescence difficult. At the beginning there are a lot of physical changes. Girls start to become women and boys men. This results in many emotional changes as well. In order to fully understand why it is so difficult to be a teenager, we must realize that adolescence also brings important mental changes. The teenager is able to think in a way that is very different from that of a child. Adolescents begin to wonder about their existence in more abstract and philosophical ways. Such questions as: Who am I? What do I want to do in my life? etc. become very important to them.

Having thalassemia can make such questions more difficult since having a chronic illness is not something that can be easily accepted and integrated into one's identity. No one likes to think that they are ill and especially that they have something which is a life-long burden. Often added complications such as diabetes, hormonal and growth problems, and the fear of a shorter life can make matters worse. Questions about one's ability to be truly independent and self-sufficient are made more difficult because of the increased physical dependence due to the treatments and the way other people view the thalassemic teenager.

Generally speaking, teenagers tend to react against what they are told by "authority" figures in order to declare their independence and their right to have their own views. Their effort, which is perfectly normal and appropriate, is to separate from their family and from what adults in general think, and formulate their own opinion, their own being. Friends of the same age become a more important source of influence, and belonging to a "peer group" is crucial for their self-esteem. In the case of thalassemia, the rebellion can take the form of refusing, or of poor "compliance" with, medical treatments, especially Desferal treatment which interferes the most with their increased social life. Although this may be a step towards emotional maturity, towards caring for your own well-being because this is what you want rather than what you are told to do, it may also be dangerous unless this stage is reached quickly. Support groups can be a great help for teenagers struggling with all these important concerns and considerations.

How about adult life? Now that thalassemics grow to adulthood, what is it that I can know that will help me?

Love and work are the two important areas of life that an adult is called upon to fulfill and that give satisfaction. When we enter into adulthood with some basic sense of who we are, of our sexual identity, and what we want to do in life the most important and difficult task we have to achieve is forming intimate relationships. We should be able to trust and be open to a few people that we have carefully chosen to be our friends, so that we do not feel isolated and lonely. Intimacy is the 6th step in emotional development. It can be difficult to achieve since in order to be able to have true friendships and a true partnership in life we must be willing and able to be very open with ourselves. This involves some risk because sometimes when we open up ourselves we get hurt. Emotional pain can be more serious than physical pain, so we often protect ourselves by not being open towards others. However, true intimacy cannot be achieved when we hide ourselves.

But can I be open about myself and not get hurt?

How easily or how much we are hurt by other people depends on how important their opinion is to us. The more we like ourselves, the less we are afraid to be open, because we feel we have fewer things to hide. We like ourselves, we feel good about ourselves. We care less about what everybody else will say, and more about what a few of our close friends think.

But can I like myself and can my friends like me since I have thalassemia?

Having thalassemia does not mean that you are not likeable as a person. Everybody has to learn how to like and accept themselves as they are. There is nothing to be ashamed of, nothing that should make us feel bad about ourselves because we have thalassemia. Everybody has strengths and weaknesses, good and bad sides. No one is all good or all bad, except in very rare cases. We all have to learn how to live with, accept, admire, and when possible or necessary, change what we have and who we are. Having thalassemia is not something we can change, but we can change how we feel about having it. It is true, and perfectly normal, that we often feel that it is too much of a burden and it makes our life more difficult. It is normal at times to feel depressed and gloomy or angry and resentful. It is true that some people may be unable to think of sharing their lives, being friends with, or employing someone with a medical problem and consequently may turn us down. It is true that life is less carefree, and we often have to wonder how soon we will die and why we have to struggle so much. However, all these concerns and difficulties do not have to make us not like ourselves, or think of ourselves as less than other people.

On the contrary, it takes a lot of strength and courage to face the challenges of dealing with thalassemia.

What kind of work should I consider?

Work is another important aspect of adult life. Whether we have thalassemia or not, choosing a career or job is not an easy task. Often our inclinations are influenced by what other people, society, and our parents consider appropriate, respectable and desirable. When choosing a job we must consider a number of factors. Primarily, being employed is essential to being self-sufficient. Financial independence is an important aspect of self-sufficiency. In order to be able to do the things we want in life we must be able to afford them and not have to depend on others for their attainment. Secondly, however, we must also seriously consider what gives us fulfillment and satisfaction. Having a job that makes us feel bored, dissatisfied, and unfulfilled for the financial security it provides is a big compromise. In adult life at least half of our time is spent at work, so having a job that makes us feel stagnant and unhappy instead of creative and productive can make our lives very miserable.

Part of the difficulty in choosing a satisfying and fulfilling job is that the choice is usually made in adolescence. At that time, however, we may not know what we really want and what makes us happy, or how the ideal we have in our mind can be reached in real life. Quite often, later on in life, people feel they have made the wrong choice and would rather be doing something else. This may cause a great crisis especially for people with a family and children. Although it is risky to leave one's job and the things one knows how to do, a change can be a very growth promoting experience, and can lead to a more satisfying and fulfilled life.

But doesn't thalassemia affect my career choice?

When choosing a career it is important to remember our limitations. For example, it would be unrealistic to decide to become a professional athlete. We must also remember that in order to have the career we want, we must have the best education available to us. Thalassemia in itself does not influence how productive or creative we can be. However everybody has to struggle very hard to find a job that is satisfying and fulfilling which also provides the necessary means for survival. We must not be afraid to go out in the job market and compete with other people for a position we want. We must make sure that we have the necessary skills and qualifications. We must also have the best medical treatment, provided at convenient times, so that our treatment does not interfere with our education or our job.

When we reach old age, or closer to our death, we will reevaluate our life and we will think of all the things we have and have not done. Our eighth, and final developmental task is ending our life with a sense of integrity for a life well spent instead of a sense of despair for a life not well spent. Many people, however, do not have the wisdom, or the foresight to realize that life will not go on forever. They should start doing all the things they want to do and that make them feel good about themselves and their lives before it is too late.

But I have been thinking about the possibility of me dying sooner than most people and it scares me a great deal.

It is normal and natural that you have such thoughts. It is also normal and natural for such thoughts to make you sad and fearful. However, death is a part of life. Every being that has been born will die. Some live for only a few moments or days, some live for many years. No one knows before hand when they will die, no matter how healthy they are.

The fact that one day we will die must not stop us from living today. Actually the idea of death can help us understand how important life is. It can help us appreciate life and all the things we have and it can make us work hard for achieving what we want to accomplish before it is too late. The better we live today the less threatened we feel about the possibility of dying tomorrow.

What is most important to remember is, that since one day we will all die we must try to make each moment and each day of our life as beautiful, satisfying, and fulfilling as we can. In order to do so, we must, at an early stage, develop an inner feeling and belief that we are capable of, and deserve, to have a happy life. Thalassemia as such is not an obstacle for achieving this way of thinking. It is the way we view it that can hinder our development.

Thalassemia Associations

For many young thalassemics it can be helpful to be close to other people with similar problems, who understand the disease, as well as the complexities in our relationships with our parents. Thalassemia Associations that bring thalassemic adolescents and young adults together can be helpful in this way. Here friendships are made, people strengthen and encourage each other (especially in relationship to taking the Desferal pump), and they support and accompany each other into the adult world. Some families and some people do not want to join a Thalassemia Association for various reasons. They may just not enjoy associations. They may be so healthy that they do not feel the need to meet other thalassemics, or they may not want people to know that thalassemia exists in the family. People themselves are the best judges of whether or not to join an association.

Thalassemics can feel guilty too, because their disease causes much trouble to their family. It is true that thalassemia puts extra pressures on the family, but it puts most pressure on you, and it is not your fault that you have it. It is just one of the many problems that arise in life that we have to face together.

Thalassemia Associations are important because they show that thalassemia is not just a problem for you or your family, it involves us all. We all gain by sharing in the struggle to cope with it in the best way possible. We play an important part by accepting the help that other people may offer, and by developing into unique and self-fulfilled individuals. Some thalassemics also help by speaking out about the services they need, by volunteering for research studies, and in many other ways.

The Thalassemia Action Group

The Thalassemia Action Group (TAG) is a patient support group sponsored by the Cooley's Anemia Foundation and run by thalassemic patients. TAG members offer each other support, understanding, and compassion. Membership programs span the needs of the very young, teenage and young adult patient population. Many parents are also involved in TAG activities. For example, an annual patient/parent conference is held where patients, families and friends gather to discuss common concerns and learn about new treatments. New TAG members are given an opportunity to meet others and develop friendships to help them better cope with their stress. TAG members also provide each other with information to maintain better health care.

Programs offered by TAG include:

- TAG newsletter
- TAGline, a telephone support network
- Scholarships for education
- Annual patient/parent conference
- Regional networking meetings

- Education and public awareness programs
- Legislative advocacy projects

TAG began in 1984 by patients who felt the need to help each other better comply with the demanding treatment regime. Through the support of TAG, patients are achieving career and other personal goals along with gaining the encouragement to continue their fight with this blood disorder.

— section by Dr. Eugenia Georganda

More Information about Thalassemia

For more information about thalassemia, the Thalassemia Action Group, or a directory of international thalassemia associations contact:

Cooley's Anemia Foundation National Office and
Thalassemia Action Group (TAG)
129-09 26th Avenue, Suite 203
Flushing, New York 11354
(800) 522-7222

Chapter 8

What You Need to Know about Being a Carrier of Cooley's Anemia (Thalassemia Trait)

What Is Thalassemia?

Thalassemia is an inherited characteristic of the blood. It reduces the amount of hemoglobin your body can make, so it can cause anemia. The trait is primarily found in people of Mediterranean, African, Southeast Asian, Asian, and Indian descent. It is rare in Northern Europeans.

There are two forms of thalassemia:

1. Thalassemia trait. People with thalassemia trait are generally healthy, but if two people with thalassemia trait both pass the trait to their child, the child will have thalassemia major. It is estimated that more than two million people in the United States carry the thalassemia trait.

2. Thalassemia major. This is a very serious blood disorder that begins early in childhood. Children who have thalassemia major cannot produce sufficient hemoglobin. They need frequent blood transfusions and medical treatment.

The World Health Organization recognizes Cooley's Anemia as the most prevalent inherited, genetic blood disorder in the world. There are over 300,000 patients worldwide.

Cooley's Anemia Foundation, Inc., 129-09 26th Avenue, Flushing, NY 11354, (718) 321-CURE, (800) 522-7222; reprinted with permission.

Thalassemia major is sometimes called Mediterranean Anemia, Cooley's Anemia, or Homozygous Beta Thalassemia.

Blood and Anemia

To understand more about thalassemia, you need to know a little about normal blood and about anemia. Thalassemia trait is sometimes confused with iron deficiency and leads to the unnecessary administration of iron.

What is blood made of?

Blood is made up of a lot of red blood cells in a clear, slightly yellow liquid called plasma. Each red blood cell only lives for about four months. It is then broken down. New red blood cells are being made all the time. The blood cells are replaced very quickly—that's why people can give blood often.

Blood is red because the red blood cells contain a substance called hemoglobin. Hemoglobin is very important because it carries oxygen from your lungs to wherever it is needed in your body.

Hemoglobin contains a lot of iron. When your red blood cells are broken down, most of the iron from the hemoglobin is used again to make new hemoglobin. You lose some iron from your body every day and you make up for it with the iron in the food you eat. In fact the main reason why people need iron in their food is to make hemoglobin.

What is anemia?

Some people have too little hemoglobin in their blood. These people have anemia. There are many different kinds of anemia. The most common kind is iron deficiency anemia. This happens when people do not have enough hemoglobin because they're not eating enough of the foods that contain iron.

Thalassemia major is a different kind of anemia. It is caused by not having enough hemoglobin, but it has nothing to do with the amount of iron you're getting from your food. It is an inherited disease.

Thalassemia Trait

What is the thalassemia trait?

People with the thalassemia trait will not become ill due to the trait, although they may be slightly anemic.

Most people with the thalassemia trait do not know that they have it. You only discover it if you have a special blood test. If you are from the Mediterranean region, you are encouraged to be tested.

The red blood cells of people with the thalassemia trait are smaller and different in shape than normal blood cells.

People with the thalassemia trait also have slightly more of a kind of hemoglobin called hemoglobin A_2 in their blood. The thalassemia trait is present at birth, it remains the same for life, and it can be handed on from parents to children. That means, it is inherited.

What does it matter if you carry the thalassemia trait?

It is important to know if you carry the thalassemia trait because two people with the thalassemia trait can have children with thalassemia major, a serious blood disease. Also, the thalassemia trait is sometimes confused with iron deficiency anemia and leads to the unnecessary administration of iron.

NORMAL RED BLOOD CELLS **THALASSEMIA TRAIT RED BLOOD CELLS**

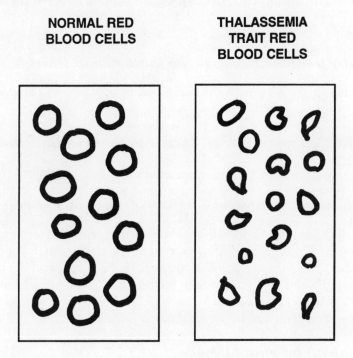

Figure 8.1. *A comparison of normal red blood cells and thalassemia trait red blood cells.*

How do you find out if you have the thalassemia trait?

You have to have a special blood test. Doctors measure the size of your red blood cells and how much hemoglobin A_2 you have in your blood.

Does a thalassemia carrier need special medical treatment?

No.

Is a thalassemia carrier more likely to get other illnesses?

No.

Is a thalassemia carrier physically or mentally weak?

No.

Does the thalassemia trait affect the sort of work you can do?

No.

Can any treatment change the thalassemia trait?

No. If you are born with the thalassemia trait you will always have it.

Can the thalassemia trait turn into thalassemia major?

No.

Do thalassemia carriers ever need iron supplements?

The best way to tell whether a thalassemia trait carrier needs iron is by special blood tests that measure the amount of iron in your blood. If you don't have these tests, the doctor may think that you are short of iron simply because you have small red cells and slight anemia, and may advise you to keep taking extra iron when you really do not need it. This will do you no good and in the long run it could be harmful.

What about pregnant women?

Pregnant women with the thalassemia trait need extra iron just as much as any other pregnant women.

Why is the thalassemia trait found in certain countries?

People with the thalassemia trait are less likely to die if they catch malaria. In the past, in countries where malaria was very common, people with the thalassemia trait survived malaria when other people died. They passed the trait onto their children so that the thalassemia trait was a great advantage and as time passed it became more common in malarial parts of the world. But now we can usually cure or prevent malaria, and the thalassemia trait is no longer an advantage. It does not go away when malaria disappears.

Many countries used to have malaria and all now have quite a large number of people with the thalassemia trait. For instance, it is estimated that two million people in the United States have the trait. In Cyprus one in seven people have the thalassemia trait (both Turkish and Greek Cypriots), and in Greece one in twelve people have the thalassemia trait. In Italy and all of the Middle East and Asia, including India, Pakistan, Hong Kong and Vietnam, the number of people with the thalassemia trait varies from one in fifty to one in ten in different areas. In Africa and the West Indies about one in fifty people have the thalassemia trait. About one in every thousand people of British origin have the trait.

Other Forms of the Thalassemia Trait

This chapter is all about the beta-thalassemia trait, but there are other forms of the thalassemia trait:

- **Delta-beta thalassemia trait and Hemoglobin Lepore trait** are very similar to the beta-thalassemia trait. If you have either of these traits, all the information in this chapter applies to you. The diagnostic tests are slightly different than those for the beta-thalassemia trait. They include measurement of hemoglobin F and a test called hemoglobin electrophoresis.

- **Alpha-thalassemia trait** may also cause mild anemia and small red blood cells. It does not cause any illness. The diagnostic tests for the alpha-thalassemia trait are different than those for the beta-thalassemia trait.

In addition to the thalassemias there are three important forms of abnormal hemoglobins. These are Hemoglobin S, Hemoglobin C, and Hemoglobin E. If someone who carries the beta-thalassemia trait marries someone who carries one of these abnormal hemoglobins, there is a risk that some of the children could have a serious anemia.

How Is the Thalassemia Trait Passed on from Parents to Their Children?

Let us consider three sorts of couples.

1. If both parents are not carriers, they cannot possibly pass on the thalassemia trait or thalassemia major to their children. All their children will have normal blood.

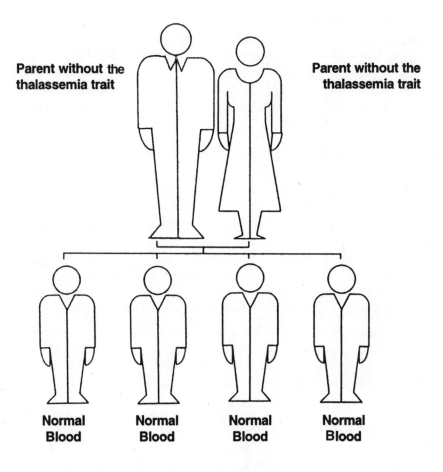

Parent without the thalassemia trait

Parent without the thalassemia trait

| Normal Blood | Normal Blood | Normal Blood | Normal Blood |

Figure 8.2. Two parents without the thalessemia trait.

2. If one parent has the thalassemia trait and one is not a carrier there is a one in two (50%) chance that each of their children will have the thalassemia trait. None of their children can have thalassemia major.

    People with the thalassemia trait can pass on the trait through many generations without realizing that it is "in the family."

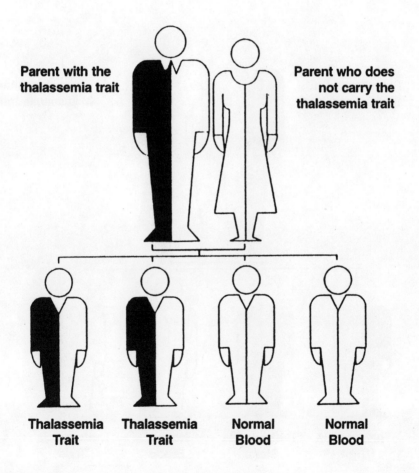

Figure 8.3. One parent with the thalessemia trait and one parent without the thalessemia trait.

3. If both parents carry the thalassemia trait, their children may have the thalassemia trait, or they may have completely normal blood, or they may have thalassemia major. In each pregnancy there is a one in four (25%) chance that their child will have normal blood, a two in four (50%) chance that the child will have the thalassemia trait, and a one in four (25%) chance that the child will have thalassemia major. The chances of having a child with thalassemia major remain one in four (25%) with each pregnancy, even if you already have a child with thalassemia major.

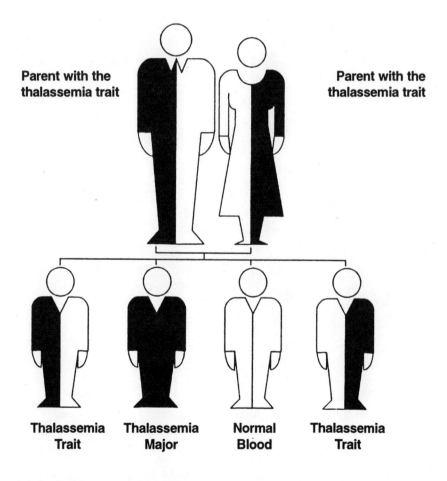

Parent with the
thalassemia trait

Parent with the
thalassemia trait

| Thalassemia | Thalassemia | Normal | Thalassemia |
| Trait | Major | Blood | Trait |

Figure 8.4. Two parents with the thalessemia trait.

Thalassemia Major

What is thalassemia major?

Thalassemia major is a serious, inherited anemia. Children with thalassemia major cannot produce sufficient hemoglobin. Because of this their bone marrow cannot produce enough red blood cells. The red blood cells that are produced are nearly empty of hemoglobin.

Children with thalassemia major are normal at birth but become anemic between the ages of three months and eighteen months. They become pale, do not sleep well, do not want to eat, and may vomit their food. If children with thalassemia major are not treated, they have miserable lives. They usually die between one and eight years of age.

Can thalassemia major be treated?

The main treatment for thalassemia major is regular blood transfusions, usually every two to four weeks.

After each blood transfusion the red blood cells in the new blood are broken down slowly over the next four months. The iron from the red blood cells stays in the body. If it is not removed, it builds up and

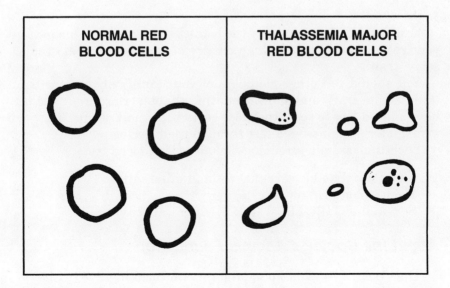

Figure 8.5. Normal red blood cells and thalassemia major red blood cells.

can damage the liver, the heart, and major organs in the body. If this iron build-up is not prevented, most people with thalassemia major die when they are about twenty years old.

At present, the only way to remove the extra iron from the body is to give infusions of a drug called Desferal under the skin from a small pump 8-10 hours every night. Desferal picks up the iron and carries it out in the urine and stool. This treatment is very successful and most children treated with blood transfusions and Desferal can now lead fairly normal lives. But the treatment is unpleasant and often upsetting. We are looking for better treatment all the time.

How can we prevent thalassemia major?

Many couples who both carry the beta-thalassemia trait decide to test each pregnancy to find out if the baby has beta-thalassemia major. Doctors can now test for thalassemia major as early as ten weeks into the pregnancy. This test, called chorionic villus sampling or CVS, is routinely done between the tenth and twelfth week. Another available option is amniocentesis routinely done between the fifteenth and nineteenth week of pregnancy. To find out more, ask your doctor to arrange for you to visit a genetic counselor.

Should my relatives have a blood test for thalassemia as well?

Yes. The fact that you carry the beta-thalassemia trait means that your relatives also have a high chance of carrying the beta-thalassemia trait.

You should tell other members of your family about your beta-thalassemia trait, and show them this chapter. Encourage them to have a blood test to see if they also carry beta-thalassemia. They can arrange for a thalassemia test through their doctor.

Each thalassemia screening includes three blood tests:

- CBC (complete blood count) without differential
- Hemoglobin electrophoresis
- Serum iron/TIBC (Total Iron Binding Capacity)

About the Cooley's Anemia Foundation

The Cooley's Anemia Foundation was formed in 1954 by the parents of thalassemia patients in the United States. The aim of the Foundation is to educate the public about the disorder, raise funds to support medical research and improve treatment options, and to encourage blood testing, counseling, and screening programs.

The Cooley's Anemia Foundation is the only national, voluntary health organization that exclusively funds medical research, patient services, public information, and professional education to combat this fatal hereditary blood disorder.

The Foundation sponsors the Thalassemia Action Group (TAG), a patient support group serving the needs of the patient population. If you want to learn more about thalassemia, please contact the Foundation.

Chapter 9

Facts about Sickle Cell Anemia

What Is Sickle Cell Anemia?

Sickle cell anemia is an inherited blood disorder, characterized primarily by chronic anemia and periodic episodes of pain.

The underlying problem involves hemoglobin, a component of the red cells in the blood. The hemoglobin molecules in each red blood cell carry oxygen from the lungs to the body organs and tissues and bring back carbon dioxide to the lungs.

In sickle cell anemia, the hemoglobin is defective. After the hemoglobin molecules give up their oxygen, some of them may cluster together and form long, rod-like structures. These structures cause the red blood cells to become stiff and to assume a sickle shape. Unlike normal red cells, which are usually smooth and donut-shaped, the sickled red cells cannot squeeze through small blood vessels. Instead, they stack up and cause blockages that deprive the organs and tissue of oxygen-carrying blood. This process produces the periodic episodes of pain and ultimately can damage the tissues and vital organs and lead to other serious medical problems. Unlike normal red blood cells, which last about 120 days in the bloodstream, sickled red cells die after only about 10 to 20 days. Because they cannot be replaced fast enough, the blood is chronically short of red blood cells, a condition called anemia.

NIH Pub. No. 96-4057, November 1996.

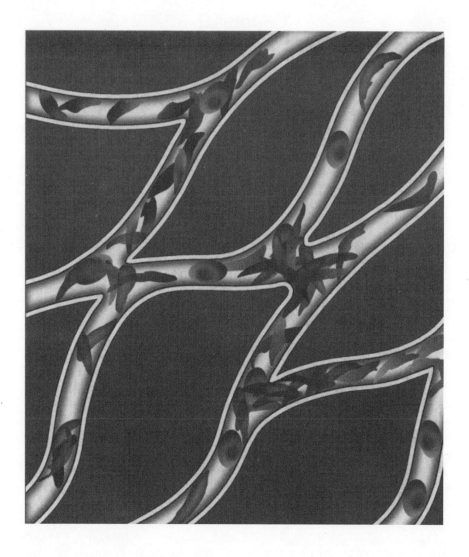

Figure 9.1. The sickle-shaped red blood cells tend to get stuck in narrow blood vessels, blocking the flow of blood.

What Causes Sickle Cell Anemia?

Sickle cell anemia is caused by an error in the gene that tells the body how to make hemoglobin. The defective gene tells the body to make the abnormal hemoglobin that results in deformed red blood cells. Children who inherit copies of the defective gene from both parents will have sickle cell anemia. Children who inherit the defective sickle hemoglobin gene from only one parent will not have the disease, but will carry the sickle cell trait. Individuals with sickle cell trait generally have no symptoms, but they can pass the sickle hemoglobin gene on to their children.

The error in the hemoglobin gene results from a genetic mutation that occurred many thousands of years ago in people in parts of Africa, the Mediterranean basin, the Middle East, and India. A deadly form of malaria was very common at that time, and malaria epidemics caused the death of great numbers of people.

Studies show that in areas where malaria was a problem, children who inherited one sickle hemoglobin gene—and who, therefore, carried the sickle cell trait—had a survival advantage: unlike the children who had normal hemoglobin genes, they survived the malaria epidemics; they grew up, had their own children, and passed on the gene for sickle hemoglobin.

As populations migrated, the sickle cell mutation spread to other Mediterranean areas, further into the Middle East, and eventually into the Western Hemisphere.

In the United States and other countries where malaria is not a problem, the sickle hemoglobin gene no longer provides a survival advantage. Instead, it may be a serious threat to the carrier's children, who may inherit two abnormal sickle hemoglobin genes and have sickle cell anemia.

How Common Is Sickle Cell Anemia?

Sickle cell anemia affects millions of people throughout the world. It is particularly common among people whose ancestors come from sub-Saharan Africa; Spanish-speaking regions (South America, Cuba, Central America); Saudi Arabia; India; and Mediterranean countries, such as Turkey, Greece, and Italy.

In this country, it affects approximately 72,000 people, most of whose ancestors come from Africa. The disease occurs in approximately 1 in every 500 African-American births and 1 in every 1,000-1,400 Hispanic-American births.

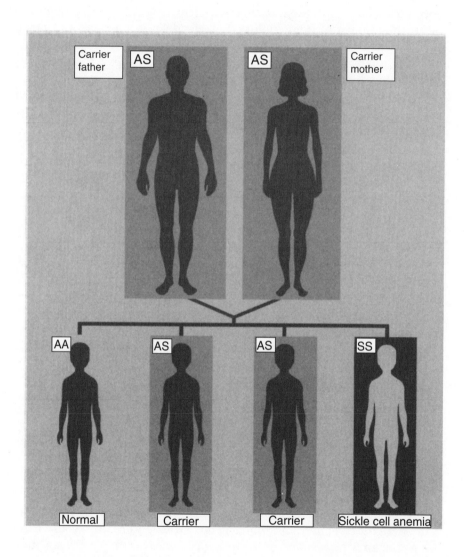

Figure 9.2. *The presence of two defective genes (SS) is needed for sickle cell anemia. If each parent carries one sickle hemoglobin gene (S) and one normal gene (A), with each pregnancy, there is a 25 percent chance of the child's inheriting two defective genes and having sickle cell anemia; a 25 percent chance of inheriting two normal genes and not having the disease; and a 50 percent chance of being an unaffected carrier like the parents.*

Approximately 2 million Americans, or 1 in 12 African Americans, carry the sickle cell trait.

What Are the Signs and Symptoms of Sickle Cell Anemia?

The clinical course of sickle cell anemia does not follow a single pattern; some patients have mild symptoms, and some have very severe symptoms. However, the basic problem is the same—the sickle-shaped red blood cells tend to get stuck in narrow blood vessels, blocking the flow of blood.

This results in the following conditions:

- **Hand-foot syndrome.** When the small blood vessels in the hands or feet are blocked, pain and swelling can result, along with fever. This may be the first symptom of sickle cell anemia in infants.

- **Fatigue, paleness**, and shortness of breath—all symptoms of anemia, or a shortage of red blood cells.

- **Pain** that occurs unpredictably in any body organ or joint, wherever the sickled blood cells block oxygen flow to the tissues. The frequency and amount of pain varies. Some patients have painful episodes (also called crises) less than once a year, and some have as many as 15 or even more episodes in a year. Sometimes the pain lasts only a few hours; sometimes it lasts several weeks. For especially severe, ongoing pain, the patient may have to be hospitalized and treated with painkillers and intravenous fluids. Pain is the principal symptom of sickle cell anemia in both children and adults.

- **Eye problems.** When the retina, the "film" at the back of the eye that receives and processes visual images, does not get enough nourishment from circulating red blood cells, it can deteriorate. Damage to the retina can be serious enough to cause blindness.

- **Yellowing of the skin and eyes.** These are signs of jaundice, resulting from the rapid breakdown of red blood cells.

- **Delayed growth and puberty** in children and often a slight build in adults. The slow rate of growth is caused by a shortage of red blood cells.

- **Infections.** In general, both children and adults with sickle cell anemia are more vulnerable to infections and have a harder time fighting them off once they start. This is the result of damage to the spleen from the sickled red cells which prevents the spleen from destroying bacteria in the blood. Infants and young children, especially, are susceptible to bacterial infections that can kill them in as little as 9 hours from onset of fever. Pneumococcal infections used to be the principal cause of death in young children with sickle cell anemia until physicians began routinely giving penicillin on a preventive basis to infants who are identified at birth or in early infancy as having sickle cell anemia.

- **Stroke.** The defective hemoglobin damages the walls of the red blood cells, causing them to stick to blood vessel walls. This can result in the development of narrowed, or blocked, small blood vessels in the brain, causing a serious, life-threatening stroke. This type of stroke occurs primarily in children.

- **Acute chest syndrome**—a life-threatening complication of sickle cell anemia, similar to pneumonia, that is caused by infection or trapped sickled cells in the lung. This is characterized by chest pain, fever, and an abnormal chest x ray.

How Is Sickle Cell Anemia Detected?

Early diagnosis of sickle cell anemia is critical so that children who have the disease can receive proper treatment.

More than 40 states now perform a simple, inexpensive blood test for sickle cell disease on all newborn infants. This test is performed at the same time and from the same blood samples as other routine newborn screening tests. Hemoglobin electrophoresis is the most widely used diagnostic test.

If the test shows the presence of sickle hemoglobin, a second blood test is performed to confirm the diagnosis. These tests also tell whether the child carries the sickle cell trait.

How Is Sickle Cell Anemia Treated?

Although there is no cure for sickle cell anemia, doctors can do a great deal to help sickle cell patients, and treatment is constantly being improved.

Basic treatment of painful crises relies heavily on pain-killing drugs and oral and intravenous fluids to reduce pain and prevent complications.

Blood transfusions are used to treat and to prevent some of the complications of sickle cell anemia. Transfusions correct anemia by increasing the number of normal red blood cells in circulation. Transfusions are used to treat spleen enlargement in children before the condition becomes life-threatening. Regular transfusion therapy also can help prevent recurring strokes in children at high risk of crippling nervous system complications.

Giving young children with sickle cell anemia oral penicillin twice a day, beginning when the child is about 2 months old and continuing until the child is at least 5 years old, can prevent pneumococcal infection and early death in these children. Recently, however, several new strains of pneumonia bacteria that are resistant to penicillin have been reported. Since the vaccines for these bacteria are ineffective in young children, studies are being planned to test new vaccines.

The first effective drug treatment for adults with severe sickle cell anemia was reported in early 1995, when a study conducted by the National Heart, Lung, and Blood Institute showed that daily doses of the anticancer drug hydroxyurea reduced the frequency of painful crises and of acute chest syndrome in these patients. Patients taking the drug also needed fewer blood transfusions. The long-term side effects of hydroxyurea and its effects in children with sickle cell anemia are still being studied.

Sickle cell anemia patients with severe chest or back pain that prevents them from breathing deeply may be able to avoid potentially serious lung complications associated with acute chest syndrome by using an incentive spirometer. This is a small plastic device, shaped like a tube, with a ball inside. The patient must breathe into it hard enough to force the ball up the tube, so using it helps the patient breathe more deeply.

Most complications of sickle cell anemia are treated as they occur. For example, laser coagulation and other types of eye surgery may be used to prevent further vision loss in patients with eye problems. Surgery may be recommended for certain kinds of organ damage— for example, to remove gallstones or replace a hip joint. Leg ulcers may be treated with cleansing solutions and zinc oxide, or with skin grafts if the condition persists.

Regular health maintenance is critical for people with sickle cell anemia. Proper nutrition, good hygiene, bed rest, protection against infections, and avoidance of other stresses all are important in maintaining good health and preventing complications. Regular visits to a physician or clinic that provides comprehensive care are necessary

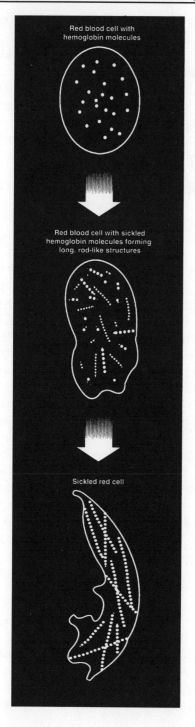

Figure 9.3. *The abnormal hemoglobin molecules tend to cluster together and form long, rod-like structures. These structures cause some red blood cells to become stiff and to assume a sickle shape.*

to identify early changes in the patient's health and ensure that the person receives immediate treatment.

Today, with good health care, many people with sickle cell anemia are in reasonably good health much of the time and living productive lives. In fact, in the past 30 years, the life expectancy of people with sickle cell anemia has increased. Many patients with sickle cell anemia now live into their midforties and beyond.

The Future of Sickle Cell Anemia Treatment

Scientists have learned a great deal about sickle cell anemia during the past 30 years—what causes it, how it affects the patient, and how to treat some of the complications. They also have begun to have success in developing drugs that will prevent the symptoms of sickle cell anemia and procedures that should ultimately provide a cure.

Some researchers are focusing on identifying drugs that will increase the level of fetal hemoglobin in the blood. Fetal hemoglobin is a form of hemoglobin that all humans produce before birth, but most stop making shortly after birth. Most humans have little fetal hemoglobin left in their bloodstream by the time they reach the age of 6 months. However, some people with sickle cell anemia continue to produce large amounts of fetal hemoglobin after birth, and studies have shown that these people have less severe cases of the disease. Fetal hemoglobin seems to prevent sickling of red cells, and cells containing fetal hemoglobin tend to survive longer in the bloodstream.

Hydroxyurea appears to work primarily by stimulating production of fetal hemoglobin. There is some evidence that administering hydroxyurea with erythropoietin, a genetically engineered hormone that stimulates red cell production, may make hydroxyurea work better. This combination approach offers the possibility that lower doses of hydroxyurea can be used to achieve the needed level of fetal hemoglobin. However, both of these drugs may produce serious side effects, so researchers continue to search for safer agents that are just as effective.

Butyrate, a simple fatty acid that is widely used as a food additive, is also being investigated as an agent that may increase fetal hemoglobin production.

Clotrimazole, an over-the-counter medication commonly used to treat fungal infections, is under investigation as a treatment to prevent the loss of water from the red blood cells that contributes to sickling. It is hoped that this medication, used alone or in conjunction with other antisickling agents, may eventually offer an effective long-term therapy for sickle cell anemia patients.

Bone marrow transplantation has been shown to provide a cure for severely affected children with sickle cell disease. Although many of the risks of this procedure have been reduced, it still is not entirely without risk. In addition, the marrow must come from a healthy matched sibling donor, and only about 18 percent of children with sickle cell anemia are likely to have a matched sibling. Researchers are working on techniques to further reduce some of the risks of bone marrow transplantation for patients with sickle cell disease.

The ultimate cure for sickle cell anemia may be gene therapy. In sickle cell anemia, the gene which switches on production of adult hemoglobin shortly before birth, is defective. Two approaches to gene therapy are being explored. Some scientists are looking into whether correcting this gene and inserting it into the bone marrow of people with sickle cell anemia will result in the production of normal adult hemoglobin. Others are looking at the possibility of turning off the defective gene and simultaneously reactivating another gene that turns on production of fetal hemoglobin. In both cases, the research is at a very early stage. Progress is being made, however, and there is a real possibility of an eventual clinical cure for sickle cell anemia.

Although the genetic defect that causes sickling was identified more than 40 years ago, until very recently, research into the development of treatments for the disease was hampered by the lack of an animal model that could be used to test experimental drugs and gene therapy. Recently, however, scientists were able to genetically engineer a line of mice that exhibit some of the characteristics of sickle cell disease in much the same way humans do. This is an important advance in the search for an effective treatment and eventual cure for sickle cell disease.

How Can Patients and Their Families and Friends Be Helped to Cope with Sickle Cell Anemia?

Sickle cell patients and their families may need help in handling the economic and psychological stresses of coping with this serious chronic disease. Sickle cell centers and clinics can provide information and counseling on handling these problems.

Parents should try to learn as much about the disease as possible so that they can recognize early signs of complications and seek early treatment.

Is It Possible to Detect Sickle Cell Anemia in an Unborn Baby?

Yes. By sampling the amniotic fluid or tissue taken from the placenta, doctors can tell whether a fetus has sickle cell anemia or sickle cell trait. This test can be done as early as the first trimester of pregnancy.

What Should Future Parents Know?

People who are planning to become parents should know whether they are carriers of the sickle cell gene, and, if they are, they may want to seek genetic counseling. The counselor can tell prospective parents what the chances are that their child will have sickle cell trait or sickle cell anemia. Accurate diagnostic tests and information are available from health departments, neighborhood health centers, medical centers and clinics that care for individuals with sickle cell anemia.

For More Information Contact

Further information about Sickle Cell Disease can be obtained from the following organizations. Full contact information, including addresses, phone numbers, e-mail addresses, and web sites, can be found in the chapter titled "Resources for Patients with Blood and Circulatory Disorders" in the end section "Additional Help and Information."

- NHLBI Information Center
- The Sickle Cell Disease Program
- Sickle Cell Disease Association of America
- National Maternal and Child Health Clearinghouse
- Agency for Health Care Policy and Research

Chapter 10

Sickle Cell Disease in Newborns and Infants

What Is Sickle Cell Disease?

Sickle cell disease is an inherited disorder of the red blood cells. Red blood cells carry oxygen to all parts of the body by using a protein called hemoglobin. Normal red blood cells contain only normal hemoglobin and are shaped like doughnuts. These cells are very flexible and move easily through small blood vessels.

But in sickle cell disease, the red blood cells contain sickle hemoglobin, which causes them to change to a curved shape (sickle shape) after oxygen is released. Sickled cells become stuck and form plugs in small blood vessels. This blockage of blood flow can damage the tissue. Because there are blood vessels in all parts of the body, damage can occur anywhere in the body.

Purpose of This Chapter

This chapter can help you understand sickle cell disease and how it can affect your child.

The best way to help your baby is to learn as much as you can about the disease, the problems it can cause, and what you can do to care for your baby. Talk about this text and your baby's health care choices with your doctor and others who know about sickle cell disease. Working together, you can give your child the best possible care.

Department of Health and Human Services (DHHS); AHCPR Publication No. 93-0564, April 1993.

You will find a description of the kinds of problems a baby with sickle cell disease may have in the following text. Remember when you read it that not all babies will have all of these problems. At the end of this chapter, you will find a list of terms often used by doctors and nurses when they talk about sickle cell disease.

Types of Sickle Cell Disease

There are several forms of sickle cell disease. The most common are sickle cell anemia, hemoglobin SC disease, and sickle-beta thalassemia. Your doctor or nurse will tell you what kind of sickle cell disease your baby has. Be sure to write down the name so that you can refer to it if your baby has to go to a new doctor or clinic.

How Are Babies Affected?

Babies with sickle cell disease may have:

- **Anemia** (a low number of red blood cells). People with anemia may tire easily.

- **Aplastic crisis.** Babies with sickle cell disease may stop making red blood cells for a short time. Signs include paleness, less activity than normal, fast breathing, and fast heartbeat. A baby with these signs must be seen quickly by the doctor.

- **Hand-and-foot syndrome.** Babies with sickle cell disease may have pain and swelling in their hands or feet.

- **Painful episodes** (mostly in the arms, hands, legs, feet, or abdomen). This happens when sickle cells plug blood vessels and block the flow of blood. Doctors call this a painful episode, event, or crisis.

- **Severe infections.** The child with sickle cell anemia is at great risk for serious infections —such as sepsis (a blood stream infection), meningitis, and pneumonia. The risk of infection is increased because the spleen does not function normally.

- **Splenic sequestration crisis.** The spleen is the organ that filters blood. In children with sickle cell disease, the spleen can enlarge rapidly from trapped red blood cells. This condition is called splenic sequestration crisis and can be life-threatening.

- **Stroke.** This happens when blood vessels in the brain are blocked by sickled red blood cells. Signs include seizure, weakness of the arms and legs, speech problems, and loss of consciousness. A baby with any of these signs must be seen quickly by a doctor.

Who Is Affected?

In the United States, most people who have sickle cell disease are African Americans. About 1 in 375 African-American children has sickle cell disease. Hispanic Americans from the Caribbean, Central America, and parts of South America may also have the disease. Sickle cell disease is also found in individuals from Turkey, Greece, Italy, the Middle East, or East India.

What Causes Sickle Cell Disease?

All forms of sickle cell disease are inherited. Children inherit genes for the disease from their parents.

Genes are substances within the father's sperm and the mother's egg that determine all of the physical characteristics of a baby. Children inherit the genes for hemoglobin from their parents. Persons who inherit both normal and sickle hemoglobin have sickle cell trait. Sickle cell trait is not a disease and does not change to disease. The individual sperm or egg from a person with sickle cell trait may contain either a gene for normal hemoglobin or a gene for sickle hemoglobin.

When both parents have sickle cell trait, for each pregnancy, the chances are:

- 1 in 4 that the baby will have only normal hemoglobin.
- 2 in 4 that the baby will have both normal and sickle hemoglobin (sickle cell trait).
- 1 in 4 that the baby will have only sickle hemoglobin (sickle cell anemia).

The inheritance of other forms of sickle cell disease can be explained by your doctor.

How Do I Know If My Baby Has Sickle Cell Disease?

All newborn babies should be tested for sickle cell disease. Many States have screening programs that test babies born in the hospital within a few days of birth. A blood sample is taken from the baby's heel for the sickle cell test, as well as screening tests for several other medical conditions.

If the test shows your baby might have sickle cell disease, the doctor will do the test again to make sure. The doctor may ask one or both parents for blood samples to test. If your baby has sickle cell disease, the doctor will tell you as soon as possible.

What If My Baby Has Sickle Cell Disease?

If your baby has sickle cell disease, the doctor will help you find the best medical care for your child. This care could be provided by your family doctor, a pediatrician (children's doctor), or a pediatric hematologist (children's blood specialist), or a special sickle cell clinic. You also may want to see a counselor who can talk with you about your chances of having another baby with sickle cell disease.

Sickle cell disease is not just a medical problem. You may have many concerns about your baby and your family—for example, how to cope with your feelings and how to pay the medical bills. Your doctor or nurse can talk with you about your concerns. They also can help you find a local social service agency to assist you. In many areas there are sickle cell support groups, as well as community organizations that offer testing, education, and support to families affected by sickle cell disease.

How Can I Help My Baby?

The best way to help your baby is to learn as much as you can about the disease and to make sure your baby gets the best health care possible. The child with sickle cell disease has special needs and must have regular medical care to stay as healthy as possible. The doctor or nurse will explain how often to bring your baby for medical care and what you can do if your baby becomes ill.

By 2 months of age, your baby should start taking penicillin by mouth twice each day. *It is very important to give the medicine exactly as the doctor tells you.* This will help prevent life-threatening infections. Penicillin should be continued until at least 5 years of age.

Also by 2 months of age, your baby will get a shot to protect against *H. influenzae,* a type of bacteria that causes an infection which can be dangerous to people with sickle cell disease. The baby also will need a shot to protect against hepatitis B, a liver disease. At age 2, your child should receive pneumococcal vaccine. Your child should have all the other shots that children normally receive.

Here are some of the most important things you need to know about caring for a baby with sickle cell disease:

- If your baby has a fever (over 101 degrees), you must get medical help right away. A fever in a child with sickle cell disease can be a sign of serious medical problems. Always take your baby's temperature when your baby appears sick. Your doctor will tell you what to do if your baby has a fever.

- If your baby is sick, you must get medical help right away. Any sign of illness in a child with sickle cell disease can be serious. Your baby needs to see the doctor quickly if the baby:

  —Is breathing fast or having a problem with breathing
  —Coughs frequently
  —Is cranky and cries more than usual
  —Screams when touched
  —Is very tired or has little energy
  —Is very weak
  —Vomits
  —Does not want to eat
  —Has diarrhea
  —Has fewer wet diapers
  —Has pain or swelling in the abdomen
  —Has swollen hands or feet
  —Has pale blue or grey lips or skin

- If any new doctor or health care provider sees your baby for any reason, explain that your baby has sickle cell disease.

- A good diet is very important for all babies. Ask your doctor or other health care provider about the right foods and liquids for your baby. Make sure your baby drinks plenty of liquids. Find out if your baby also should have vitamins or iron.

- Make sure your baby does not become overheated or chilly. Keep your baby warm. Cold baths or cold air can slow the baby's blood flow and cause problems.

Questions to Ask

You should always feel free to ask any question about sickle cell disease and how it affects you and your family. Here are some questions you may want to ask the doctor, nurse, counselor, or social worker.

- What does my baby have? How did he or she get it?

- What do I have? How did I get it? How will it affect me and my family?

- How often does my baby need to see you?

- What medicine does my baby need? What do I need to know about giving it?

- What should my baby eat and drink?

- Is there anything my baby should not do?

- How can I tell if my baby gets sick?

- What should I do, and who should I call, if my baby gets sick?

- What other help is available to my family?

Additional Resources

To learn more about sickle cell disease and how to cope with it, contact the following organizations. Full contact information, including addresses, phone numbers, e-mail addresses and web sites, is given in the chapter titled "Resources" in the end section "Additional Help and Information."

- California State Department of Health, Children's Medical Services Branch

- Cincinnati Comprehensive Sickle Cell Center, Children's Hospital Medical Center

- Clinical Center Communications

- Education Programs Associates

- Howard University, Comprehensive Sickle Cell Center

- March of Dimes

- Mid-South Sickle Cell Center, Le Bonheur Children's Medical Center

- Mississippi State Department of Health, Genetics Division

- National Association for Sickle Cell Disease

- National Maternal and Child Health Clearinghouse

- New York State Department of Health, Newborn Screening Program
- Northern California Comprehensive Sickle Cell Center
- Texas Department of Health, Newborn Screening Program

This is not a complete list. Check with your state or local health department or sickle cell agency for more information.

Common Sickle Cell Terms

Your doctor, nurse, or other caregiver may use these terms in talking with you about sickle cell disease and your child.

Acute chest syndrome. A serious condition caused by infection or trapped red blood cells in the lungs. Fast or difficult breathing, chest pain, and coughing are signs of acute chest syndrome in the child with sickle cell disease. A child with acute chest syndrome usually will have to go to the hospital for treatment.

Anemia. A reduced number of red blood cells. Anemia occurs in persons with sickle cell disease because sickled red blood cells do not live as long as normal red blood cells. A child with sickle cell disease cannot make red blood cells fast enough to keep up with the rapid breakdown, so the person with sickle cell disease has fewer red blood cells than normal and is anemic.

Aplastic crisis. Occurs when a child's bone marrow temporarily stops producing red blood cells. A child with aplastic crisis may appear pale and be tired and less active than usual.

Capillaries. Tiny blood vessels where sickle-shaped blood cells may get trapped and cause problems.

Gene. The biological units that are passed from both parents to a child. Genes determine all of the child's characteristics—for example, hair, eye, and skin color, foot size, height—and whether the child will have sickle cell disease or another inherited disease.

Haemophilus influenzae. A type of bacteria that causes infection and can lead to serious problems in the child with sickle cell disease. Babies must receive a special vaccine beginning at 2 months of age to protect them from this condition.

Hand-and-foot syndrome. Pain and swelling of the hands and feet caused by sickle-shaped red blood cells that plug blood vessels in the hands and feet. Often this will be the baby's first problem caused by sickle cell disease.

Hemoglobin. A molecule found in red blood cells that carries oxygen from the lungs to other parts of the body.

Pain event or painful episode. Pain caused by plugging of blood vessels by sickled blood cells. Pain is most often felt in the arms, legs, back, and abdomen. The pain may last only a few hours or as long as a week or two. The pain may be mild or so severe that pain medicine is needed. The number of pain events a person has may vary greatly.

Sepsis. The presence of infection in the blood stream.

Sickle cell anemia. The most common form of sickle cell disease. Other types of sickle cell disease include hemoglobin SC disease and sickle beta-thalassemia; there are also other, less common types of sickle cell disease.

Sickle cell disease. A group of inherited disorders in which anemia is present and sickle hemoglobin is produced.

Sickle cell trait. The condition in which a person has both normal and sickle hemoglobin in the red cells as a result of inheriting a normal hemoglobin gene and a gene for sickle hemoglobin. Sickle cell trait is not a disease and does not change to sickle cell disease. Persons with sickle cell trait may pass the sickle gene to their children.

Sickled cells. In children with sickle cell disease, hemoglobin molecules in red blood cells stick to one another and cause the red cells to become crescent or sickle shaped. Sickled cells cannot pass easily through tiny blood vessels.

Splenic sequestration crisis. Occurs when a large portion of the child's blood becomes trapped in the spleen. Early signs include paleness, an enlarged spleen, and pain in the abdomen.

Streptococcus pneumoniae. A bacteria that causes a very serious type of pneumonia in children with sickle cell disease. Twice daily doses of penicillin by mouth, starting at about 2 months of age, can help to prevent this life-threatening infection in children with sickle cell anemia and sickle beta-thalassemia.

For More Information

The information in this chapter was taken from the *Clinical Practice Guideline on Sickle Cell Disease: Screening, Diagnosis, Management, and Counseling in Newborns and Infants*. The guideline was written by a panel of experts sponsored by the Agency for Health Care Policy and Research. Other guidelines on common health problems also are being developed.

For more information about guidelines, contact:

Agency for Health Care Policy and Research
Publications Clearinghouse
P. O. Box 8547
Silver Spring, MD 20907

Or call (800) 358-9295; for callers outside the U.S. only: (301) 495-3453, weekdays, 9 a.m. to 5 p.m., Eastern time.

Chapter 11

The Multicenter Study of Hydroxyurea in Sickle Cell Anemia

What Was MSH?

MSH was a study in which about 150 patients with sickle cell anemia, treated with hydroxyurea (HU), were compared with 150 patients treated with a capsule that looked identical but contained only starch (placebo), to see if HU could lessen the number of painful crises.

What Is a "Painful Crisis" in a Patient with Sickle Cell Anemia?

A painful crisis is a sudden attack of pain, which may be mild or extremely severe, often occurring in bones and joints in adults. For this study, which was limited to patients with moderately severe disease (at least 3 attacks/year), a crisis was a visit to a medical facility for pain not due to another disease, lasting at least 4 hours, and treated with injections of a narcotic pain-killer.

Why Was an Early "Clinical Alert" Put Out?

To get information from the study to doctors and patients as quickly as possible; to be sure that physicians and patients knew that the drug has to be used very carefully, if it is to be used safely; and to be sure that the drug is not used inappropriately (as for treatment of acute attacks, or without careful monitoring).

National Heart, Lung, and Blood Institute, January 30, 1995.

What Were the Most Important Findings in the Study?

Sickle cell anemia patients treated with HU had about half as many painful crises; had longer periods between crises; had fewer attacks of acute chest syndrome (a pneumonia-like problem); had to be hospitalized less often; had to be transfused less often; and had no significant bad effects from treatment.

Most HU treated patients did continue to have some crises, and all had to get their blood counts checked every 2-4 weeks. Taking capsules during an acute attack did not stop the attacks. HU works slowly, and a decrease in the frequency of crises was not seen until about 6-8 weeks after starting. Good effects of treatment only last while patients continue to take their capsules.

Is Hydroxyurea a "Cure" for Sickle Cell Disease?

No, but it can help some patients. It can prevent attacks from occurring, but is of no help in actually treating a painful crisis once it has started.

Were There Any Deaths in the Study?

Yes, but numbers in the HU and placebo groups did not differ significantly. No deaths were related to use of HU.

Is Hydroxyurea Ever Dangerous?

It can be very dangerous if the patient and his/her blood count are not followed carefully. If, and only if, they are watched closely, it is not dangerous when prescribed by a physician experienced in the use of such treatments.

Are There Any Unclear/Undefined Risks?

This study did not address these problems directly, but there might be a risk to the baby if a pregnant woman took HU. Problems which developed in animals were seen at doses about 10 times as large as those we used. There also might possibly be a risk if a man were taking HU at the time of conception. In our study, treatment was stopped if any patient or his partner became pregnant during the study, and all babies were normal at birth. If there is a risk, and we aren't sure there is, we don't know if the risk would continue after one stopped taking the drug.

There might be a risk of leukemia or cancer from long-term therapy (greater than 5 years) at doses similar to those we used, but there are no data which support that possibility in patients with sickle cell anemia. No patients in our 2-year study developed cancer or leukemia. We actually began testing HU about 10 years ago, and the first 2 patients we treated are doing well, although they still dohave crises. We do not know if the drug is safe in growing children.

Are There Any Unclear/Undefined Benefits?

Our study did not address these questions, but long-term treatment might prevent development of such long-term problems as kidney failure, problems with the hip and shoulder joints, and perhaps ankle ulcers. There was no evidence that HU helped these conditions once they had developed.

Must Patients Be Evaluated Before Starting Treatment?

Definitely. They must understand the possible benefits, the possible short and long-term risks, and what they must do if treatment is to be safe. Our study was carried out in adult patients with more than 3 crises per year; patients with less than 3 crises per year must understand that the MSH study results do not necessarily apply to them.

Are There Any Special Things That Patients Must Do?

They must take the drug regularly, every day, only as directed by their doctors, and they must not continue to take the drug without having their blood counts checked regularly.

How Often Must Patients Have Blood Tests?

At the beginning of treatment, about every 2 weeks. Later that interval can be lengthened, and some patients followed for 5 or more years need tests every other month.

How Often Must Patients See a Doctor?

At the beginning, every 2 weeks. Later, if the patient is feeling well, visits as well as blood counts can be less frequent, but they must be done regularly. The exact schedule will vary from patient to patient.

Will All Patients with Sickle Cell Anemia Benefit from Using Hydroxyurea?

Probably not. We don't know for sure which patients are most likely to benefit, but the results we obtained came from severely affected patients, and we think that treatment with HU should probably be reserved for patients with frequent crises.

There are patients with other types of sickle cell disease—hemoglobin SC disease for example—who did not participate in the trial.

Could Hydroxyurea Help Such Patients?

Since most patients with hemoglobin SC disease have fewer crises than the patients in our study, they probably would not think that the inconvenience of frequent blood counts, and the possible risks of treatment, were worth the possible gain. A few patients with Hb SC disease do have frequent crises, and they theoretically could benefit from treatment with hydroxyurea.

Can Hydroxyurea Save a Patient's Life?

No, in an acute situation, like a stroke or heart, lung or kidney failure. It cannot make such problems go away, any more than it can make an on-going painful crisis go away. By preventing future sickling, it might prolong patients' lives, but we have not used the drug long enough to know if that is really true.

Is the Drug Safe or Effective in Children?

We don't know; all of our patients were adults.

Is Hydroxyurea a New Drug?

No, it has been available for treating other diseases for many years.

What Is the Correct Dose?

Our study was designed to test whether maximum tolerated doses were effective, but did not examine the question of whether lower doses might also work. Based on present knowledge, we recommend using maximum tolerated doses, with careful observation for beneficial effects at lower doses. Each patient's dose must be adjusted individually over the course of several months. In long-term use, doses are about 1-15 mg/lb/day taken by mouth as a single daily dose. We suggest starting with a single daily dose of no more than 7 mg/lb (15 mg/kg), which is usually two 500 mg capsules/day, and carefully working up or down to find a dose which produces maximum benefit with minimum depression of blood counts. At first, counts must be checked every 2 weeks. Other dosage regimens are being investigated, and might eventually be shown to be superior.

Is the Drug Readily Available?

It is available in the United States, but has not been approved for use in sickle cell anemia by the FDA. Doctors can prescribe it for sickle cell patients, but patients must understand that it is still a very new drug for this disease. Because it is new, insurance companies may not be obligated to pay for it under certain prescription programs.

How Much Does It Cost?

In pharmacies, the price of 100 capsules is $121-164; it can be purchased from AARP by mail for $117/100 capsules. Most patients take 2-3 capsules/day, which would cost about $100/month.

How Does the Drug Work?

It may work by increasing the amount of fetal (baby) hemoglobin in red blood cells, but we aren't sure. We think it makes red cells less likely to sickle, or less likely to plug-up blood vessels, or both, but we aren't sure.

What Led to the Discovery?

Basic research in sickling and the way hemoglobin is made in the test tube, which led to experiments in animals, and then to early trials in patients. The first research on the subject began more than 30 years ago, but has accelerated greatly in the past 10 years or so.

Are There New Developments on the Horizon?

Several other drugs under investigation (erythropoietin, butyrate and related compounds) may work together with hydroxyurea to make it more effective, but those studies are still in progress. Bone marrow transplantation can really cure the disease, but the risks are high, and only a small number of young patients are good candidates for that form of experimental therapy. Some day gene therapy may provide a safe and effective cure, and that will be some years in the future.

What Is the Next Step for Patients with Sickle Cell Anemia?

If patients think they might be interested in hydroxyurea treatment, they should discuss it with their doctors. Consultation with a blood specialist (a hematologist) might be helpful in some situations. In every case, the patient must understand the risks of treatment, the need for frequent blood counts, the cost of the drug, and the fact that HU cannot treat crises once they have started.

Where Can My Doctor Get More Information?

By calling the Sickle Cell Disease Scientific Research Group (301-435-0055) to get the name of one of the clinics which participated in the study closest to you.

Chapter 12

New Hope for People with Sickle Cell Anemia

In tropical regions of the world where the parasite-borne disease malaria is prevalent, people with a single copy of a particular genetic mutation have a survival advantage. Over time, people from these regions have migrated, had children, and in some cases married each other. Some of their children inherit two copies of the mutation.

While inheriting one copy of the mutation confers a benefit, inheriting two copies is a tragedy. Children born with two copies of the genetic mutation have sickle cell anemia, a painful disease that affects the red blood cells and is curable only in rare instances.

A recent clinical trial sponsored by the National Heart, Lung, and Blood Institute (NHLBI) found that the drug Hydrea (hydroxyurea) significantly reduced painful episodes in adults with a severe form of sickle cell anemia. NHLBI is a component of the National Institutes of Health (NIH).

Hydrea is approved by the Food and Drug Administration to treat certain types of cancer. On the basis of the new clinical trial findings, FDA is encouraging Hydrea's manufacturer, Bristol-Myers Squibb, to apply for approval of the drug to treat sickle cell anemia.

"FDA will consider it a priority application so that sickle cell anemia can be added to the indications for Hydrea, if the data show that [the drug] is indeed safe and effective," said Anthony Murgo, M.D., a medical officer in the division of oncology at FDA's Center for Drug Evaluation and Research.

FDA Consumer, May 1996.

Genetic Defect Changes Cell Shape

The genetic defect that causes sickle cell anemia affects hemoglobin, a component of red blood cells. Hemoglobin's job is to carry oxygen to all the cells and tissues of the body. Red blood cells that contain normal hemoglobin are soft and round. Their soft texture enables them to squeeze through the body's small blood vessels.

People with sickle cell anemia, however, have a type of abnormal hemoglobin called hemoglobin S. (Normal hemoglobin is called hemoglobin A.) A genetic error makes the hemoglobin molecules stick together in long, rigid rods after they release oxygen. These rods cause the red blood cells to become hard and sickle-shaped, unable to squeeze through tiny blood vessels. The misshapen cells can get stuck in the small blood vessels, causing a blockage that deprives the body's cells and tissues of blood and oxygen.

When this happens "it's like having mini heart attacks throughout the entire body," said Duane R. Bonds, M.D., leader of the sickle cell disease scientific research group at NHLBI in Bethesda, MD.

"A heart attack is painful because the blood flow to the heart is interrupted. In sickle cell anemia, the blood flow can be interrupted to any of the major organs, causing severe pain and organ damage at the site of the blood flow blockage."

These painful "crises," as they are called, damage the lungs, kidneys, liver, bones, and other organs and tissues. Recurrence of these episodes is the most disabling feature of sickle cell anemia. They can cause leg ulcers, blindness, and many other health problems, depending upon where in the body the blood flow blockage occurs. A blockage in the brain can cause a stroke, which may result in paralysis or death.

The body, recognizing that the sickled cells are abnormal, destroys them at a faster rate than it can replace them. This causes a type of anemia, a shortage of red blood cells. Symptoms of anemia include extreme fatigue and susceptibility to infection.

Penicillin Treatment

An important breakthrough occurred in 1986 when an NHLBI-sponsored study found that young children with sickle cell anemia who took penicillin twice a day by mouth had much lower rates of *S. pneumoniae* infection than a similar group of children who received a placebo.

In 1987, an expert panel convened by NHLBI recommended that all infants born in the United States be screened for sickle cell anemia so that children with the disease could be identified early and offered treatment with penicillin. Forty-two states now have newborn screening programs, according to Bonds. NHLBI also recommends that affected infants get daily penicillin therapy beginning by the age of 3 months.

In the first year of life, children with sickle cell anemia are protected from blood flow blockages by the presence of fetal hemoglobin.

"Fetal hemoglobin is the hemoglobin that all of us produce before we're born," explained Bonds. Fetal hemoglobin physically blocks hemoglobin S, preventing it from forming the long, rigid rods that lead to sickling of the red blood cells. Several weeks before birth, however, the fetus' bone marrow usually begins to shut down the production of fetal hemoglobin and starts making adult hemoglobin instead. At birth, an infant's red blood cells contain roughly equal amounts of fetal and adult hemoglobin.

By the time the child is 6 months old, it has usually stopped making any fetal hemoglobin. As the level of fetal hemoglobin in the child's blood falls, explained Bonds, there is no longer anything to prevent the red blood cells from becoming sickle-shaped and getting stuck in the blood vessels, causing a painful crisis.

The symptoms of a painful crisis may be relieved by giving patients fluids and painkillers, said Lilia Talarico, M.D., a medical officer in the division of gastrointestinal and hematologic drug products in FDA's Center for Drug Evaluation and Research. However, no FDA-approved treatment is currently available to prevent painful crises from occurring.

Life Expectancy Improves

Despite the absence of an effective treatment, life expectancy for individuals with sickle cell anemia has improved, said Bonds, as a result of early identification through neonatal screening, early initiation of penicillin therapy, close medical monitoring, and early intervention to relieve the symptoms of a painful episode. A recent study found that half of all patients with sickle cell anemia survive into their 40s.

Rates of early death are highest among those with a severe form of the disease. "Between 10 and 15 percent of patients will have three or more painful crises per year," said Bonds. "The more crises you have per year, the greater your chances of dying prematurely. Your organs become more damaged when they are chronically not receiving enough blood and oxygen."

Some people continue to produce fetal hemoglobin throughout their lives. A study of the life expectancy of people with sickle cell anemia found that adults with high levels of fetal hemoglobin lived longer than those who had low levels.

People with sickle cell anemia who suffer strokes or infections, who are pregnant, or who must undergo surgery may be treated with blood transfusions. Risks of this treatment include the possibility of acquiring a viral illness such as hepatitis and the possibility of organ damage caused by iron overload.

Sickle cell anemia can be cured by a bone marrow transplant, which replaces the defective red blood cells with healthy cells from a donor. But a transplant is not a realistic option for most people with sickle cell anemia, according to Bonds, because of a shortage of compatible donors and because of the risks presented by the drug regimen that is required to prepare a patient for a transplant.

"First you give drugs to kill off the patient's marrow, then you do the transplant to replace the marrow." But the powerful drugs given to kill the patient's bone marrow can be dangerous for someone who has had a stroke or is at risk for stroke, she said.

In January 1995, NHLBI announced the successful conclusion of a five-year, multicenter trial of Hydrea in the treatment of sickle cell anemia. The study involved 299 patients ages 18 and older who were recruited at 21 medical centers in the United States.

All patients had experienced at least three painful crises in the year before they entered the trial. Half of the patients received Hydrea and half received a placebo. Neither the patients nor their doctors knew who was taking the drug and who was taking the placebo. Patients who took Hydrea had roughly half as many painful crises as those who took the inactive pill.

The trial had been scheduled to conclude in May 1995. However, scientists involved found the results so compelling that they stopped the study early and notified doctors of the results so that all patients who might benefit could be offered the treatment. A report of the trial's findings was published in the May 1995 *New England Journal of Medicine*.

Hydrea Studies

Hydrea is approved by FDA to treat certain types of leukemia and other cancers. Doctors have been interested in Hydrea for the treatment of sickle cell anemia for about 10 years, since pilot studies in humans showed that the drug could increase the level of fetal hemoglobin in red blood cells.

Because Hydrea is already on the market for other uses, it was unnecessary for FDA to issue a Treatment IND (investigational new drug) to make the drug available to patients with sickle cell anemia, said FDA's Murgo. A Treatment IND is a mechanism used by FDA to make investigational new drugs available to patients while they are under study.

As with other approved medications, doctors may prescribe Hydrea for sickle cell anemia if in their professional judgment a patient will benefit from the treatment.

"We are excited about the report [of the Hydrea clinical trial]," said Murgo. "But until the manufacturer [of the drug] submits the detailed data for us to review, [the agency] cannot approve the drug to treat sickle cell anemia."

Bonds, who was the project officer for the multicenter study, cautioned that Hydrea treatment is not appropriate for every patient.

"We only recommend it for patients over 18 who have had at least three painful crises in the previous year. The patients have to be monitored very carefully. They must have a blood test every two weeks to ensure that their blood count is not depressed to a level where they might be at risk for infection or bleeding."

Hydrea should not be prescribed for patients who are likely to become pregnant or who are unable to follow instructions regarding treatment, said Murgo.

Many questions about Hydrea in the treatment of sickle cell anemia remain unanswered, said Bonds. Doctors do not know what the most effective and least toxic dose of the drug is or whether taking it for many years presents health risks.

Some doctors prescribe Hydrea to treat polycythemia vera, a disease in which the number of red blood cells increases abnormally. Some evidence suggests that the drug may cause leukemia in a few of these patients, both Murgo and Bonds said.

However, they added, patients with polycythemia vera already have a higher-than-average risk of getting leukemia, so it is unclear whether the leukemia is caused by Hydrea or whether the patients would have developed it anyway.

NHLBI is planning a five-year follow-up study of patients who took part in the Hydrea trial to see whether any of them develop leukemia or other problems that may result from long-term use of the drug. Another study, which began in January 1995, is looking at the safety and effectiveness of Hydrea in children ages 5 to 15 who have sickle cell anemia.

Research continues on other possible ways of reducing the occurrence of painful sickle cell episodes by increasing the production of fetal hemoglobin. For example, NIH scientists are studying whether a combined regimen of Hydrea and erythropoietin, a hormone that increases the production of red blood cells, is less toxic and more effective than Hydrea alone. (Erythropoietin is licensed by FDA to treat anemia in certain patients.) Studies are also under way to determine the safety and efficacy of butyrate, an experimental drug that can stimulate production of fetal hemoglobin.

NHLBI recently funded three centers that will try to develop gene therapy for sickle cell anemia, said Bonds. "If you could replace the abnormal genes, you could cure the disease. However, there are significant technical problems involved in making gene therapy work."

Because of these problems, gene therapy is unlikely to be a reality for many years, she said. Nevertheless, she said she is optimistic that new, effective treatments for sickle cell anemia will be developed in the future.

"I like to tell people that [the results of the Hydrea study] will one day be likened to [the discovery of] insulin or penicillin. Those drugs were the first major breakthroughs for the treatment of diabetes and severe bacterial infections, although other agents have since [been introduced] to treat those diseases."

— by Eleanor Mayfield

Eleanor Mayfield is a writer in Silver Spring, MD

Chapter 13

Hereditary Hemochromatosis

Introduction

"Iron is a paradoxical nutrient; a minute amount is essential to life but in quantities in excess of need can be toxic." In normal individuals, although the mechanism of iron absorption is poorly understood, it is known that variations in absorption occur in response to iron needs. As we shall see, there are individuals in whom this mechanism is at fault.

Iron is also a unique nutrient which has earned its reputation as a "one-way" nutrient, i.e., the body has no way of ridding itself of excess iron once absorbed, except by blood loss. And so, we may now begin to understand what happens in individuals when the absorption mechanism fails to exclude unneeded iron.

A normal adult has about 4 grams of total body iron, an amount equivalent to the weight of a teaspoonful of water, three-fourths of which is in the hemoglobin of blood. In hemochromatosis, both the hereditary and the acquired types, there is a considerably increased amount of body iron. In the hereditary type, which will be discussed first, the total iron is increased to 20–40 grams or more.

What Is Hereditary Hemochromatosis (HH)?

It is a genetic disorder in which there is an increased absorption of dietary iron above needs. It is caused by an abnormal H gene.

A gene is a code for a family likeness, a trait, a characteristic. There may be hundreds of thousands of genes, located on the 23 pairs of genetic material (called chromosomes) that we inherit at the time of conception, 2 pair from each parent which makes each one of us so unique.

Individuals inheriting one H gene and one normal gene are called carriers. Although their iron-absorption rate is somewhat higher than normal, they do not seem to accumulate enough iron to cause organ damage. When two carriers marry, however, each of their children has a 25% chance of inheriting two abnormal genes, or two normal genes, or a 50% chance of inheriting one H and one normal gene and become carriers, as their parents.

Individuals inheriting two H genes absorb excessive iron above their needs from infancy on. Since the body has no way of getting rid of excess iron once it is absorbed, except by blood loss, the iron slowly accumulates in the liver, heart, pancreas, and other hormonal glands, and joints. Since it takes decades for enough iron to accumulate and cause organ damage, symptoms are delayed in men until their 30s to 50s; years later in women, generally, because of the protective effect of their blood loss through menstruation and child-bearing.

What Are the Symptoms of HH?

They vary considerably among patients. The symptoms, unfortunately, resemble those in other conditions, making early diagnosis difficult. These symptoms may include fatigue, weakness, weight loss, abdominal discomfort or pain, joint pains, backache, itchiness, frequent infections. A tanned appearance not due to sun exposure occurs frequently. More specific (late) symptoms and signs depend on the organs that are affected the most, such as liver dysfunction with or without cirrhosis; heart irregularities, shortness of breath or chest pain; cancers; diabetic symptoms of thirst, frequency of urination, and weight loss; or other hormonal deficiencies, such as decreased body hair and libido; and joint pains.

Who May Be at Risk of Having HH?

1. Individuals whose routine laboratory screening blood tests (see below) are repeatedly abnormal.

2. Blood relatives of patients, especially siblings.

3. Individuals with symptoms and signs of HH, as described above.

Because you may have one or more such symptoms, do not overreact and conclude that you have HH, because there are many other causes for such symptoms.

What to Do If You Suspect You May Have HH

See your family physician or visit a clinic, and convey your suspicions. The minimal cost of the screening tests, referred to in the next paragraph, are worth the benefits of easing your mind or, if you should prove to have HH, the benefits of early diagnosis and treatment to prevent the serious complications of HH.

How Is Diagnosis Made?

The initial screening tests are:

1. A fasting transferrin saturation test, which is the ratio of serum iron to total iron-binding capacity.

2. A ferritin test.

The first test is better since the second can be normal. When either test is abnormal when repeated, a liver biopsy is essential for diagnosis.

Screening of Relatives

After a diagnosis of a patient, all first-degree relatives should also be screened for HH. This should include:

1. A check-up by a physician.

2. Laboratory tests, including the two screening tests referred to above.

3. HLA typing, discussed below.

HLA Typing

This refers to finding out one's tissue type. From recent genetic advances in the late 1970s, we know:

1. That HH is significantly associated with specific HLA types in families with the disorder,

2. That HH is a recessive disorder, which means that two H genes must be inherited to iron-load and damage organs, and

3.   That both the H gene and the HLA-type genes are located to-
     gether on the pair of chromosomes numbered 6.

The practical value of this knowledge is that, since each sibling
has a 25% chance of inheriting a pair of H genes, it follows that all
siblings with the same HLA type as his sibling have also inherited
two H genes and are therefore at risk of progressive iron-loading organs. Early treatment of such family members is vital to prevent organ damage. HLA-typing will also identify siblings who may be
carriers, or who are normal and need not worry.

How Common Is HH?

Until the mid-1970s, HH was considered to be rare, estimated to
affect only about 20,000 Americans. With the application of newer
genetic knowledge to studies of families with the disorder in Europe,
Australia, and North America, it is now estimated that there may be
over 1,500,000 Americans affected, with a carrier population between
25,000,000 and 30,000,000. This makes HH *THE* most common genetic disorder now known.

Is There a Treatment?

Yes, a simple and harmless one. By removing one pint of blood
(called a phlebotomy), as in a routine blood donation, once or more
times a week, the bone marrow is stimulated to make more blood, and
excess body iron is gradually removed. Depending upon the amount
of iron accumulated, treatment may take one to two years. Once the
excess iron has been removed, blood-lettings are done only three to
four times a year for life, so as to prevent reaccumulation of iron, as
abnormal iron absorption is a life-long event.

Additional specific treatment may be essential to treat the various
existing complications, such as diabetes, heart problems, arthritis, etc.

Is There Any Special Diet to Follow?

Since you're losing more iron from your phlebotomies than you're
absorbing from your diet, you may eat a balanced diet of meats, fish,
dairy, eggs, legumes, fruits, vegetables, and nuts and raisins.

Avoid alcohol, vitamin supplements, especially Vitamin C which
can increase iron toxicity. One glass of juice daily is all the Vitamin
C you need.

Prevention of HH

The old adage of "an ounce of prevention is worth a pound of cure" applies especially to HH. Although it is not possible to prevent inheriting the H gene, it is possible to prevent the complications of HH by early diagnosis, in a number of ways:

1. Routine periodic screening while enjoying good health.

2. Screening of all blood relatives of patients.

3. Routine autopsies, with special iron stains of the liver, heart, and pancreas. Many families have been unexpectedly identified to have HH following the incidental discovery of HH of a relative at post-mortem examination.

Prognosis

There is good evidence that with the removal of excess body iron, patients feel better, stronger, their tan color lessens, liver size decreases, diabetes improves, heart function improves; also, there have been recorded cases of improvement of liver cirrhosis. Without phlebotomy treatments, progressive iron accumulation and organ damage continues.

Acquired Hemochromatosis

Acquired hemochromatosis is secondary to a primary medical condition. Such patients are under medical care and their physicians are aware of their iron-loading tendencies. Their treatments are necessarily individualized. This form of iron-loading is not due to the inheritance of the H gene but is due to:

1. Many transfusions of blood (over 80) given to patients with chronic anemias (congenital or acquired) so as to sustain their lives. Treatment includes iron-removal via injection of iron-chelators.

2. Increased iron absorption secondary to genetic or acquired disease such as some Thalassemias, porphyrias, sideroblastic anemias, liver injuries due to chronic hepatitis, alcoholic, viral, and other cirrhoses.

3. There are reports of iron-loading due to long-term abuse of iron supplements; these are treated with phlebotomies.

Goals of the Hemochromatosis Foundation, Inc.

1. To increase national awareness that hemochromatosis is not only the most common genetic disorder, but that it is probably the only genetic disorder which, if diagnosed early and treated adequately, is compatible with a healthy and full life span.

2. To encourage routine screening for HH whenever possible: during routine exams by physicians in their offices, hospitals, clinics, at fairs, and in blood banks.

   A recent pilot study of 10,000 apparently healthy men and women blood donors resulted in the diagnosis of 5/1,000 donors affected with HH, together with many blood relatives, who are now being treated prophylactically.

3. To encourage pathologists to include iron studies of all autopsies. A diagnosis at death will result in screening and diagnosing affected younger, living blood relatives.

4. To encourage government funding for studies of the prevalence of HH among Americans.

5. To encourage government funding for research aimed at identifying the genetic defect or defects causing the increased iron absorption, and at understanding the toxic effects of iron on tissues.

6. To increase awareness of governmental agencies and food industries of the potential harm from unneeded extra-dietary iron.

7. To encourage government-funded monitoring and evaluation of the results of exposure of the affected, as well as carriers and normal individuals, to iron supplements, to iron-fortified foods, to alcohol, and to megadoses of Vitamin C, which increases iron absorption.

Services Now Available

1. Educational booklets for professionals, for the public, and for HH families.

2. Referral of patients to physicians knowledgeable about hemochromatosis, or to research centers when necessary.

3.   Assistance to physicians on how to monitor the treatment of HH when requested.

4.   Emotional support to patients and families.

5.   Video teaching tapes available for purchase.

6.   Periodic teaching conferences for patients and physicians.

7.   Biennial international conferences; first one sponsored by The New York Academy of Sciences (1987).

8.   Quarterly newsletter *Hemochromatosis Awareness*.

—by M. A. Krikker, M.D.

Chapter 14

Immune Thrombocytopenic Purpura

What Is Immune Thrombocytopenic Purpura?

Immune Thrombocytopenic Purpura (ITP) is a disorder of the blood. Immune refers to the immune system's involvement in this disorder. Antibodies, part of the body's immunologic defense against infection, attach to blood platelet, cells that help stop bleeding, and cause their destruction. Thrombocytopenia refers to decrease in blood platelet. Purpura refers to the purplish-looking areas of the skin and mucous membranes (such as the lining of the mouth) where bleeding has occurred as a result of decreased platelet.

Some cases of ITP are caused by drugs, and others are associated with infection, pregnancy, or immune disorders such as systemic lupus erythematosus. About half of all cases are classified as "idiopathic," meaning the cause is unknown.

What Are the Symptoms of ITP?

The main symptom is bleeding which can include bruising ("ecchymosis") and tiny red dots on the skin or mucous membranes ("petechiae"). In some instances bleeding from the nose, gums, digestive or urinary tracts may also occur. Rarely, bleeding within the brain occurs.

NIH Publication No. 90-2114, September 1990.

How Is ITP Diagnosed?

The physician will take a medical history and perform a thorough physical examination. A careful review of medications the patient is taking is important because some drugs can be associated with thrombocytopenia. A complete blood count will be done. A low platelet count will establish thrombocytopenia as the cause of purpura. Often the next procedure is a bone marrow examination to verify that there are adequate platelet-forming cells (megakaryocyte) in the marrow and to rule out other diseases such as metastatic cancer (cancer that has spread to the bone marrow) and leukemia, cancer of the blood cells themselves). Another blood sample may be drawn to check for other conditions sometimes associated with thrombocytopenia such as lupus and infection.

Acute and Chronic Form of Thrombocytopenic Purpura

Acute (temporary) thrombocytopenic purpura is most commonly seen in young children. Boys and girls are equally affected. Symptoms often, but do not necessarily, follow a viral infection. About 85 percent of children recover within 1 year and the problem doesn't return.

Thrombocytopenic purpura is considered chronic when it has lasted more than 6 months. The onset of illness may be at any age. Adults more often have the chronic disorder and females are affected two to three times more than males. The onset of illness may be at any age.

How Is ITP Treated?

If the doctor thinks a drug is the cause of the thrombocytopenia, standard treatment involves discontinuing the drug's use. Infection, if present, is treated vigorously since control of the infection may result in a return of the platelet count to normal.

The treatment of idiopathic thrombocytopenic purpura is determined by the severity of the symptoms. In some cases, no therapy is needed. In most cases, drugs that alter the immune system's attack on the platelet are prescribed. These include corticosteroids (i.e., prednisone) and/or intravenous infusions of immune globulin. Another treatment that usually results in an increased number of platelet is removal of the spleen, the organ that destroys antibody-coated platelets. Other drugs such as vincristine, azathioprine (Imuran), Danazol, cyclophosphamide, and cyclosporine are prescribed for patients only in the severe case where other treatments have not shown benefit since these drugs have potentially harmful side effects.

Except in certain situations (e.g., internal bleeding and preparation for surgery), platelet transfusions usually are not beneficial and, therefore, are seldom performed. Because all therapies can have risks, it is important that over-treatment (treatment based solely on platelet counts and not on symptoms) be avoided. In some instances lifestyle adjustments may be helpful for prevention of bleeding due to injury. These would include use of protective gear such as helmets and avoidance of contact sports in symptomatic patients or when platelet counts are less than 50,000. Otherwise, patients usually can carry on normal activities, but final decisions about activity should be made in consultation with the patient's hematologist.

Where Can I Obtain Further Information on ITP?

Blood specialists (hematologist) are experts in the diagnosis and treatment of these disorders. These doctors practice in most mid-and large-size cities. A majority of medical centers have hematology divisions in their medicine or pediatrics departments, and patients who need evaluation, treatment, or information can often be referred there.

Additional information can be obtained from the National Organization for Rare Disorder at P.O. Box 8923, New Fairfield, Connecticut 06812; telephone (203) 746-6518.

Part Three

Leukemias

Chapter 15

Leukemia: An Overview

MedicineNet *Power Points about Leukemia*

- Leukemia is a cancer of the blood cells.

- While the exact cause(s) of leukemia is not known, risk factors have been identified.

- Leukemias are grouped by how quickly the disease develops (acute or chronic) as well as by the type of blood cell that is affected.

- People with leukemia are at significantly increased risk for developing infections, anemia, and bleeding.

- Diagnosis of leukemia is supported by findings of the medical history and examination, and examining blood under a microscope. Leukemia cells can also be detected and further classified with a bone marrow aspiration and/or biopsy.

- Treatment of leukemia depends on the type of leukemia, certain features of the leukemia cells, the extent of the disease, and prior history of treatment, as well as the age and health of the patient.

- Most patients with leukemia are treated with chemotherapy. Some patients also may have radiation therapy and/or bone marrow transplantation.

The information provided below has been modified from that furnished by the National Institutes of Health and the National Cancer Institute of the United States of America

What Is Leukemia?

Leukemia is a type of cancer. Cancer is a group of more than 100 diseases that have two important things in common. One is that certain cells in the body become abnormal. Another is that the body keeps producing large numbers of these abnormal cells.

Leukemia is cancer of the blood cells. Each year, nearly 27,000 adults and more than 2,000 children in the United States learn that they have leukemia. To understand leukemia, it is helpful to know about normal blood cells and what happens to them when leukemia develops.

Normal Blood Cells

The blood is made up of fluid called plasma and three types of cells. Each type has special functions.

White blood cells (also called WBCs or leukocytes) help the body fight infections and other diseases.

Red blood cells (also called RBCs or erythrocytes) carry oxygen from the lungs to the body's tissues and take carbon dioxide from the tissues back to the lungs. The red blood cells give blood its color.

Platelets (also called thrombocytes) help form blood clots that control bleeding.

Blood cells are formed in the bone marrow, the soft, spongy center of bones. New (immature) blood cells are called blasts. Some blasts stay in the marrow to mature. Some travel to other parts of the body to mature.

Normally, blood cells are produced in an orderly, controlled way as the body needs them. This process helps keep us healthy.

Leukemia Cells

When leukemia develops, the body produces large numbers of abnormal blood cells. In most types of leukemia, the abnormal cells are white blood cells. The leukemia cells usually look different from normal blood cells, and they do not function properly.

What Are Possible Causes of Leukemia?

At this time, we do not know what causes leukemia. Researchers are trying to solve this problem. Scientists know that leukemia occurs in males more often than in females and in white people more often than in black people. However, they cannot explain why one person gets leukemia and another does not.

By studying large numbers of people all over the world, researchers have found certain risk factors that increase a person's chance of developing leukemia. For example, exposure to large amounts of high-energy radiation increases the risk of contracting leukemia. Such radiation was produced by the atomic bomb explosions in Japan during World War II. In nuclear power plants, strict safety rules protect workers and the public from exposure to harmful amounts of radiation.

Some research suggests that exposure to electromagnetic fields is a possible risk factor for leukemia. (Electromagnetic fields are a type of low-energy radiation that comes from power lines and electric appliances.) However, more studies are needed to prove this link.

Certain genetic conditions can increase the risk for leukemia. One such condition is Down's syndrome. Children born with this syndrome are more likely to get leukemia than other children.

Workers exposed to certain chemicals over a long period of time are at higher risk for leukemia. Benzene is one of these chemicals. Also, some of the drugs used to treat other types of cancer may increase a person's risk of developing leukemia. However, this risk is very small when compared with the benefits of chemotherapy.

Scientists have identified a virus that seems to increase the risk for one very uncommon type of leukemia. However, this virus has no known association with common forms of leukemia. Scientists throughout the world continue to study viruses and other possible risk factors for leukemia. By learning what causes this disease, researchers hope to better understand how to prevent and treat it.

What Are the Types of Leukemia?

There are several types of leukemia. They are grouped in two ways. One way is by how quickly the disease develops and gets worse. The other way is by the type of blood cell that is affected.

Leukemia is either acute or chronic. In acute leukemia, the abnormal blood cells are blasts that remain very immature and cannot carry out their normal functions. The number of blasts increases rapidly, and the disease becomes worse quickly. In chronic leukemia, some blast cells are present, but in general, these cells are more mature and can carry out some of their normal functions. Also, the number of blasts increases less rapidly than in acute leukemia. As a result, chronic leukemia worsens gradually.

Leukemia can arise in either of the two main types of white blood cells—lymphoid cells or myeloid cells. When leukemia affects lymphoid cells, it is called lymphocytic leukemia. When myeloid cells are affected, the disease is called myeloid or myelogenous leukemia.

These are the most common types of leukemia:

- Acute lymphocytic leukemia (ALL) is the most common type of leukemia in young children. This disease also affects adults, especially those age 65 and older.

- Acute myeloid leukemia (AML) occurs in both adults and children. This type of leukemia is sometimes called acute nonlymphocytic leukemia (ANLL).

- Chronic lymphocytic leukemia (CLL) most often affects adults over the age of 55. It sometimes occurs in younger adults, but it almost never affects children.

- Chronic myeloid leukemia (CML) occurs mainly in adults. A very small number of children also develop this disease.

- Hairy cell leukemia is an uncommon type of chronic leukemia.

What Are Symptoms of Leukemia?

Leukemia cells are abnormal cells that cannot do what normal blood cells do. They cannot help the body fight infections. For this reason, people with leukemia often develop infections and have fevers.

Also, people with leukemia often have less than the normal amount of healthy red blood cells and platelets. As a result, there are not enough red blood cells to carry oxygen through the body. With this condition, called anemia, patients can look pale and feel weak and tired. When there are not enough platelets, patients bleed and bruise easily.

Like all blood cells, leukemia cells travel through the body. Depending on the number of abnormal cells and where these cells collect, patients with leukemia can have a number of symptoms.

In acute leukemia, symptoms appear and worsen quickly. People with this disease go to their doctor because they feel sick. In chronic leukemia, symptoms may not appear for a long time. When symptoms do appear, they generally are mild at first and get worse gradually. Doctors often find chronic leukemia during a routine checkup—before there are any symptoms.

These are some of the common symptoms of leukemia:

- Fever, chills, and other flu-like symptoms;
- Weakness and fatigue;
- Frequent infections;
- Loss of appetite and/or weight;
- Swollen or tender lymph nodes, liver, or spleen;
- Easy bleeding or bruising;
- Tiny red spots (called petechiae) under the skin;
- Swollen or bleeding gums;
- Sweating, especially at night; and/or
- Bone or joint pain.

In acute leukemia, the abnormal cells can collect in the brain or spinal cord (also called the central nervous system or CNS). The result may be headaches, vomiting, confusion, loss of muscle control, and seizures. Leukemia cells also can collect in the testicles and cause swelling. Some patients develop sores in the eyes or on the skin. Leukemia also can affect the digestive tract, kidneys, lungs, or other parts of the body.

In chronic leukemia, the abnormal blood cells may gradually collect in various parts of the body. Chronic leukemia can affect the skin, central nervous system, digestive tract, kidneys, and testicles.

How Is Leukemia Diagnosed?

To find the cause of a person's symptoms, the doctor asks about the patient's medical history and does a physical exam. In addition to checking general signs of health, the doctor feels for swelling in the liver, the spleen, and in the lymph nodes under the arms, in the groin, and in the neck.

Blood tests also help in the diagnosis. A sample of blood is examined under a microscope to see what the cells look like and to determine the number of mature cells and blasts. Although blood tests may reveal that a patient has leukemia, they may not show what type of leukemia it is.

To check further for leukemia cells or to tell what type of leukemia a patient has, a hematologist, oncologist, or pathologist examines a sample of bone marrow under a microscope. The doctor withdraws the sample by inserting a needle into a large bone (usually the hip) and removing a small amount of liquid bone marrow. This procedure is called bone marrow aspiration. A bone marrow biopsy is performed with a larger needle and removes a small piece of bone and bone marrow.

If leukemia cells are found in the bone marrow sample, the patient's doctor orders other tests to find out the extent of the disease. A spinal tap (lumbar puncture) checks for leukemia cells in the fluid that fills the spaces in and around the brain and spinal cord (cerebrospinal fluid). Chest x-rays can reveal signs of disease in the chest.

How Is Leukemia Treated?

Treatment for leukemia is complex. It varies with the type of leukemia and is not the same for all patients. The treatment plan is tailored to fit each patient's needs. The treatment depends not only on the type of leukemia but also on certain features of the leukemia cells, the extent of the disease, and whether the leukemia has been treated before. It also depends on the patient's age, symptoms, and general health.

Whenever possible, patients should be treated at a medical center that has doctors who have experience in treating leukemia. If this is not possible, the patient's doctor should discuss the treatment plan with a specialist at such a center. The patient's doctor may be able to suggest a doctor who specializes in adult or childhood leukemia. Doctors who treat adult leukemia are oncologists and hematologists. Pediatric oncologists and hematologists treat childhood leukemia. Also, patients and their doctors can call the Cancer Information Service to request up-to-date treatment information from the National Cancer Institute's PDQ data base.

Acute leukemia needs to be treated right away. The goal of treatment is to bring about a remission. Then, when there is no evidence of the disease, more therapy may be given to prevent a relapse. Many people with acute leukemia can be cured.

Chronic leukemia patients who do not have symptoms may not require immediate treatment. However, they should have frequent checkups so the doctor can see whether the disease is progressing. When treatment is needed, it can often control the disease and its symptoms. However, chronic leukemia can seldom be cured.

Many patients and their families want to learn all they can about leukemia and the treatment choices so they can take an active part in decisions about medical care. The doctor is the best person to answer these questions. When discussing treatment, the patient (or, in the case of a child, the patient's family) may want to talk with the doctor about research studies of new treatment methods.

When a person is diagnosed with leukemia, shock and stress are natural reactions. These feelings may make it difficult to think of every question to ask the doctor. Taking notes or, if the doctor agrees, using a tape recorder can make it easier to remember the answers. Some people find that it also helps to have a family member or friend with them—to take part in the discussion, to take notes, or just to listen. Patients do not need to ask all their questions or remember all the answers at one time. They will have other chances for the doctor to explain things that are not clear and to ask for more information.

Methods of Treatment

Most patients with leukemia are treated with chemotherapy. Some also may have radiation therapy and/or bone marrow transplantation (BMT) or biological therapy. In some cases, surgery to remove the spleen (an operation called a splenectomy) may be part of the treatment plan.

Chemotherapy is the use of drugs to kill cancer cells. Depending on the type of leukemia, patients may receive a single drug or a combination of two or more drugs.

Some anticancer drugs can be taken by mouth. Most are given by IV injection (injected into a vein). Often, patients who need to have many IV treatments receive the drugs through a catheter. One end of this thin, flexible tube is placed in a large vein, often in the upper chest. Drugs are injected into the catheter, rather than directly into a vein, to avoid the discomfort of repeated injections and injury to the skin.

Anticancer drugs given by IV injection or taken by mouth enter the bloodstream and affect leukemia cells in most parts of the body. However, the drugs often do not reach cells in the central nervous system because they are stopped by the blood-brain barrier. This protective barrier is formed by a network of blood vessels that filter blood going to the brain and spinal cord. To reach leukemia cells in the central nervous system, doctors use intrathecal chemotherapy. In this type of treatment, anticancer drugs are injected directly into the cerebrospinal fluid.

Intrathecal chemotherapy can be given in two ways. Some patients receive the drugs by injection into the lower part of the spinal column.

Others, especially children, receive intrathecal chemotherapy through a special type of catheter called an Ommaya reservoir. This device is placed under the scalp, where it provides a pathway to the cerebrospinal fluid. Injecting anticancer drugs into the reservoir instead of into the spinal column can make intrathecal chemotherapy easier and more comfortable for the patient.

Chemotherapy is given in cycles: a treatment period followed by a recovery period, then another treatment period, and so on. In some cases, the patient has chemotherapy as an outpatient at the hospital, at the doctor's office, or at home. However, depending on which drugs are given and the patient's general health, a hospital stay may be necessary.

Radiation therapy is used along with chemotherapy for some kinds of leukemia. Radiation therapy (also called radiotherapy) uses high-energy rays to damage cancer cells and stop them from growing. The radiation comes from a large machine. Radiation therapy for leukemia can be given in two ways. For some patients, the doctor may direct the radiation to one specific area of the body where there is a collection of leukemia cells, such as the spleen or testicles. Other patients may receive radiation that is directed to the whole body. This type of radiation therapy, called total-body irradiation, usually is given before a bone marrow transplant.

Bone marrow transplantation can also be used for some patients. The patient's leukemia-producing bone marrow is destroyed by high doses of drugs and radiation and is then replaced by healthy bone marrow. The healthy bone marrow can come from a donor, or it can be marrow that has been removed from the patient and stored before the high-dose treatment. If the patient's own bone marrow is used, it may first be treated outside the body to remove leukemia cells. Patients who have a bone marrow transplant usually stay in the hospital for several weeks. Until the transplanted bone marrow begins to produce enough white blood cells, patients have to be carefully protected from infection.

Biological therapy involves treatment with substances that affect the immune system's response to cancer. Interferon is a form of biological therapy that is used for some types of leukemia.

Clinical Trials

Many patients with leukemia take part in clinical trials (treatment studies). Clinical trials help doctors find out whether a new treatment is both safe and effective. They also help doctors answer questions about how the treatment works and what side effects it causes.

Patients who take part in studies may be among the first to receive treatments that have shown promise in research. In many studies, some of the patients receive the new treatment, while others receive standard treatment so that doctors can compare different treatments. Patients who take part in a trial make an important contribution to medical science. Although these patients take certain risks, they may have the first chance to benefit from improved treatment methods.

Doctors are studying new treatments for all types of leukemia. They are working on new drugs, new drug combinations, and new schedules of chemotherapy. They also are studying ways to improve bone marrow transplantation.

Many clinical trials involve various forms of biological therapy. Interleukins and colony-stimulating factors are forms of biological therapy being studied to treat leukemia. Doctors are also studying ways to use monoclonal antibodies in the treatment of leukemia. Often, biological therapy is combined with chemotherapy or bone marrow transplantation.

Patients with leukemia (or their families) should talk with the doctor if they are interested in taking part in a clinical trial.

Supportive Care

Leukemia and its treatment can cause a number of complications and side effects. Patients receive supportive care to prevent or control these problems and to improve their comfort and quality of life during treatment.

Because leukemia patients develop infections very easily, they may receive antibiotics and other drugs to help protect them from infections. They are often advised to stay out of crowds and away from people with colds and other infectious diseases. If an infection develops, it can be serious and should be treated promptly. Patients may need to stay in the hospital to treat the infection.

Anemia and bleeding are other problems that often require supportive care. Transfusions of red blood cells may be given to help reduce the shortness of breath and fatigue that anemia can cause. Platelet transfusions can help reduce the risk of serious bleeding.

Dental care also is very important. Leukemia and chemotherapy can make the mouth sensitive, easily infected, and likely to bleed. Doctors often advise patients to have a complete dental exam before treatment begins. Dentists can show patients how to keep their mouth clean and healthy during treatment.

What Are the Side Effects of Treatment for Leukemia?

It is hard to limit the effects of therapy so that only leukemia cells are destroyed. Because treatment also damages healthy cells and tissues, it causes side effects.

The side effects of cancer treatment vary. They depend mainly on the type and extent of the treatment. Also, each person reacts differently. Side effects may even be different from one treatment to the next. Attempts are made to plan the patient's therapy to keep side effects to a minimum.

Doctors and nurses can explain the side effects of treatment and can suggest medicine, diet changes, or other ways to deal with them. The National Cancer Institute booklets *Chemotherapy and You* and *Radiation Therapy and You* also have helpful information about cancer treatment and coping with side effects.

Chemotherapy

The side effects of chemotherapy depend mainly on the drugs the patient receives. In addition, as with other types of treatment, side effects may vary from person to person. Generally, anticancer drugs affect dividing cells. Cancer cells divide more often than healthy cells and are more likely to be affected by chemotherapy. Still, some healthy cells also may be damaged. Healthy cells that divide often, including blood cells, cells in hair roots, and cells in the digestive tract, are likely to be damaged. When chemotherapy affects healthy cells, it can lower patients' resistance to infection, and patients may have less energy and bruise or bleed easily. They may lose their hair. They can also have nausea, vomiting, and mouth sores. Most side effects go away gradually during the recover periods between treatments or after treatment stops.

Some anticancer drugs can affect a patient's fertility. Women's periods may become irregular or stop, and women may have symptoms of menopause, such as hot flashes and vaginal dryness. Men may stop producing sperm. Because these changes can be permanent, some men choose to have their sperm frozen and stored. Most children treated for leukemia appear to have normal fertility when they grow up. However, depending on the drugs and doses used and on the age of the patient, some boys and girls may not be able to have children when they mature.

Radiation Therapy

Patients receiving radiation therapy can become very tired. Resting is important, but doctors usually suggest that patients remain as active as they can.

When radiation is directed to the head, patients often lose their hair. Radiation can cause the scalp or the skin in the treated area to become red, dry, tender, and itchy. Patients will be shown how to keep the skin clean. They should not use any lotion or cream on the treated area without consulting with the doctor. Radiation therapy can also cause nausea, vomiting, and loss of appetite. These side effects are temporary, and doctors and nurses can often suggest ways to control them until the treatment is over.

However, some side effects may be lasting. Children (especially young ones) who receive radiation to the brain may develop problems with learning and coordination. For this reason, doctors use the lowest possible doses of radiation, and they give this treatment only to children who cannot be treated successfully with chemotherapy alone.

Also, radiation to the testicles is likely to affect both fertility and hormone production. Most boys who have this form of treatment are not able to have children later on. Some may need to take hormones.

Bone Marrow Transplantation

Patients who have a bone marrow transplant face an increased risk of infection, bleeding, and other side effects of the large doses of chemotherapy and radiation they receive. In addition, graft-versus-host disease (GVHD) may occur in patients who receive bone marrow from a donor. In GVHD, the donated marrow reacts against the patient's tissues (most often the liver, the skin, and the digestive tract). GVHD can be mild or very severe. It can occur any time after the transplant (even years later). Drugs may be given to reduce the risk of GVHD and to treat the problem if it occurs.

Nutrition for Cancer Patients

Some cancer patients find it hard to eat well. They may lose their appetite. In addition, the common side effects of therapy, such as nausea, vomiting, or mouth sores, can make eating difficult. For some patients, foods taste different. Also, people may not feel like eating when they are uncomfortable or tired.

Eating well means getting enough calories and protein to help prevent weight loss and regain strength. Patients who eat well during cancer treatment often feel better and have more energy. In addition, they may be better able to handle the side effects of treatment.

Doctors, nurses, and dietitians can offer advice for healthy eating during cancer treatment. Patients and their families also may want to read the National Cancer Institute booklets *Eating Hints for Cancer*

Patients and *Managing Your Child's Eating Problems During Cancer Treatment*, which contain many useful suggestions.

What Happens after Treatment for Leukemia?

Regular follow-up exams are very important after treatment for leukemia. The doctor will continue to check the patient closely to be sure that the cancer has not returned. Checkups usually include exams of the blood, bone marrow, and cerebrospinal fluid. From time to time, the doctor does a complete physical exam.

Cancer treatment may cause side effects many years later. For this reason, patients should continue to have regular checkups and should also report health changes or problems to their doctor as soon as they appear.

Living with a serious disease is not easy. Cancer patients and those who care about them face many problems and challenges. Coping with these difficulties is easier when people have helpful information and support services. Several useful booklets are available from the Cancer Information Service. These including *Taking Time: Support for People with Cancer and the People Who Care About Them* and *Young People With Cancer: A Handbook for Parents.*

Cancer patients may worry about holding their job, caring for their family, or keeping up with other responsibilities. Parents of children with leukemia may worry about whether their children will be able to take part in normal school or social activities, and the children themselves may be upset about not being able to join in activities with their friends. Worries about tests, treatments, hospital stays, and medical bills are also common. Doctors, nurses, and other members of the health care team can answer questions about treatment, working, or other activities. Also, meeting with a social worker, counselor, or a member of the clergy can be helpful to patients who want to talk about their feelings or discuss their concerns.

Friends and relatives can be very supportive. Also, many patients find it helps to discuss their concerns with others who have cancer. Cancer patients often get together in support groups, where they can share what they have learned about coping with cancer and the effects of treatment. In addition to groups for adults with cancer, special support groups for children with cancer or their parents are available in many cities. It is important to keep in mind, however, that each patient is different. Treatments and ways of dealing with cancer that work for one person may not be right for another—even if they both have the same kind of cancer. It is a good idea to discuss the advice of friends and family members with the doctor.

Often, a social worker at the hospital or clinic can suggest groups that can help with rehabilitation, emotional support, financial aid, transportation, or home care. For example, the American Cancer Society, the Leukemia Society of America, and the Candlelighters Childhood Cancer Foundation have many services for patients and their families. The Cancer Information Service also has information on resources in local areas.

What Does the Future Hold for Patients with Leukemia?

Researchers are finding better ways to treat leukemia, and the chances of recovery keep improving. Still, it is natural for patients and their families to be concerned about the future.

Sometimes people use rates of survival and other statistics to try to figure out whether a patient will be cured or how long the patient will live. It is important to remember, however, that statistics are averages based on large numbers of patients. They cannot be used to predict what will happen to a certain patient because no two cancer patients are alike. Treatments and responses vary greatly. The doctor who takes care of the patient is in the best position to discuss the chance of recovery (prognosis). Patients and their families should feel free to ask the doctor about the prognosis, but they should keep in mind that not even the doctor knows exactly what will happen. Doctors often talk about surviving cancer, and they may use the term remission rather than cure. Even though many leukemia patients are cured, doctors use these terms because the disease can recur.

What Resources Are Available to Patients with Leukemia?

Information about cancer is available from many sources, including the ones listed below. You may wish to check for additional information at your local library or bookstore and from support groups in your community.

Cancer Information Service (CIS)
1-800-4-CANCER

The Cancer Information Service, a program of the National Cancer Institute, is a nationwide telephone service for cancer patients, their families and friends, the public, and health care professionals. The staff can answer questions in English and Spanish and can send booklets about cancer. They also know about local resources and services. One toll-free number, 1-800-4-CANCER (1-800-422-6237), connects callers with the office that serves their area.

American Cancer Society (ACS)
1599 Clifton Road, N.E.
Atlanta, GA 30329
1-800-ACS-2345

The American Cancer Society is a voluntary organization with a national office and local units all over the country. It supports research, conducts educational programs, and offers many services to patients and their families. To obtain free booklets about services and activities in local areas, call the Society's toll-free number, 1-800-ACS-2345 (1-800-227-2345), or the number listed under "American Cancer Society" in the white pages of the telephone book.

Candlelighters Childhood Cancer Foundation (CCCF)

Candlelighters is a national organization of parents whose children have or have had cancer. It operates a patient information service and publishes newsletters and other materials for parents and young people. Local chapters sponsor family support groups. The national office, at 1-800-366-CCCF (1-800-366-2223), can supply the telephone numbers of local chapters.

Leukemia Society of American (LSA)

The Leukemia Society of America supports cancer research and provides information and financial help to patients with leukemia. It also offers support groups for patients and their families and provides referrals to other sources of help in the community. Publications are available by calling 1-800-955-4LSA (1-800-955-4572) toll free. For information about services offered in local areas, call the number listed under Leukemia Society of America in the white pages of the telephone book.

Chapter 16

Adult Acute Lymphocytic Leukemia

What Is Adult Acute Lymphocytic Leukemia?

Adult acute lymphocytic leukemia (also called acute lymphoblastic leukemia or ALL) is a disease in which too many infection-fighting white blood cells, called lymphocytes, are found in the blood and bone marrow. Lymphocytes are made by the bone marrow and by other organs of the lymph system. The bone marrow is the spongy tissue inside the large bones in the body. The bone marrow makes red blood cells (which carry oxygen and other materials to all tissues of the body), white blood cells (which fight infection), and platelets (which make the blood clot). Normally, the bone marrow makes cells, called blasts, that develop (mature) into several different types of blood cells that have specific jobs to do in the body.

Lymphocytes are found in the lymph which is a colorless, watery fluid present in the lymph vessels. The lymph vessels are part of the lymph system, which is made up of thin tubes that branch, like blood vessels, into all parts of the body. Along the network of vessels are groups of small, bean-shaped organs called lymph nodes. Clusters of lymph nodes are found in the underarm, pelvis, neck, and abdomen. The spleen (an organ in the upper abdomen that makes lymphocytes

National Cancer Institute (NCI), PDQ database at http://cancernet.nci.nih. gov/pdq.htm, updated October 1997. The PDQ computer system gives up-to-date information on cancer and its prevention, detection, treatment, and supportive care for people with cancer and their families, and for doctors, nurses, and other health care professionals.

and filters old blood cells from the blood), the thymus (a small organ beneath the breastbone), and the tonsils (an organ in the throat) are also part of the lymph system.

Lymphocytes fight infection by making substances called antibodies, which attack germs and other harmful bacteria in the body. In ALL, the developing lymphocytes do not mature and become too numerous. These immature lymphocytes are then found in the blood and the bone marrow. They also collect in the lymph tissues and make them swell. Lymphocytes may crowd out other blood cells in the blood and bone marrow. If the bone marrow cannot make enough red blood cells to carry oxygen, then anemia may develop. If the bone marrow cannot make enough platelets to make the blood clot normally, then bleeding or bruising may develop more easily. The cancerous lymphocytes can also invade other organs, the spinal cord, and the brain.

Leukemia can be acute (progressing quickly with many immature cancer cells) or chronic (progressing slowly with more mature looking leukemia cells). ALL progresses quickly and can occur in adults and children. Treatment is different for adults than it is for children. (For more information on childhood ALL, refer to the chapter in this book on childhood acute lymphocytic leukemia. Separate chapters are also included about chronic lymphocytic leukemia, chronic myelogenous leukemia, adult or childhood acute myeloid leukemia, and hairy-cell leukemia).

ALL is often difficult to diagnose. The early signs may be similar to the flu or other common diseases. A doctor should be seen if the following signs or symptoms won't go away: fever, persistent weakness or tiredness, aching in the bones or joints, or swollen lymph nodes.

If there are symptoms, a doctor may order blood tests to count the number of each of the different kinds of blood cells. If the results of the blood tests are not normal, a doctor may do a bone marrow biopsy. During this test, a needle is inserted into a bone and a small amount of bone marrow is taken out and looked at under the microscope. A doctor may also do a spinal tap in which a needle is inserted through the back to take a sample of the fluid that surrounds the brain and spine. The fluid is then looked at under a microscope to see if leukemia cells are present. A doctor can then tell what kind of leukemia is present and plan the best treatment.

The chance of recovery (prognosis) depends on how the leukemia cells look under a microscope, how far the leukemia has spread, and the patient's age and general health.

Stages of Adult Acute Lymphocytic Leukemia

There is no staging for ALL. Your choice of treatment depends on whether a patient has been treated before.

Untreated

Untreated ALL means that no treatment has been given except to treat symptoms. There are too many white blood cells in the blood and bone marrow, and there may be other signs and symptoms of leukemia.

In Remission

Remission means that treatment has been given and that the number of white blood cells and other blood cells in the blood and bone marrow is normal. There are no signs or symptoms of leukemia.

Recurrent/Refractory

Recurrent disease means that the leukemia has come back after going into remission. Refractory disease means that the leukemia has failed to go into remission following treatment.

How Adult Acute Lymphocytic Leukemia Is Treated

There are treatments for all patients with ALL. The primary treatment of ALL is chemotherapy. Radiation therapy may be used in certain cases. Bone marrow transplantation is being studied in clinical trials.

Chemotherapy uses drugs to kill cancer cells. Chemotherapy may be taken by pill, or it may be put into the body by a needle in a vein or muscle. Chemotherapy is called a systemic treatment because the drug enters the bloodstream, travels through the body, and can kill cancer cells throughout the body. Chemotherapy may sometimes be put into the fluid that surrounds the brain by inserting a needle in the brain or back (intrathecal chemotherapy).

Radiation therapy uses x-rays or other high-energy rays to kill cancer cells and shrink tumors. Radiation for ALL usually comes from a machine outside the body (external radiation therapy).

There are two phases of treatment for ALL. The first stage is called induction therapy. The purpose of induction therapy is to kill as many of the leukemia cells as possible and make patients go into remission. Once in remission with no signs of leukemia, patients enter a second phase of treatment (called continuation therapy), which tries to kill any remaining leukemia cells. A patient may receive chemotherapy for up to several years to stay in remission.

Radiation therapy or chemotherapy to the brain may be given to patients if leukemia cells have spread to the brain. Patients may also receive central nervous system (CNS) prohylaxis, another type of therapy, to prevent leukemia cells from growing in the brain during induction therapy and remission.

Bone marrow transplantation is used to replace bone marrow with healthy bone marrow. First, all of the bone marrow in the body is destroyed with high doses of chemotherapy with or without radiation therapy. Healthy marrow is then taken from another person (a donor) whose tissue is the same as or almost the same as the patient's. The donor may be a twin (the best match), a brother or sister, or a person who is not related. The healthy marrow from the donor is given to the patient through a needle in the vein, and the marrow replaces the marrow that was destroyed. A bone marrow transplant using marrow from a relative or person not related to the patient is called an allogeneic bone marrow transplant.

Another type of bone marrow transplant, called autologous bone marrow transplant, is being studied in clinical trials. To do this type of transplant, bone marrow is taken from the patient and treated with drugs to kill any cancer cells. The marrow is frozen to save it. Next, high-dose chemotherapy is given with or without radiation therapy to destroy all of the remaining marrow. The frozen marrow that was saved is then thawed and given to the patient through a needle in a vein to replace the marrow that was destroyed.

A greater chance for recovery occurs if the doctor chooses a hospital that does more than five bone marrow transplants per year.

Treatment by Stage

Treatment of adult ALL depends on the type of disease, the patient's age, and overall condition.

Standard treatment may be considered based on its effectiveness in past studies, or participation in a clinical trial may be considered. Not all patients are cured with standard therapy, and some standard treatments may have more side effects than are desired. For these reasons, clinical trials are designed to find better ways to treat cancer patients and are based on the most up-to-date information. Clinical trials are ongoing in most parts of the country for most stages of ALL. For more information, call the Cancer Information Service at 1-800-4-CANCER (1-800-422-6237); TTY at 1-800-332-8615.

Untreated Adult Acute Lymphocytic Leukemia

Treatment will probably be systemic chemotherapy. This may be intrathecal chemotherapy alone or combined with either radiation therapy to the brain or high doses of systemic chemotherapy to treat or prevent leukemia in the brain. Treatment may also include blood transfusions, antibiotics, and instructions to keep the body and teeth especially clean. Clinical trials are testing new drugs.

Adult Acute Lymphocytic Leukemia in Remission

Treatment may be one of the following:

1. Clinical trials of short-term, high-dose chemotherapy followed by long-term, low-dose chemotherapy.

2. Clinical trials of allogeneic bone marrow transplantation.

3. Clinical trials of autologous bone marrow transplantation.

4. Intrathecal chemotherapy alone or combined with either radiation to the brain or high doses of systemic chemotherapy to prevent leukemia cells from growing in the brain (CNS prophylaxis).

Recurrent Adult Acute Lymphocytic Leukemia

Radiation therapy may be given to reduce symptoms. Patients may also choose to take part in a clinical trial of bone marrow transplantation.

To Learn More Call
1-800-4-CANCER

To learn more about adult ALL, call the National Cancer Institute's Cancer Information Service at 1-800-4-CANCER (1-800-422-6237); TTY at 1-800-332-8615. By dialing this toll-free number, trained information specialists can help answer your questions.

The Cancer Information Service also has a variety of booklets about cancer that are available to the public and can be sent on request.

The following booklets about leukemia may be helpful:

What You Need To Know About Leukemia
Research Report: Bone Marrow Transplantation

The following general booklets on questions related to cancer may also be helpful:

Taking Time: Support for People with Cancer and the People Who Care About Them
What Are Clinical Trials All About?
Chemotherapy and You: A Guide to Self-Help During Treatment
Radiation Therapy and You: A Guide to Self-Help During Treatment
Eating Hints for Cancer Patients
Advanced Cancer: Living Each Day
When Cancer Recurs: Meeting the Challenge Again
What You Need To Know About Cancer

There are many other places where people can get materials and information about cancer treatment and services. The social service office at a hospital can be checked for local and national agencies that help with getting information about finances, getting to and from treatment, getting care at home, and dealing with problems.

For more information from the National Cancer Institute, please write to this address:

National Cancer Institute
Office of Cancer Communications
31 Center Drive, MSC 2580
Bethesda, MD 20892-2580

If you want to know more about cancer and how it is treated, or if you wish to know about clinical trials for your type of cancer, you can call the NCI's Cancer Information Service at 1-800-422-6237, toll free. A trained information specialist can talk with you and answer your questions.

Chapter 17

Childhood Acute Lymphocytic Leukemia

Description

What Is Childhood Acute Lymphocytic Leukemia?

Childhood acute lymphocytic leukemia (also called acute lympho-blastic leukemia or ALL) is a disease in which too many underdevel-oped infection-fighting white blood cells, called lymphocytes, are found in a child's blood and bone marrow. ALL is the most common form of leu-kemia in children, and the most common kind of childhood cancer.

Lymphocytes are made by the bone marrow and by other organs of the lymph system. The bone marrow is the spongy tissue inside the large bones in the body. The bone marrow makes red blood cells (which carry oxygen and other materials to all tissues of the body), white blood cells (which fight infection), and platelets (which make the blood clot). Normally, the bone marrow makes cells called blasts that de-velop (mature) into several different types of blood cells that have specific jobs to do in the body.

The lymph system is made up of thin tubes that branch, like blood vessels, into all parts of the body. Lymph vessels carry lymph, a col-orless, watery fluid that contains lymphocytes. Along the network of

National Cancer Institute (NCI), PDQ database at http://cancernet.nci.nih. gov/pdq.htm, updated April 1998. The PDQ computer system gives up-to-date information on cancer and its prevention, detection, treatment, and supportive care for people with cancer and their families, and for doctors, nurses, and other health care professionals.

vessels are groups of small, bean-shaped organs called lymph nodes. Clusters of lymph nodes are found in the underarm, pelvis, neck, and abdomen. The spleen (an organ in the upper abdomen that makes lymphocytes and filters old blood cells from the blood), the thymus (a small organ beneath the breastbone), and the tonsils (an organ in the throat) are also part of the lymph system.

Lymphocytes fight infection by making substances called antibodies, which attack germs and other harmful bacteria in the body. In ALL, the developing lymphocytes become too numerous and do not mature. These immature lymphocytes are then found in the blood and the bone marrow. They also collect in the lymph tissues and make them swell. Lymphocytes may crowd out other blood cells in the blood and bone marrow. If your child's bone marrow cannot make enough red blood cells to carry oxygen, your child may have anemia. If your child's bone marrow cannot make enough platelets to make the blood clot normally, your child may bleed or bruise easily. The cancerous lymphocytes can also invade other organs, the spinal cord, and the brain.

Leukemia can be acute (progressing quickly with many immature cancer cells) or chronic (progressing slowly with more mature-looking leukemia cells). Acute lymphocytic leukemia progresses quickly, and can occur in both children and adults. Treatment is different for adults than it is for children. For information on adult ALL, see the PDQ patient information statement on adult acute lymphocytic leukemia. Separate PDQ patient information statements are also available for chronic lymphocytic leukemia, chronic myelogenous leukemia, adult or childhood acute myeloid leukemia, and hairy cell leukemia.

Early signs of ALL may be similar to those of the flu or other common diseases, such as a fever that won't go away, feeling weak or tired all the time, aching bones or joints, or swollen lymph nodes. If your child has symptoms of leukemia, his or her doctor may order blood tests to count the number of each of the different kinds of blood cells. If the results of the blood tests are not normal, a bone marrow biopsy may be performed. During this test, a needle is inserted into a bone in the hip and a small amount of bone marrow is removed and examined under the microscope, enabling the doctor to determine what kind of leukemia your child has and plan the best treatment.

Your child's doctor may also do a spinal tap, in which a needle is inserted through the back to remove a sample of the fluid that surrounds the brain and spine. The fluid is then examined under a microscope to see if leukemia cells are present.

Your child's chance of recovery (prognosis) depends on your child's age at diagnosis, the number of white blood cells in the blood (the white blood cell count) at diagnosis, how far the disease has spread, the biologic characteristics of the leukemia cells, and how well the leukemia cells respond to treatment.

Stage Explanation

Stages of Childhood Acute Lymphocytic Leukemia

There is no staging for childhood acute lymphocytic leukemia. The treatment depends on whether or not the patient has been previously treated for leukemia.

Untreated

Untreated acute lymphocytic leukemia (ALL) means that no treatment has been given except to alleviate symptoms. There are too many white blood cells in the blood and bone marrow, and there may be other signs and symptoms of leukemia.

In Remission

Remission means that treatment has been given and that the number of white blood cells and other blood cells in the blood and bone marrow is normal. There are no signs or symptoms of leukemia.

Recurrent/refractory

Recurrent disease means that the leukemia has come back (recurred) after going into remission. Refractory disease means that the leukemia failed to go into remission following treatment.

Treatment Option Overview

How Childhood Acute Lymphocytic Leukemia Is Treated

There are treatments for all patients with childhood acute lymphocytic leukemia (ALL). The primary treatment for ALL is chemotherapy. Radiation therapy may be used in certain cases. Bone marrow transplantation is being studied in clinical trials.

Chemotherapy uses drugs to kill cancer cells. Chemotherapy drugs may be taken by mouth, or may be put into the body by a needle in a vein or muscle. Chemotherapy is called a systemic treatment because the drug enters the bloodstream, travels through the body, and can kill cancer cells throughout the body. For ALL, chemotherapy drugs may sometimes be injected (usually through the spine) into the fluid that surrounds the brain and spinal cord; this is known as intrathecal chemotherapy.

Radiation therapy uses x-rays or other high-energy rays to kill cancer cells and shrink tumors. Radiation for ALL usually comes from a machine outside the body (external beam radiation therapy).

Bone marrow transplantation is a newer type of treatment. First, high doses of chemotherapy with or without radiation therapy are given to destroy all of the bone marrow in the body. Healthy marrow is then taken from another person (a donor) whose tissue is the same as or almost the same as the patient's. The donor may be a twin (the best match), a brother or sister, or another person not related. The healthy marrow from the donor is given to the patient through a needle in a vein, and the marrow replaces the marrow that was destroyed. A bone marrow transplant using marrow from a relative or person not related is called an allogeneic bone marrow transplant.

An even newer type of bone marrow transplant, called autologous bone marrow transplant, is being studied in clinical trials. During this procedure, bone marrow is taken from the patient and may be treated with drugs to kill any cancer cells. The marrow is frozen to save it. The patient is then given high-dose chemotherapy with or without radiation therapy to destroy all of the remaining marrow. The frozen marrow that was saved is thawed and given through a needle in a vein to replace the marrow that was destroyed.

There are generally four phases of treatment for ALL. The first phase, remission induction therapy, uses chemotherapy to kill as many of the leukemia cells as possible to cause the cancer to go into remission. Once a child goes into remission and there are no signs of leukemia, a second phase of treatment, called consolidation or intensification therapy, is given. Consolidation therapy uses high-dose chemotherapy to attempt to kill any remaining leukemia cells. The third phase, called central nervous system (CNS) prophylaxis, is preventive therapy using intrathecal and/or high-dose systemic chemotherapy to the central nervous system (CNS) to kill any leukemia cells present there, or to prevent the spread of cancer cells to the brain and spinal cord even if no cancer has been detected there. Radiation therapy to the brain may also be given, in addition to chemotherapy, for this purpose. CNS prophylaxis is often given in conjunction with consolidation/intensification therapy. The fourth phase of treatment, called maintenance therapy, uses chemotherapy for several years to maintain the remission.

Treatment by Stage

Treatment for childhood acute lymphocytic leukemia depends on the prognostic group to which your child is assigned based primarily on your child's age and white blood cell count at diagnosis.

Your child may receive treatment that is considered standard based on its effectiveness in a number of patients in past studies, or you may choose to have your child take part in a clinical trial. Not all patients are cured with standard therapy and some standard treatments may have more side effects than are desired. For these reasons, clinical trials are designed to test new treatments and to find better ways to treat cancer patients. Clinical trials are ongoing in most parts of the country for most stages of childhood ALL. For more information, call the Cancer Information Service at 1-800-4-CANCER (1-800-422-6237); TTY at 1-800-332-8615.

Untreated Childhood Acute Lymphocytic Leukemia

Your child's treatment will probably be remission induction chemotherapy to kill cancer cells and cause the leukemia to go into remission. Induction chemotherapy is almost always successful in inducing remission. Intrathecal and/or high-dose systemic chemotherapy, with or without radiation therapy to the brain, may also be given to prevent the spread of cancer cells to the brain and spinal cord. Clinical trials are testing new ways of inducing remission.

Childhood Acute Lymphocytic Leukemia in Remission

Your child's treatment will probably be intensive chemotherapy to kill any remaining cancer cells. Intrathecal and/or high doses of systemic chemotherapy, with or without radiation therapy to the brain, may also be given during this phase of treatment to prevent the spread of cancer cells to the brain and spinal cord. Following intensification therapy, chemotherapy generally continues until the child has been in continuous remission for several years.

Recurrent Childhood Acute Lymphocytic Leukemia

Treatment depends on the type of treatment your child received before, how soon the cancer came back following treatment, and whether the leukemia cells are found outside the bone marrow. Your child's treatment will probably be systemic chemotherapy or bone marrow transplantation. You may want to consider entering your child into a clinical trial of new chemotherapy drugs or bone marrow transplantation.

To Learn More

To learn more about childhood acute lymphocytic leukemia, call the National Cancer Institute's Cancer Information Service at 1-800-4-CANCER (1-800-422-6237); TTY at 1-800-332-8615. By dialing this toll-free number, you can speak with someone who can answer your questions.

The Cancer Information Service can also send you booklets. The following booklets about leukemia may be helpful to you:

What You Need To Know About Leukemia
Research Report: Bone Marrow Transplantation

The following booklets on childhood cancer may also be helpful to you:

Young People with Cancer: A Handbook for Parents
Talking with Your Child About Cancer
When Someone in Your Family Has Cancer
Managing Your Child's Eating Problems During Cancer Treatment

The following general booklets related to questions on cancer may also be helpful:

What You Need To Know About Cancer
Taking Time: Support for People with Cancer and the People Who Care About Them
What Are Clinical Trials All About?
Chemotherapy and You: A Guide to Self-Help During Treatment
Radiation Therapy and You: A Guide to Self-Help During Treatment

There are many other places you can get material about cancer treatment and services to help you. You can check the social service office at your hospital for local and national agencies that help with your finances, getting to and from treatment, care at home, and dealing with your problems.

You can also write to the National Cancer Institute at this address:

National Cancer Institute
Office of Cancer Communications
31 Center Drive, MSC 2580
Bethesda, MD 20892-2580

If you want to know more about cancer and how it is treated, or if you wish to know about clinical trials for your type of cancer, you can call the NCI's Cancer Information Service at 1-800-422-6237, toll free. A trained information specialist can talk with you and answer your questions.

Chapter 18

Chronic Lymphocytic Leukemia

What Is Chronic Lymphocytic Leukemia?

Chronic lymphocytic leukemia (CLL) is a disease in which too many infection-fighting white blood cells, called lymphocytes, are found in the body. Lymphocytes are made in the bone marrow and by other organs of the lymph system. The bone marrow is the spongy tissue inside the large bones in the body. The bone marrow makes red blood cells (which carry oxygen and other materials to all tissues of the body), white blood cells (which fight infection), and platelets (which make the blood clot). Normally, bone marrow cells, called blasts, develop (mature) into several different types of blood cells that have specific jobs to do in the body.

The lymph system is made up of thin tubes that branch, like blood vessels, into all parts of the body. Lymph vessels carry lymph, a colorless, watery fluid that contains lymphocytes. Along the network of vessels are groups of small, bean-shaped organs called lymph nodes. Clusters of lymph nodes are found in the underarm, pelvis, neck, and abdomen. The spleen (an organ in the upper abdomen that makes lymphocytes and filters old blood cells from the blood), the thymus (a

National Cancer Institute (NCI), PDQ database at http://cancernet.nci.nih. gov/pdq.htm, updated November 1997. The PDQ computer system gives up-to-date information on cancer and its prevention, detection, treatment, and supportive care for people with cancer and their families, and for doctors, nurses, and other health care professionals.

197

small organ beneath the breastbone), and the tonsils (an organ in the throat) are also part of the lymph system.

Lymphocytes fight infection by making substances called antibodies, which attack germs and other harmful things in the body. In CLL, the developing lymphocytes do not mature correctly and too many are made. The lymphocytes may look normal, but they cannot fight infection as well as they should. These immature lymphocytes are then found in the blood and the bone marrow. They also collect in the lymph tissues and make them swell. Lymphocytes may crowd out other blood cells in the blood and bone marrow. Anemia may develop if the bone marrow cannot make enough red blood cells to carry oxygen. If the bone marrow cannot make enough platelets to make the blood clot normally, bleeding or bruising may occur easily.

Leukemia can be acute (progressing quickly with many immature cells) or chronic (progressing slowly with more mature, normal looking cells). Chronic lymphocytic leukemia progresses slowly and usually occurs in people 60 years of age or older. In the first stages of the disease there are often no symptoms. As time goes on, more and more lymphocytes are made and symptoms begin to appear. A doctor should be seen if the lymph nodes swell, the spleen or liver becomes larger than normal, a feeling of fatigue persists, or bleeding occurs easily.

If there are symptoms, a doctor will do a physical examination and may order blood tests to count the number of each of the different kinds of blood cells. More blood tests may be done if the results of the blood tests are not normal. The doctor may also do a bone marrow biopsy. During this test, a needle is inserted into a bone and a small amount of bone marrow is taken out and looked at under the microscope. The doctor can then tell what kind of leukemia the patient has and plan the best treatment.

The chance of recovery (prognosis) depends on the stage of the disease, and the patient's age and general health.

There are separate chapters in this book on acute lymphocytic leukemia (adult and childhood), acute myeloid leukemia (adult and childhood), chronic myelogenous leukemia, and hairy cell leukemia.

Stages of Chronic Lymphocytic Leukemia

Once chronic lymphocytic leukemia has been found (diagnosed), more tests may be done to find out if leukemia cells have spread to other parts of the body. This is called staging. A doctor needs to know the stage of the disease to plan treatment. The following stages are used for chronic lymphocytic leukemia:

Stage 0

There are too many lymphocytes in the blood, but there are usually no other symptoms of leukemia. Lymph nodes and the spleen and liver are not swollen and the number of red blood cells and platelets is normal.

Stage I

There are too many lymphocytes in the blood and lymph nodes are swollen. The spleen and liver are not swollen and the number of blood cells and platelets is normal.

Stage II

There are too many lymphocytes in the blood, and lymph nodes, the liver, and spleen are swollen.

Stage III

There are too many lymphocytes in the blood and there are too few red blood cells (anemia). Lymph nodes and the liver or spleen may be swollen.

Stage IV

There are too many lymphocytes in the blood and too few platelets, which make it hard for the blood to clot. The lymph nodes, liver, or spleen may be swollen, and there may be too few red blood cells (anemia).

Refractory

Refractory means that the leukemia does not respond to treatment.

How Chronic Lymphocytic Leukemia Is Treated

There are treatments for all patients with chronic lymphocytic leukemia. Three kinds of treatment are used:

- chemotherapy (using drugs to kill cancer cells)
- radiation therapy (using high-dose x-rays or other high-energy rays to kill cancer cells)
- treatment for complications of the leukemia, such as infection.

The use of biological therapy (using the body's immune system to fight cancer) is being tested in clinical trials. Surgery may be used in certain cases.

Chemotherapy uses drugs to kill cancer cells. Chemotherapy may be taken by pill, or it may be put into the body by a needle in the vein or muscle. Chemotherapy is called a systemic treatment because the drug enters the bloodstream, travels through the body, and can kill cancer cells throughout the body.

Radiation therapy uses x-rays or other high-energy rays to kill cancer cells and shrink tumors. Radiation for CLL usually comes from a machine outside the body (external radiation therapy).

If the spleen is swollen, a doctor may take out the spleen in an operation called a splenectomy. This is only done in rare cases.

Biological therapy tries to get the body to fight cancer. It uses materials made by the body or made in a laboratory to boost, direct, or restore the body's natural defenses against disease. Biological therapy is sometimes called biological response modifier (BRM) therapy or immunotherapy.

Because infection often occurs in patients with CLL, a special substance called immunoglobulin, which contains antibodies, may be given to prevent infections.

Sometimes a special machine is used to filter the blood to take out extra lymphocytes. This is called leukapheresis.

Bone marrow transplantation is used to replace the bone marrow with healthy bone marrow. First, all of the bone marrow in the body is destroyed with high doses of chemotherapy with or without radiation therapy. Healthy marrow is then taken from another person (a donor) whose tissue is the same as or almost the same as the patient's. The donor may be a twin (the best match), a brother or sister, or another person not related. The healthy marrow from the donor is given to the patient through a needle in the vein, and the marrow replaces the marrow that was destroyed. A bone marrow transplant using marrow from a relative or person not related to the patient is called an allogeneic bone marrow transplant.

Another type of bone marrow transplant, called autologous bone marrow transplant, is being studied in clinical trials. To do this type of transplant, bone marrow is taken from the patient and treated with drugs to kill any cancer cells. The marrow is frozen to save it. Next, the patient is given high-dose chemotherapy with or without radiation therapy to destroy all of the remaining marrow. The frozen marrow that was saved is then thawed and given back to the patient through a needle in a vein to replace the marrow that was destroyed.

Treatment by Stage

Treatment of chronic lymphocytic leukemia depends on the stage of the disease, and the patient's age and overall health.

Standard treatment may be considered because of its effectiveness in patients in past studies, or participation in a clinical trial may be considered. Most patients with chronic lymphocytic leukemia are not cured with standard therapy and some standard treatments may have more side effects than are desired. For these reasons, clinical trials are designed to find better ways to treat cancer patients and are based on the most up-to-date information. Clinical trials are ongoing in most parts of the country for most stages of chronic lymphocytic leukemia. To know more about clinical trials, call the Cancer Information Service at 1-800-4-CANCER (1-800-422-6237); TTY at 1-800-332-8615.

Stage 0 Chronic Lymphocytic Leukemia

If the patient has stage 0 CLL, treatment may not be needed or chemotherapy may be given. A doctor will follow the patient closely so treatment can be started if the leukemia gets worse.

Stage I Chronic Lymphocytic Leukemia

Treatment may be one of the following:

1. If there are no symptoms, no treatment may be needed. A doctor will follow the patient closely so treatment can be started if the leukemia gets worse.

2. External radiation therapy to swollen lymph nodes.

3. Chemotherapy.

Stage II Chronic Lymphocytic Leukemia

Treatment may be one of the following:

1. If there are few or no symptoms, no treatment may be needed. A doctor will follow the patient closely so treatment can be started if the leukemia gets worse.

2. Chemotherapy.

3. Clinical trials of biological therapy.

4. External radiation therapy to the spleen.

Stage III Chronic Lymphocytic Leukemia

Treatment may be one of the following:

1. Chemotherapy.

2. Clinical trials of bone marrow transplantation.

3. Surgery to remove the spleen (splenectomy).

4. External radiation therapy to the spleen.

5. External radiation therapy to the whole body (whole body radiation).

6. Clinical trials of biological therapy.

Stage IV Chronic Lymphocytic Leukemia

Treatment may be one of the following:

1. Chemotherapy.

2. Clinical trials of bone marrow transplantation.

3. Surgery to remove the spleen (splenectomy).

4. External radiation therapy to the spleen.

5. External radiation therapy to the whole body (whole body radiation).

6. Clinical trials of biological therapy.

Refractory Chronic Lymphocytic Leukemia

Treatment depends on many factors; patients may wish to consider entering a clinical trial of new chemotherapy drugs and bone marrow transplantation.

To Learn More Call 1-800-4-CANCER

To learn more about chronic lymphocytic leukemia, call the National Cancer Institute's Cancer Information Service at 1-800-4-CANCER (1-800-422-6237); TTY at 1-800-332-8615. By dialing this toll-free number, trained information specialists can answer your questions.

The Cancer Information Service also has booklets that are available to the public and can be sent on request. The following booklets about leukemia may be helpful:

What You Need To Know About Leukemia
Research Report: Bone Marrow Transplantation

The following general booklets on questions related to cancer may also be helpful:

What You Need To Know About Cancer
Taking Time: Support for People with Cancer and the People Who Care About Them
What Are Clinical Trials All About?
Chemotherapy and You: A Guide to Self-Help During Treatment
Radiation Therapy and You: A Guide to Self-Help During Treatment
Eating Hints for Cancer Patients
Advanced Cancer: Living Each Day
When Cancer Recurs: Meeting the Challenge Again

There are many other places where people can get materials and information about cancer treatment and services. The social service office at a hospital can be checked for local and national agencies that help with getting information about finances, getting to and from treatment, getting care at home, and dealing with problems.

For more information from the National Cancer Institute, please write to this address:

National Cancer Institute
Office of Cancer Communications
31 Center Drive, MSC 2580
Bethesda, MD 20892-2580

If you want to know more about cancer and how it is treated, or if you wish to know about clinical trials for your type of cancer, you can call the NCI's Cancer Information Service at 1-800-422-6237, toll free. A trained information specialist can talk with you and answer your questions.

Chapter 19

Chronic Myelogenous Leukemia

What Is Chronic Myelogenous Leukemia?

Chronic myelogenous leukemia (also called CML or chronic granulocytic leukemia) is a disease in which too many white blood cells are made in the bone marrow. The bone marrow is the spongy tissue inside the large bones in the body. The bone marrow makes red blood cells (which carry oxygen and other materials to all tissues of the body), white blood cells (which fight infection), and platelets (which make the blood clot).

Normally, bone marrow cells, called blasts, develop (mature) into several different types of blood cells that have specific jobs to do in the body. CML affects the blasts that are developing into white blood cells, called granulocytes. The blasts do not mature and become too numerous. These immature blast cells are then found in the blood and the bone marrow. In most people with CML, the genetic material (chromosomes) in the leukemia cells have a feature that is not normal called a Philadelphia chromosome. This chromosome usually doesn't go away, even after treatment.

Leukemia can be acute (progressing quickly with many immature blasts) or chronic (progressing slowly with more mature looking cancer

National Cancer Institute (NCI), PDQ database at http://cancernet.nci. nih.gov/pdq.htm, updated November 1997. The PDQ computer system gives up-to-date information on cancer and its prevention, detection, treatment, and supportive care for people with cancer and their families, and for doctors, nurses, and other health care professionals.

cells). Chronic myelogenous leukemia progresses slowly and usually occurs in people who are middle-aged or older, although it also can occur in children. In the first stages of CML, most people don't have any symptoms of cancer. A doctor should be seen if any of the following symptoms appear: tiredness that won't go away, a feeling of no energy, fever, not feeling hungry, or night sweats. Also, the spleen (the organ in the upper abdomen that makes other types of white blood cells and filters old blood cells from the blood) may be swollen.

If there are symptoms, a doctor may order blood tests to count the number of each of the different kinds of blood cells. If the results of the blood test are not normal, the doctor may order more blood tests. A bone marrow biopsy may also be done. During this test, a needle is inserted into a bone and a small amount of bone marrow is taken out and looked at under the microscope. The doctor can then tell what kind of leukemia the patient has and plan the best treatment.

Separate chapters containing patient information on acute lymphocytic leukemia (adult and childhood), acute myeloid leukemia (adult and childhood), and hairy cell leukemia are also available in this book.

Stages of Chronic Myelogenous Leukemia

Once chronic myelogenous leukemia (CML) has been found (diagnosed), more tests may be done to find out if leukemia cells have spread into other parts of the body such as the brain. This is called staging. CML progresses through different phases and these phases are the stages used to plan treatment. The following stages are used for chronic myelogenous leukemia:

Chronic Phase

There are few blast cells in the blood and bone marrow and there may be no symptoms of leukemia. This phase may last from several months to several years.

Accelerated Phase

There are more blast cells in the blood and bone marrow and fewer normal cells.

Blastic Phase

More than 30% of the cells in the blood or bone marrow are blast cells. The blast phase of CML is sometimes called "blast crisis." Sometimes

blast cells will form tumors outside of the bone marrow in places such
as the bone or lymph nodes. Lymph nodes are small, bean-shaped
structures that are found throughout the body. They produce and store
infection-fighting cells.

Meningeal

Leukemia cells are found in the fluid that surrounds the brain and/
or spinal cord. Meningeal CML can occur during the accelerated phase
or the blastic phase.

Refractory

Leukemia cells do not decrease even though treatment is given.

How Chronic Myelogenous Leukemia Is Treated

There are treatments for all patients with chronic myelogenous
leukemia. Three kinds of treatment are used:

- chemotherapy (using drugs to kill cancer cells)
- radiation therapy (using high-dose x-rays or other high-energy
  rays to kill cancer cells)
- bone marrow transplantation (killing the bone marrow and replacing it with healthy marrow).

The use of biological therapy (using the body's immune system to
fight cancer) is being tested in clinical trials. Surgery may be used in
certain cases to relieve symptoms.

Chemotherapy uses drugs to kill cancer cells. Chemotherapy may
be taken by pill, or it may be put into the body by a needle in the vein
or muscle. Chemotherapy is called a systemic treatment because the
drug enters the bloodstream, travels through the body, and can kill
cancer cells throughout the body. Chemotherapy also can be put directly into the fluid around the brain and spinal cord through a tube
inserted into the brain or back. This is called intrathecal chemotherapy.

Radiation therapy uses x-rays or other high-energy rays to kill
cancer cells and shrink tumors. Radiation for CML usually comes from
a machine outside the body (external radiation therapy) and is sometimes used to relieve symptoms or as part of therapy given before a
bone marrow transplant.

Bone marrow transplantation is used to replace the patient's bone marrow with healthy bone marrow. First, all of the bone marrow in the body is destroyed with high doses of chemotherapy with or without radiation therapy. Healthy marrow is then taken from another person (a donor) whose tissue is the same as or almost the same as the patient's. The donor may be a twin (the best match), a brother or sister, or another person not related. The healthy marrow from the donor is given to the patient through a needle in the vein, and the marrow replaces the marrow that was destroyed. A bone marrow transplant using marrow from a relative or person not related to the patient is called an allogeneic bone marrow transplant.

Another type of bone marrow transplant, called autologous bone marrow transplant, is being tested in clinical trials. To do this type of transplant, bone marrow is taken from the patient and treated with drugs to kill any cancer cells. The marrow is then frozen to save it. The patient is given high-dose chemotherapy with or without radiation therapy to destroy all of the remaining marrow. The frozen marrow that was saved is then thawed and given back to the patient through a needle in a vein to replace the marrow that was destroyed.

A greater chance for recovery occurs if a doctor chooses a hospital that does more than five bone marrow transplants per year.

Biological therapy tries to get the body to fight cancer. It uses materials made by the body or made in a laboratory to boost, direct, or restore the body's natural defenses against disease. Biological therapy is sometimes called biological response modifier (BRM) therapy or immunotherapy.

If the spleen is swollen, a doctor may take out the spleen in an operation called a splenectomy.

Treatment by Stage

Standard treatment may be considered because of its effectiveness in patients in past studies or participation in a clinical trial may be considered. Most patients are not cured with standard therapy and some standard treatments may have more side effects than are desired. For these reasons, clinical trials are designed to find better ways to treat cancer patients and are based on the most up-to-date information. Clinical trials are ongoing in most parts of the country for patients with CML of any phase. To know more about clinical trials, call the Cancer Information Service at 1-800-4-CANCER (1-800-422-6237); TTY at 1-800-332-8615.

Chronic Phase Chronic Myelogenous Leukemia

Treatment may be one of the following:

1. Bone marrow transplantation.
2. Biological therapy.
3. Chemotherapy to lower the number of white blood cells.
4. Surgery to remove the spleen (splenectomy).

Accelerated Phase Chronic Myelogenous Leukemia

Treatment may be one of the following:

1. Bone marrow transplantation.
2. Chemotherapy to lower the number of white blood cells.
3. Transfusions of blood or blood products to relieve symptoms.

Blastic Phase Chronic Myelogenous Leukemia

Treatment may be one of the following:

1. Chemotherapy.
2. Bone marrow transplantation.
3. Clinical trials are testing new chemotherapy drugs and new combinations of drugs.
4. Radiation therapy to relieve symptoms caused by tumors formed in the bone.

Meningeal Chronic Myelogenous Leukemia

Treatment may be one of the following:

1. Intrathecal chemotherapy.
2. Radiation therapy to the brain.

Refractory Chronic Myelogenous Leukemia

The treatment depends on many factors. A patient may wish to consider entering a clinical trial. If the patient has had a bone marrow transplant, the treatment may be biological therapy or white blood cells from the bone marrow donor may be given to the patient through a vein.

To Learn More Call 1-800-4-CANCER

To learn more about chronic myelogenous leukemia, call the National Cancer Institute's Cancer Information Service at 1-800-4-CANCER

(1-800-422-6237); TTY at 1-800-332-8615. By dialing this toll-free number, trained information specialists can answer your questions.

The Cancer Information Service also has booklets about cancer that are available to the public and can be sent on request. The following booklets about leukemia may be helpful:

What You Need To Know About Leukemia
Research Report: Bone Marrow Transplantation

The following general booklets on questions related to cancer may also be helpful:

Taking Time: Support for People with Cancer and the People Who Care About Them
What Are Clinical Trials All About?
Chemotherapy and You: A Guide to Self-Help During Treatment
Radiation Therapy and You: A Guide to Self-Help During Treatment
Eating Hints for Cancer Patients
What You Need To Know About Cancer
Advanced Cancer: Living Each Day
When Cancer Recurs: Meeting the Challenge Again

There are many other places where people can get material and information about cancer treatment and services. The social service office at a hospital can be checked for local and national agencies that help with getting information about finances, getting to and from treatment, getting care at home, and dealing with problems.

For more information from the National Cancer Institute, please write to this address:

National Cancer Institute
Office of Cancer Communications
31 Center Drive, MSC 2580
Bethesda, MD 20892-2580

If you want to know more about cancer and how it is treated, or if you wish to know about clinical trials for your type of cancer, you can call the NCI's Cancer Information Service at 1-800-422-6237, toll free. A trained information specialist can talk with you and answer your questions.

Chapter 20

Adult Acute Myeloid Leukemia

Description

What Is Adult Acute Myeloid Leukemia?

Adult acute myeloid leukemia (AML) is a disease in which cancer (malignant) cells are found in the blood and bone marrow. AML is also called acute nonlymphocytic leukemia or ANLL. The bone marrow is the spongy tissue inside the large bones in the body. The bone marrow makes red blood cells (which carry oxygen and other materials to all tissues of the body), white blood cells (which fight infection), and platelets (which make the blood clot).

Normally, the bone marrow makes cells called blasts that develop (mature) into several different types of blood cells that have specific jobs to do in the body. AML affects the blasts that are developing into white blood cells called granulocytes. In AML, the blasts do not mature and become too numerous. These immature blast cells are then found in the blood and the bone marrow.

Leukemia can be acute (progressing quickly with many immature blasts) or chronic (progressing slowly with more mature looking cancer cells). Acute myeloid leukemia progresses quickly. AML can occur in adults or children. (For more information on the treatment of childhood

National Cancer Institute (NCI), PDQ database at http://cancernet.nci.nih. gov/pdq.htm, updated October 1997. The PDQ computer system gives up-to-date information on cancer and its prevention, detection, treatment, and supportive care for people with cancer and their families, and for doctors, nurses, and other health care professionals.

AML, refer to the PDQ patient information statement on childhood acute myeloid leukemia. Separate PDQ statements are also available for chronic lymphocytic leukemia, chronic myelogenous leukemia, adult acute lymphocytic leukemia, and hairy-cell leukemia).

AML is often difficult to diagnose. The early signs may be similar to the flu or other common diseases. A doctor should be seen if the following signs or symptoms won't go away: fever, weakness or tiredness, or achiness in the bones or joints.

If there are symptoms, a doctor may order blood tests to count the number of each of the different kinds of blood cells. If the results of the blood tests are not normal, a doctor may do a bone marrow biopsy. During this test, a needle is inserted into a bone and a small amount of bone marrow is taken out and looked at under a microscope. A doctor can then tell what kind of leukemia is present and plan the best treatment.

The chance of recovery (prognosis) depends on the type of AML and the patient's age and general health.

Stage Explanation

Stages of Adult Acute Myeloid Leukemia

There is no staging for AML. The choice of treatment depends on whether the patient has been treated.

Untreated

Untreated AML means no treatment has been given except to treat symptoms. There are too many white blood cells in the blood and bone marrow, and there may be other signs and symptoms of leukemia. Rarely, tumor cells can appear as a solid tumor called an isolated granulocytic sarcoma or chloroma.

In Remission

Treatment has been given, and the number of white blood cells and other blood cells in the blood and bone marrow is normal. There are no signs or symptoms of leukemia.

Recurrent/refractory

Recurrent disease means the leukemia has come back after going into remission. Refractory disease means the leukemia has not gone into remission following treatment.

Treatment Option Overview

How Adult Acute Myeloid Leukemia Is Treated

There are treatments for all patients with AML. The primary treatment of AML is chemotherapy. Radiation therapy may be used in certain cases. Bone marrow transplantation and biological therapy are being studied in clinical trials.

Chemotherapy is the use of drugs to kill cancer cells. Drugs may be given by mouth, or they may be put into the body by a needle in a vein or muscle. Chemotherapy is called a systemic treatment because the drug enters the bloodstream, travels through the body, and can kill cancer cells throughout the body. Chemotherapy may sometimes be put into the fluid that surrounds the brain through a needle in the brain or back (intrathecal chemotherapy).

Radiation therapy uses x-rays or other high-energy rays to kill cancer cells and shrink tumors. Radiation for AML usually comes from a machine outside the body (external radiation therapy).

If the leukemia cells have spread to the brain, radiation therapy to the brain or intrathecal chemotherapy will be given.

There are two phases of treatment for AML. The first stage is called induction therapy. The purpose of induction therapy is to kill as many of the leukemia cells as possible and make patients go into remission. Once in remission with no signs of leukemia, patients enter a second phase of treatment (called continuation therapy), which tries to kill any remaining leukemia cells. Chemotherapy may be given for several years to keep a patient in remission.

Bone marrow transplantation is used to replace the bone marrow with healthy bone marrow. First, all of the bone marrow in the body is destroyed with high doses of chemotherapy with or without radiation therapy. Healthy marrow is then taken from another person (a donor) whose tissue is the same as or almost the same as the patient's. The donor may be a twin (the best match), a brother or sister, or a person who is not related. The healthy marrow from the donor is given to the patient through a needle in the vein, and the marrow replaces the marrow that was destroyed. A bone marrow transplant using marrow from a relative or from a person who is not related is called an allogeneic bone marrow transplant.

Another type of bone marrow transplant, called autologous bone marrow transplant, is being studied in clinical trials. To do this type of transplant, bone marrow is taken from the patient and treated with drugs to kill any cancer cells. The marrow is then frozen to save it. Next, high-dose chemotherapy is given with or without radiation therapy to destroy all of the remaining marrow. The frozen marrow that was saved is then thawed and given to the patient through a needle in a vein to replace the marrow that was destroyed.

Another type of autologous transplant is called a peripheral blood stem cell transplant. The patient's blood is passed through a machine that removes the stem cells (immature cells from which all blood cells develop), then returns the blood to the patient. This procedure is called leukapheresis and usually takes 3 or 4 hours to complete. The stem cells are treated with drugs to kill any cancer cells and then frozen until they are transplanted to the patient. This procedure may be done alone or with an autologous bone marrow transplant.

A greater chance for recovery occurs if the doctor chooses a hospital that does more than five bone marrow transplantations per year.

Biological therapy tries to get the body to fight cancer. It uses materials made by the patient's body or made in a laboratory to boost, direct, or restore the body's natural defenses against disease. Biological therapy is sometimes called biological response modifier therapy or immunotherapy.

Treatment by Stage

Treatment for adult AML depends on the type of AML, the patient's age and overall health.

Standard treatment may be considered based on its effectiveness in past studies, or participation in a clinical trial may be considered. Not all patients are cured with standard therapy, and some standard treatments may have more side effects than are desired. For these reasons, clinical trials are designed to find better ways to treat cancer patients and are based on the most up-to-date information. Clinical trials are ongoing in most parts of the country for most stages of adult AML. For more information, call the Cancer Information Service at 1-800-4-CANCER (1-800-422-6237); TTY at 1-800-332-8615.

Untreated Adult Acute Myeloid Leukemia

Treatment will probably be systemic chemotherapy. If leukemia cells are found in the brain, intrathecal chemotherapy may be given. Clinical trials are testing new drugs.

Adult Acute Myeloid Leukemia in Remission

Treatment may be one of the following:

1. Systemic chemotherapy. Clinical trials are testing new chemotherapy drugs and new ways of giving the drugs.

2. Clinical trials of bone marrow or peripheral stem cell transplantation.

Recurrent Adult Acute Myeloid Leukemia

Radiation therapy may be given to reduce symptoms. Patients may also choose to take part in clinical trials of new chemotherapy drugs or bone marrow transplantation.

To Learn More

To learn more about adult acute myeloid leukemia, call the National Cancer Institute's Cancer Information Service at 1-800-4-CANCER (1-800-422-6237); TTY at 1-800-332-8615. By dialing this toll-free number, trained information specialists can help answer your questions.

The Cancer Information Service also has a variety of booklets that are available to the public and can be sent on request. The following booklets about leukemia may be helpful:

What You Need To Know About Leukemia
Research Report: Bone Marrow Transplantation

The following general booklets on questions related to cancer may also be helpful:

What You Need To Know About Cancer
Taking Time: Support for People with Cancer and the People Who Care About Them
What Are Clinical Trials All About?
Chemotherapy and You: A Guide to Self-Help During Treatment
Radiation Therapy and You: A Guide to Self-Help During Treatment Eating Hints for Cancer Patients
Advanced Cancer: Living Each Day
When Cancer Recurs: Meeting the Challenge Again

There are many other places where people can get information about cancer treatment and services. The social service office at a hospital can be checked for local and national agencies that help with getting information about finances, getting to and from treatment, getting care at home, and dealing with problems.

For more information from the National Cancer Institute, please write to this address:

National Cancer Institute
Office of Cancer Communications
31 Center Drive, MSC 2580
Bethesda, MD 20892-2580

If you want to know more about cancer and how it is treated, or if you wish to know about clinical trials for your type of cancer, you can call the NCI's Cancer Information Service at 1-800-422-6237, toll free. A trained information specialist can talk with you and answer your questions.

Chapter 21

Childhood Acute Myeloid Leukemia

Description

What Is Childhood Acute Myeloid Leukemia?

Childhood acute myeloid leukemia (AML) is a cancer of the blood-forming tissue, primarily the bone marrow and lymph nodes. AML is also called acute nonlymphocytic leukemia or acute myelogenous leukemia, and is divided into several subtypes. It is less common than acute lymphocytic leukemia (also called acute lymphoblastic leukemia or ALL), another form of leukemia that occurs in children.

All types of blood cells are produced by the bone marrow. The bone marrow is the spongy tissue inside the large bones of the body. The bone marrow makes red blood cells (which carry oxygen and other materials to all tissues of the body), white blood cells (which fight infection), and platelets (which help make the blood clot).

The bone marrow controls the production of normal cells. In leukemia, the process breaks down and the bone marrow starts producing large numbers of abnormal cells of only one type of cell, usually one of the white cells. These abnormal, immature cells, called blasts, then flood the blood stream and lymph system, and may invade vital organs such as the brain, testes, ovaries, or skin. AML tumor cells

National Cancer Institute (NCI), PDQ database at http://cancernet.nci.nih.gov/pdq.htm, updated April 1998. The PDQ computer system gives up-to-date information on cancer and its prevention, detection, treatment, and supportive care for people with cancer and their families, and for doctors, nurses, and other health care professionals.

rarely can appear as a solid tumor (called an isolated granulocytic sarcoma or chloroma).

Leukemia can be acute (progressing quickly with many immature blasts) or chronic (progressing slowly with more mature-looking cancer cells). Acute myeloid leukemia progresses quickly, and can occur in both children and adults. Treatment is different for adults than it is for children. For information about the treatment of adult AML, see the chapter on adult acute myeloid leukemia. Separate PDQ information statements are also available for chronic lymphocytic leukemia, chronic myelogenous leukemia, adult and childhood acute lymphocytic leukemia, and hairy cell leukemia.

If your child has symptoms of leukemia, your child's doctor may order blood tests to count the number of each of the different kinds of blood cells. If the results of the blood tests are not normal, a bone marrow biopsy may be performed. During this test, a needle is inserted into a bone in the hip and a small amount of bone marrow is removed and examined under a microscope, enabling the doctor to determine what kind of leukemia your child has and plan the best treatment. Chromosomal analysis may also be performed.

Stage Explanation

Stages of Childhood Acute Myeloid Leukemia

There is no staging for acute myeloid leukemia (AML), since AML is always spread throughout the bloodstream. Treatment depends on whether or not the patient has been previously treated for leukemia.

Untreated

Untreated AML means no treatment has been given except to alleviate or the leukemia may appear as a tumor called a chloroma.

In Remission

Remission means that remission induction treatment has been given and that the number of white blood cells and other cells in the blood and bone marrow is approaching normal. There are no signs or symptoms of leukemia.

Recurrent/refractory

Recurrent means that the leukemia has come back (recurred) after going into remission. Refractory means that the leukemia failed to go into remission following treatment.

Treatment Option

How Childhood Acute Myeloid Leukemia Is Treated

There are treatments for all patients with childhood acute myeloid leukemia (AML). The primary treatment for AML is chemotherapy, sometimes followed by bone marrow transplantation. Radiation therapy may be used in certain cases. Biological therapy is also being studied in clinical trials.

Chemotherapy is the use of drugs to kill cancer cells. Chemotherapy drugs may be taken by mouth or injected into a vein (intravenous injection) or a muscle. Chemotherapy is called a systemic treatment because the drug enters the bloodstream, travels through the body, and can kill cancer cells throughout the body. Chemotherapy may sometimes be injected into the fluid that surrounds the brain and spinal cord (intrathecal chemotherapy).

Radiation therapy uses x-rays or other high-energy rays to kill cancer cells and shrink tumors. Radiation for AML usually comes from a machine outside the body (external radiation therapy).

Bone marrow transplantation, a newer type of treatment, is used to replace the patient's bone marrow with healthy bone marrow. First, high doses of chemotherapy with or without radiation therapy are given to destroy all of the bone marrow in the body. Healthy marrow is then taken from another person (a donor) whose tissue is the same as or almost the same as the patient's. The donor may be a twin (the best match), a brother or sister, or another person not related. The healthy marrow from the donor is given to the patient through a needle in a vein, and the healthy marrow replaces the marrow that was destroyed. A bone marrow transplant using marrow from a relative or person not related is called an allogeneic bone marrow transplant.

A newer type of bone marrow transplant, called autologous bone marrow transplant, is being studied in clinical trials. During this procedure, bone marrow is taken from the patient and may be treated with drugs to kill any cancer cells. The marrow is then frozen to save it. Next, the patient is given high-dose chemotherapy, with or without radiation therapy, to destroy all of the remaining marrow. The frozen marrow that was saved is then thawed and returned to the patient to replace the marrow that was destroyed.

Biological therapy attempts to stimulate or restore the ability of the patient's immune system to fight cancer. It uses substances produced by the patient's own body or made in a laboratory to boost, direct, or restore the body's natural defenses against disease. Biological therapy is sometimes called biological response modifier therapy or immunotherapy.

There are two or three phases of treatment for AML. The first phase, remission induction therapy, uses chemotherapy to kill as many of the leukemia cells as possible and cause the leukemia to go into remission. Once the leukemia goes into remission and there are no signs of leukemia, postremission therapy is given. The purpose of postremission therapy is to kill any remaining leukemia cells. Postremission therapy is divided into two phases, postremission consolidation and postremission intensification. Your child may receive either or both phases of postremission therapy.

As preventive therapy, your child may also receive central nervous system (CNS) prophylaxis, which consists of intrathecal and/or high-dose systemic chemotherapy to the central nervous system (CNS) to kill any leukemia cells present there, or to prevent the spread of cancer cells to the brain and spinal cord even if no cancer has been detected there. Radiation therapy to the brain may also be given, in addition to chemotherapy, for this purpose.

Unwanted effects can result from treatment long after it ends, so it is important that your child continue to be seen by his or her doctor. Chemotherapy can later lead to heart, kidney, and hearing problems. Radiation therapy may later lead to problems with growth and development, and with sight.

Treatment by Stage

Treatment for childhood AML depends on the type of leukemia. The best treatment is given by cancer doctors with experience in treating children with leukemia, and is given at hospitals where leukemia patients are often treated.

Your child may receive treatment that is considered standard based on its effectiveness in a number of patients in past studies, or you may choose to have your child take part in a clinical trial. Not all patients are cured with standard therapy, and some standard treatments may have more side effects than are desired. For these reasons, clinical trials are designed to test new treatments and to find better ways to treat cancer patients, and are based on the most up-to-date information. Clinical trials are ongoing in most parts of the country for most types of childhood AML. If you want more information, call the Cancer Information Service at 1-800-4-CANCER (1-800-422-6237); TTY at 1-800-332-8615.

Untreated Childhood Acute Myeloid Leukemia

Your child's treatment will probably be remission induction chemotherapy to kill cancer cells and cause the leukemia to go into remission. Induction chemotherapy is usually successful in inducing remission. Intrathecal chemotherapy with or without radiation therapy to the brain may be given to prevent the spread of cancer cells to the brain and spinal cord. Biological therapy may be added to treatment to help your child recover more quickly from the side effects of induction therapy.

Clinical trials are currently testing chemotherapy with or without bone marrow transplantation.

Childhood Acute Myeloid Leukemia in Remission

Treatment will consist of additional chemotherapy or bone marrow transplantation. Central nervous system prophylaxis and/or maintenance chemotherapy may also be given in some cases.

Clinical trials are currently testing bone marrow transplantation, as well as different chemotherapy treatments and ways to decrease resistance to chemotherapy drugs.

Recurrent Childhood Acute Myeloid Leukemia

Treatment depends on the type of treatment your child received before. You may want to consider entering your child into a clinical trial. Treatments currently being studied in clinical trials include new chemotherapy drugs, bone marrow transplantation, and biological therapy.

Unwanted side effects can result from treatment long after it ends, so it is important that your child continue to be seen by his or her doctor. Chemotherapy can later lead to heart problems, as well as kidney and hearing problems. Radiation therapy may interfere with a child's growth and may increase the risk of hormonal dysfunction and cataract formation.

To Learn More

To learn more about childhood acute myeloid leukemia, call the National Cancer Institute's Cancer Information Service at 1-800-4-CANCER (1-800-422-6237); TTY at 1-800-332-8615. By dialing this toll-free number, you can speak with someone who can answer your questions.

The Cancer Information Service can also send you booklets. The following booklets about leukemia may be helpful to you:

What You Need To Know About Leukemia
Research Report: Bone Marrow Transplantation

The following booklets on childhood cancer may also be helpful to you:

Young People with Cancer: A Handbook for Parents
Talking with Your Child About Cancer
When Someone in Your Family Has Cancer
Managing Your Child's Eating Problems During Cancer Treatment

The following general booklets related to questions on cancer may also be helpful:

What You Need To Know About Cancer
Taking Time: Support for People with Cancer and the People Who Care About Them
What Are Clinical Trials All About?
Chemotherapy and You: A Guide to Self-Help During Treatment
Radiation Therapy and You: A Guide to Self-Help During Treatment

There are many other places you can get material about cancer treatment and services to help you. You can check the social service office at your hospital for local and national agencies that help with your finances, getting to and from treatment, care at home, and dealing with your problems.

You can also write to the National Cancer Institute at this address:

National Cancer Institute
Office of Cancer Communications
31 Center Drive, MSC 2580
Bethesda, MD 20892-2580

If you want to know more about cancer and how it is treated, or if you wish to know about clinical trials for your type of cancer, you can call the NCI's Cancer Information Service at 1-800-422-6237, toll free. A trained information specialist can talk with you and answer your questions.

Chapter 22

Hairy Cell Leukemia

Description

What Is Hairy Cell Leukemia?

Hairy cell leukemia is a disease in which cancer (malignant) cells are found in the blood and bone marrow. The disease is called hairy cell leukemia because the cancer cells look "hairy" when examined under a microscope.

Hairy cell leukemia affects white blood cells called lymphocytes. Lymphocytes are made in the bone marrow and other organs. The bone marrow is the spongy tissue inside the large bones in the body. The bone marrow makes red blood cells (which carry oxygen and other materials to all tissues of the body), white blood cells (which fight infection), and platelets (which make the blood clot). Lymphocytes also are made in the spleen (an organ in the upper abdomen that makes lymphocytes and filters old blood cells from the blood), the lymph nodes (small bean-shaped organs throughout the body), and other organs.

When hairy cell leukemia develops, the leukemia cells may collect in the spleen, and the spleen swells. There also may be too few normal white blood cells in the blood because the leukemia cells invade

National Cancer Institute (NCI), PDQ database at http://cancernet.nci.nih.gov/pdq.htm, updated January 1998. The PDQ computer system gives up-to-date information on cancer and its prevention, detection, treatment, and supportive care for people with cancer and their families, and for doctors, nurses, and other health care professionals.

223

the bone marrow, and the marrow cannot produce enough normal white blood cells. This may result in an infection. A doctor should be seen if the following symptoms occur: constant tiredness, the spleen is larger than normal, or the development of an infection that won't go away.

If there are symptoms, a doctor will order blood tests to count the number of each of the different types of blood cells. If the results of the blood tests are not normal, more blood tests may have to be done. The doctor may also do a bone marrow biopsy. During this test, a needle is inserted into a bone and a small amount of bone marrow is taken out and looked at under the microscope. The doctor can then tell what kind of leukemia the patient has and plan the best treatment.

The chance of recovery (prognosis) depends on how many cancer cells are in the blood and bone marrow, and the patient's age and general health.

There are separate PDQ patient information summaries on acute lymphocytic leukemia (adult and childhood), acute myeloid leukemia (adult and childhood), chronic lymphocytic leukemia, and chronic myelogenous leukemia.

Stage Explanation

Stages of Hairy Cell Leukemia

There is no staging system for hairy cell leukemia. Patients are grouped together based on whether they have been treated for their leukemia or not.

Untreated Hairy Cell Leukemia

No treatment has been given for the leukemia. Treatment may have been given for infections or other side effects of the leukemia.

Progressive Hairy Cell Leukemia, Post-splenectomy

Surgery has been done to remove the spleen (splenectomy), but the leukemia is getting worse.

Refractory Hairy Cell Leukemia

The leukemia has been treated but no longer responds to the treatment.

Treatment Option Overview

How Hairy Cell Leukemia Is Treated

Some people with hairy cell leukemia have few symptoms and may not need treatment right away. There are treatments for all patients with hairy cell leukemia that is causing symptoms. Three kinds of treatment are used:

- surgery
- chemotherapy (using drugs to kill cancer cells)
- biological therapy (using the body's immune system to fight cancer)

Bone marrow transplants are being tested in clinical trials.

If the spleen is swollen, the doctor may take out the spleen in an operation called a splenectomy.

Chemotherapy uses drugs to kill cancer cells. Chemotherapy may be taken by pill, or it may be put into the body by a needle in the vein, muscle, or under the skin. Chemotherapy is called a systemic treatment because the drug enters the bloodstream, travels through the body, and can kill cancer cells throughout the body.

Biological therapy tries to get the body to fight the cancer. It uses materials made by the body or made in a laboratory to boost, direct, or restore the body's natural defenses against disease. Biological therapy is sometimes called biological response modifier (BRM) therapy or immunotherapy. Interferon, a substance made by the body to fight off foreign materials, is often used to treat hairy cell leukemia.

Bone marrow transplantation is used to replace the bone marrow with healthy bone marrow. First, all of the bone marrow in the body is destroyed with high doses of chemotherapy with or without radiation therapy. Healthy marrow is then taken from another person (a donor) whose tissue is the same as or almost the same as the patient's. The donor may be a twin (the best match), a brother or sister, or another unrelated person. The healthy marrow from the donor is given to the patient through a needle in the vein, and the marrow replaces the marrow that was destroyed. Bone marrow transplants using marrow from a relative or unrelated person is called an allogeneic bone marrow transplant.

Treatment by Stage

Standard treatment may be considered because of its effectiveness in patients in past studies, or participation in a clinical trial may be considered. Not all patients are cured with standard therapy and some standard treatments may have more side effects than are desired. For these reasons, clinical trials are designed to find better ways to treat cancer patients and are based on the most up-to-date information. Clinical trials are ongoing in most parts of the country for patients with hairy cell leukemia. To learn more about clinical trials, call the Cancer Information Service at 1-800-4-CANCER (1-800-422-6237); TTY at 1-800-332-8615.

Untreated Hairy Cell Leukemia

Treatment may be one of the following:

1. If there are no symptoms, treatment may not be needed. The doctor will follow the patient closely so treatment can be started if the leukemia gets worse.

2. Biological therapy.

3. Chemotherapy.

4. Surgery to remove the spleen (splenectomy).

Progressing Hairy Cell Leukemia, Initial Treatment

Treatment may be one of the following:

1. Chemotherapy. Clinical trials are testing new chemotherapy drugs.

2. Biological therapy.

3. Bone marrow transplantation in some cases.

4. Surgery to remove the spleen (splenectomy).

Refractory Hairy Cell Leukemia

If the patient has not responded to biological therapy, chemotherapy may be given. The patient may also wish to take part in a clinical trial of new chemotherapy drugs.

To Learn More

To learn more about hairy cell leukemia, call the National Cancer Institute's Cancer Information Service at 1-800-4-CANCER (1-800-

422-6237); TTY at 1-800-332-8615. By dialing this toll-free number, trained information specialists can answer your questions.

The Cancer Information Service also has booklets about cancer that are available to the public and can be sent on request. The following general booklets on questions related to cancer may be helpful:

What You Need To Know About Cancer
Taking Time: Support for People with Cancer and the People Who Care About Them
What Are Clinical Trials All About?
Chemotherapy and You: A Guide to Self-Help During Treatment
Radiation Therapy and You: A Guide to Self-Help During Treatment Eating Hints for Cancer Patients
Advanced Cancer: Living Each Day
When Cancer Recurs: Meeting the Challenge Again
Research Report: Bone Marrow Transplantation

There are many other places where people can get materials and information about cancer treatment and services. The social service office at a hospital can be checked for local and national agencies that help with getting information about finances, getting to and from treatment, getting care at home, and dealing with problems.

For more information from the National Cancer Institute, please write to this address:

National Cancer Institute
Office of Cancer Communications
31 Center Drive, MSC 2580
Bethesda, MD 20892-2580

If you want to know more about cancer and how it is treated, or if you wish to know about clinical trials for your type of cancer, you can call the NCI's Cancer Information Service at 1-800-422-6237, toll free. A trained information specialist can talk with you and answer your questions.

Part Four

Bleeding Disorders

Chapter 23

Hemophilia

Background

Hemophilia is the oldest known hereditary bleeding disorder. There are two types of hemophilia, A and B (Christmas Disease). Both are caused by low levels or complete absence of a blood protein essential for clotting. Patients with hemophilia A lack the blood clotting protein, factor VIII, and those with hemophilia B lack factor IX. There are about 20,000 hemophilia patients in the United States. Each year, about 400 babies are born with this disorder. Approximately 85% have hemophilia A and the remainder have hemophilia B. The severity of hemophilia is related to the amount of the clotting factor in the blood. About 70% of hemophilia A patients have less than one percent of the normal amount and, thus, have severe hemophilia. A small increase in the blood level of the clotting factor, up to five percent of normal, results in mild hemophilia with rare bleeding except after injuries or surgery. Enormous strides made in assuring the safety of the blood supply and in the genetic aspects of hemophilia research allow us now to focus on issues which will improve the quality of life of the hemophilia patient and, ultimately, develop a cure.

Information in this chapter was taken from "Hemophilia," National Heart, Lung, and Blood Institute (NHLBI) at http://www.nhlbi.nih.gov/nhlbi/glood/other/gp/hemophel.htm dated May 13, 1996 and "Hemophilia Update: 1997" NHLBI hemo-97.htm dated February 5, 1997.

Challenges

The most important challenges facing the hemophilia patient, health care provider, and research community today are:

1. Safety of products used for treatment;
2. Management of the disease including inhibitor formation, irreversible joint damage, and life-threatening hemorrhage; and
3. Progress toward a cure.

Safety of Products Used for Treatment

In the past 10 to 15 years, advances in screening of blood donors, laboratory testing of donated blood, and techniques to inactivate viruses in blood and blood products have remarkably increased the safety of blood products used to treat hemophilia. Although treatment-related infection with the AIDS virus or most of the hepatitis viruses is a thing of the past, these measures do not completely avoid viruses such as hepatitis A and parvovirus. These infections are rare; nevertheless, they can pose a threat. Researchers are working to improve procedures to destroy these viruses.

There is a great deal of concern about Creutzfeldt-Jakob disease (CJD), a rare transmissible nervous system disease that is inevitably fatal, being transmitted through transfusion. The infection of many hemophilia patients with the AIDS virus before the virus was discovered has elicited a great deal of concern in the hemophilia community about CJD and its potential transmission through blood-derived treatment products. A disorder related to CJD, bovine spongiforme encephalopathy or "mad cow disease," and its suspected relationship to an especially severe form of CJD, has generated considerable interest recently in Britain. No one has ever detected the transmission of CJD disease through blood or blood products, although a number of CJD victims have been blood donors, even within weeks of coming down with the disease. Collaborative studies are underway by the National Heart, Lung, and Blood Institute and the National Institute of Neurological Disorders and Stroke to determine, in experimental animals, if the CJD agent(s) can be transmitted by blood.

To ensure absolute safety from transfusion-transmitted viruses and other agents, hemophiliacs may now be treated with factor VIII which has been produced through biotechnology. This product, recombinant factor VIII, is manufactured by a process entirely free of blood products. It, thus, contains only the factor VIII necessary to treat the disease and none of the other components of blood or attendant unwanted agents. Although the cost of this product exceeds that of the blood-derived product, it is clearly the treatment of choice for those, such as newborns, who have not yet been exposed to blood products. A factor IX product has also been produced by such a process and is currently in clinical trials. Once this product is shown to be safe and effective, all hemophiliacs will have available a treatment for bleeding which is totally free of any contaminating agents.

Management of the Disease

While current treatment has greatly improved the outlook for most hemophiliacs, the development of antibodies (inhibitors) that block the activity of the clotting factors has complicated treatment for some patients. Approximately 15 percent of severe hemophilia A patients and 2.5 percent of hemophilia B patients develop such antibodies after exposure to transfused factors. When inhibitors are present in large amounts, the patient may require very high and expensive quantities of transfused clotting factors to stem bleeding, and, in some instances, even that may not be effective. The factor VIII products produced through biotechnology have been found to cause inhibitors in only about 5 percent of patients and are, thus, safer in this respect. Nevertheless, these inhibiting antibodies will remain a concern for hemophilia patients unless our ability to understand and control the immune system is improved. A number of NHLBI-supported scientists are directing research at this problem.

The major cause of disability in hemophilia patients is chronic joint disease—"arthropathy"—caused by uncontrolled bleeding into the joints. Life-threatening hemorrhage is a constant risk. Traditional treatment of hemophilia in the United States has involved "on-demand" treatment, meaning that patients are treated with factor replacement only after bleeding symptoms are recognized. These bleeds ultimately result in severely impaired joints. Several European countries are treating hemophiliacs by periodic infusion (prophylaxis) regardless of bleeding status. This approach maintains the factor level high enough that bleeding, joint destruction, and life-threatening hemorrhage are almost entirely avoided. There are, nevertheless, serious disadvantages such as the need for frequent infusions, the requirement for almost continuous access to veins by catheters, and the considerable cost of factor. In the United States, it is estimated that most patients on prophylaxis which is begun in the first few years of life will easily exceed the common life-time insurance cap of

$1,000,000 by the second decade of life. The treatment decisions are not easy ones.

Progress toward a Cure

Although treatment for hemophilia has become safer, therapeutic products are still not risk free. The ultimate goal is to offer a cure for the disease. Hemophilia is known to be caused by defects in the genes for factor VIII and factor IX. The challenge is to transfer normal genes into a patient so that they will produce the normal clotting protein. A small amount of active factor produced by the patient's own body will correct the disease. Although much remains to be studied before such treatment can be offered to patients, there have been a number of studies done in animals such as mice and dogs in which a factor VIII or IX gene has been inserted and has produced the proper blood product for periods that exceed one year. Major issues that remain to be resolved include the low level of production of the clotting factor, reduction of immune reactions that stop the production after a period, and development of ways to insert the gene directly into the body without manipulating cells outside the body. Until recently, dogs with naturally occurring hemophilia were used for testing of gene therapy techniques; however, the number of such animals is very limited. Recently, a mouse model of hemophilia produced through genetic technology was announced. The availability of this small animal will accelerate the development of technologies for ultimate use in humans.

Prospects

It is clear that tremendous progress has been made to reduce the exposure of hemophilia patients to transfusion-transmitted disease through making the blood supply safer and by providing replacement products from sources not involving blood. However, concern remains for hemophiliacs still dependent on blood products and the threat of agents which may contaminate the blood supply and are not avoided or inactivated with currently available techniques. It is also known from international studies that crippling joint involvement can be avoided through periodic and regular transfusion. The expense, danger of indwelling catheters, and inconvenience of the treatment regimen are all negative factors. All of these issues will become less important, even irrelevant, if the disease can be cured. At the present time, there are sufficient indications that gene therapy will ultimately be this cure. The technology for gene therapy is not as simple as was first thought. Yet because of its special characteristics, hemophilia will likely be among the first genetic diseases to be successfully treated.

Hemophilia Updated: 1997

Advances in treatment over the last three decades have permitted a near-normal lifestyle and life-span for many individuals with hemophilia. The introduction of factor VIII concentrate products in the 1970s allowed treatment at home and largely replaced the need for transfusion of whole blood or plasma in the hospital. An unfortunate result of increased freedom from bleeding as a cause of disability and death was infection with hepatitis from products made from pooled plasma. This culminated in the early 1980s with the unexpected and devastating infection of about 70% of severe hemophiliac patients with HIV, the cause of AIDS. Since then, the development and improvement of methods for inactivating viruses with lipid envelopes in plasma, including factor VIII and IX concentrates, has improved the safety of transfused products to the point where the threat of infection with HIV, hepatitis B (HBV) or hepatitis C (HCV) viruses has been essentially eliminated.

Safety of Products Used in Treatment

A number of major efforts focused at different levels in the production of replacement products for hemophiliacs have resulted in a substantially lower risk of transfusion-transmitted agents for the hemophilia community. Blood donors are carefully screened to eliminate those likely to have been exposed to hepatitis or HIV. In addition, the plasma used to prepare factor concentrates and factor concentrate products are tested for known bacterial and viral contaminants to eliminate transmission by transfusion. Finally, solvent/detergent and heat treatment processes are in use to inactivate viruses in plasma pools utilized in the preparation of clotting factors. As a result of these practices, millions of doses of coagulation factor concentrates have been infused since 1987 without a single documented case of HIV, HCV, or HBV. In further efforts, research supported by the National Heart, Lung, and Blood Institute (NHLBI) is underway to develop tests for HIV and hepatitis nucleic acids to replace the current antibody tests. Successful implementation will more than double safety of transfusion. The NHLBI is using still another approach to augment safety of transfused products, that is through the support of research to inactivate non-enveloped viruses such as parvovirus B-19 and hepatitis A virus that might contaminate plasma and plasma derivatives. These viruses are not inactivated by solvent/detergent treatment and tend to be heat stable. A recently developed photochemical treatment appears to be effective against viruses in this class. It is expected that this newer viral elimination procedure, in combination with established virucidal procedures, will further ensure the safety of coagulation factor concentrates.

Over the last few years, improved procedures have led to high purity plasma-derived factor VIII and factor IX products which appear to be safer when subjected to viral inactivation procedures than were the previous lower potency materials. "First generation" recombinant factor VIII, produced without human plasma, became available in 1992. This added a measure of safety especially from non-enveloped viruses, although the need for human albumen to stabilize the factor left a tiny and currently hypothetical risk of human infectious agent transmission. The first recombinant factor IX preparation is now in clinical trials. It is a "second generation" product which is manufactured and packaged without any human or animal plasma proteins. A similarly produced factor VIII concentrate is under development.

Although most individuals with hemophilia can use replacement products repeatedly without problems, about 20% develop neutralizing antibodies that make the product less effective. Antibody inhibitors are more likely to occur in individuals with severe hemophilia. At this time, it is not possible to predict who will develop the antibody inhibitors, but there is some evidence for genetic predisposition for an immune response. The treatment for people with inhibitors can be complex and expensive. Often more than one approach is tried before the bleeding is arrested. The decreased ability to control bleeding in the joints can lead to earlier development of arthritis. In some cases, immune tolerance can be induced which allows standard treatment to again be effective. Studies are being conducted to avoid or modify the immune response and to prepare recombinant factor VIII proteins with reduced antigenicity.

The Goal

The goal of having all hemophilia treatment products completely free of human blood products with no possibility of transmitting infectious agents from human donors has not yet been achieved. Despite the advances described above, approximately 60% of hemophilia treatment is still with blood-derived products. Therefore, vigilance in maintaining the safety of the blood supply remains critical. Current screening of donors, testing of donated blood and inactivating enveloped viruses have essentially removed the danger of transmitting HIV, HBV, and HCV by hemophilia treatment concentrates. There remains a small risk from non-enveloped viruses, such as hepatitis A and parvovirus, that escape current inactivation procedures. These infections are rarely transmitted by plasma products and generally result in self-limited relatively mild illnesses, unless the patient also has immune deficiency. There is now concern about Creutzfeldt-Jakob Disease (CJD), a rare nervous system disease. At this time the transmission of CJD through blood or blood products is theoretical although the possibility is being reevaluated by combined efforts of NIH, CDC, and FDA. Results from some critical studies should be available later this year. In the meantime, the FDA has made recommendations that plasma not be taken from donors at increased risk for developing CJD and that products made from pools that include plasma from one or more donors who developed CJD at some time after donating be quarantined and destroyed.

Future Directions

Gene therapy providing continuous production of the deficient clotting factor could be the next major advance in hemophilia treatment. Studies that explore different viral and non-viral gene transfer methods for the delivery of the factor VIII and factor IX gene continue. Efficient expression and secretion of biologically functional protein is critical to the development of effective gene therapy. Basic research studies are unraveling the complex mechanisms that control the production of modified genes which increase the expression levels and enhance biological activity of these coagulation factors. Significant progress has been made in obtaining, modifying and inserting hemophilia genes in animals. Mice with hemophilia, deficient in either the factor VIII or factor IX gene, which exhibit bleeding problems seen in the human deficiency are now available. These small animal models provide valuable tools for testing multiple gene therapy procedures more rapidly than in the larger animal models available previously. Important needs remain to increase the level and duration of gene expression in animals before these procedures are ready for human use.

Conclusion

In summary, the current high level of safety of the blood supply has resulted from many years of targeted efforts to eliminate transfusion-transmitted agents at various stages—from improved methods of donor selection, through products that are purer and have been subjected to better viral inactivation methods, and through the development and marketing of first and second generation recombinant products that are increasingly free of human plasma proteins. Continued vigilance is necessary to guard against the introduction of new agents into the blood supply. Despite improved factor replacement treatment, the morbidity and mortality of hemophilia from arthropathy and critical hemorrhage will continue unless a cure can be effected. The promise of gene therapy as that cure still exists although the transfer of results in small and large animals to man constitute formidable problems. The original goal of availability before the turn of the century may have been overly optimistic. Nevertheless, slow and careful progress continues to be made toward this critical goal.

Chapter 24

Hemophilia Treatments, Symptoms, and Complications

What Is Hemophilia?

More than 15,000 people in the US have hemophilia (either hemophilia A or hemophilia B). A person with hemophilia has a missing or low supply of one of the factors needed for normal blood clotting. Depending on the level of these factors in the blood, hemophilia may be mild, moderate, or severe. About 60% of persons with hemophilia are of the severe type. They are at risk for bleeding after dental work, surgery, and trauma. They also may suffer internal bleeding with no trauma or injury and without apparent cause. Repeated joint bleeds can lead to other health problems and disabilities, including chronic joint problems and loss of range of motion. About 15% of persons with hemophilia have moderate hemophilia. These people are at risk for bleeding after surgery or trauma, joint problems, and rarely, spontaneous bleeds. Twenty-five percent of people with hemophilia have mild hemophilia. Their disease may be so mild that it may go undetected until bleeding occurs after trauma or surgery.

The hemophilia gene is carried by females on one of their X chromosomes and may be passed to their male offspring. This is why hemophilia is called an X-linked genetic condition. Female carriers of hemophilia have one X chromosome with a working (normal) gene and one X chromosome with a nonworking (defective) gene. There is a 50%

chance the carrier will pass the hemophilia gene on to male offspring. In other words, there is a 50% chance that each of her male children will have hemophilia. There also is a 50% chance the carrier will pass the hemophilia gene on to her female offspring, meaning that there is a 50% chance each of her daughters win also be carriers.

In about a third of all cases there is no family history of the disease, and hemophilia occurs as the result of a new or spontaneous mutation. In such situations, the presence of the hemophilia gene may only become apparent when the mother is tested for carrier status after she gives birth to a son with hemophilia.

Any male who inherits the defective X chromosome has hemophilia. This is because males, unlike females, have only one X chromosome.

The Y chromosome is mainly involved in determining gender and does not contain genes for the production of clotting factors. Boys born to a father with hemophilia and a mother who is not a carrier will not have the disease. This is because boys get the X chromosome from their mother and Y chromosome from their father. However, all daughters born to men with hemophilia will inherit the fathers hemophilia gene. This is because they get one X chromosome from their mother and one X chromosome from their father. They thus will be carriers.

Some female carriers have no health problems or symptoms related to carrying the hemophilia gene. These women are known as asymptomatic carriers. However, other female carriers have low factor levels that are associated with bleeding problems. These symptomatic carriers may suffer excessive menstrual bleeding, bruising, nosebleeds, and bleeding after surgery, dental work, or childbirth. Stress, exercise, medicines, and changing hormone levels during menstruation and during and after pregnancy all may effect the bleeding patterns of symptomatic carriers. Female carriers who have excessive bleeding should be evaluated by a doctor skilled in treating bleeding disorders. Local hemophilia agencies can offer information about medical and other community resources.

History of Treatment

Each time internal bleeding occurs in a person with hemophilia, treatment with an infusion of a clotting factor may be required to replace the missing protein needed to form a blood clot. The infusion will stop the bleeding. However, because the infused clotting factor remains active for only a short time, serious bleeds may require repeated infusions to stop the bleeding. Many people with severe hemophilia use clotting factor on a regular basis to prevent or avoid bleeding episodes. This preventive use of factor is known as prophylaxis and is described in the section called "New Approaches to Treatment."

Until 1965, the only available treatment for hemophilia, other than using rest and ice, was whole blood or fresh-frozen plasma transfusions that could only be given in hospitals. These transfusions were only partly effective because the body cannot hold the large amounts of fluid needed to provide enough clotting factor to control bleeding fully. As a result of this insufficient treatment, joint damage in persons with severe hemophilia often was serious enough to require the use of wheelchairs or crutches at an early age.

In 1965, a medical breakthrough ended the need for high-volume whole plasma transfusions for persons with hemophilia A. At that time, Dr. Judith Graham Pool discovered cryoprecipitate, the factor-rich component of blood. Cryoprecipitate is the blood fraction containing concentrated factor VIII. Cryoprecipitate allowed for easier, more effective, and more efficient treatment because less fluid had to be transfused into the patient.

By the early 1970s, clotting factors VIII and IX became widely available in a new concentrated, freeze-dried form. This made it possible for people to self-infuse at home, work, and school. That meant fewer hospitalizations, more flexibility, and better opportunities for preventive treatment.

Since the late 1970s, much progress has been made in the treatment of hemophilia. Examples of these improvements include the availability of:

- new clotting factor products and drugs such as desmopressin acetate (also known as DDAVP, used to treat mild-to-moderate hemophilia A and von Willebrand disease)

- new, synthetic (not derived from plasma) clotting products that take advantage of recombinant technologies

- better screening methods to detect and remove viruses and other agents from factor concentrates and blood products

- improved surgical options

- advanced genetic testing methods

- medically supervised home-infusion therapy

- prophylactic treatment

New Approaches to Treatment

Prophylaxis

An important improvement in bleeding disorders treatment involves the use of clotting factor on a regular basis to prevent bleeds before they occur. The prophylactic (preventive) use of clotting factor offers a number of benefits to persons with bleeding disorders. Such use might help to reduce or prevent joint disease, lower the number of hospitalizations, reduce time lost from work or school, increase independence, and improve quality of life. Talk with your healthcare provider to find out more about prophylaxis in order to decide if this is the best treatment choice for you or your child.

Genetically Engineered Factor Products

Recombinant factors are products created through an advanced method called recombinant DNA technology. "Recombinant" has been "recombined" in the laboratory by breaking up and splicing together DNA from several different types of organisms. When producing clotting factor, this process, known as genetic engineering, does not use blood. Thus the risk of human blood-borne viruses and contaminants is avoided. This is why recombinant clotting factors are the safest factor products available today. Recombinant factor VIII was first approved by the U.S. Food and Drug Administration (FDA) in 1993. In early 1997, the FDA licensed a recombinant factor IX product.

Hemophilia Complications

HIV Infection

People who are treated with blood and blood products might be exposed to blood-borne viruses and contaminants. From the late 1970s to the mid-1980s, about half of all people with hemophilia became infected with HIV through blood products. Many of these persons have developed AIDS. The AIDS epidemic has placed great health, economic, ethical, and emotional burdens on affected families and the wider bleeding disorders community.

Since 1985, new viral screening and purification methods have made the blood supply safer than ever. HIV transmission by any factor VIII or IX product in the United States has not occurred since 1986 due to viral inactivation (viral killing) methods used to treat blood products. These include heat treatment, solvent-detergent cleansing, and monoclonal purification. These advances are described in more detail below.

Hepatitis

Hepatitis is an inflammation of the liver that occurs when the liver is injured or infected. It can range from an asymptomatic to a life-threatening condition. Symptoms may include fatigue, nausea, vomiting, muscle and joint aches, liver tenderness and enlargement, and weight loss.

Hepatitis can be caused by any substance that damages the liver, including alcohol, drugs, chemicals, or viruses, or a combination of any of these. Hepatitis caused by viruses is called viral hepatitis and can be transmitted through blood and blood products. There are six different viruses now known to cause hepatitis A, B, C, D, E, and G. Hepatitis A, B, and C account for almost 95% of all cases of viral hepatitis. The other strains are uncommon.

Today's factor products are much safer than those of the past, though there is still some risk of getting hepatitis from clotting factor. Screening methods to identify donors with hepatitis have become more sensitive, greatly lowering the chances of transmitting one of the hepatitis viruses. Also, new viral inactivation methods now are being used on clotting factor products that make them much safer to use. As of 1997, there have been no reports of hepatitis C transmission through clotting factor treated with these new processes. Hepatitis B and D also are killed by these methods. There is no known case of hepatitis E transmission through blood products. Small numbers of people with hemophilia have been exposed to hepatitis G, probably through blood products. Hepatitis A has been found in solvent detergent-treated clotting factor, in part because hepatitis A can resist the viral-killing methods now being used. Transmission of hepatitis A remains a risk for people with bleeding disorders who use plasma-derived products. However, hepatitis A may be prevented by immunization with a vaccine.

Today's blood safety measures, though highly advanced, are not perfect. Whole blood and blood components, including packed red blood cells, plasma, platelets, and cryoprecipitate, cannot be treated with current virus-killing methods. This is because these methods would damage or inactivate important blood components, making these blood products useless. According to recent figures, for each unit of blood the risk of getting hepatitis C is less than 1 in 1,000 while the risk of getting hepatitis B is 1 in 50,000. As a health precaution, it is advised that persons with bleeding disorders get vaccines against both hepatitis A and hepatitis B. They also should be tested for hepatitis C on a yearly basis. There is, however, no vaccine for hepatitis C.

Joint Problems

Joint and muscle bleeds are less common among persons with von Willebrand disease and mild hemophilia. However, such bleeds pose major problems for people with moderate and severe hemophilia. A frequent complication of hemophilia is joint damage or hemophilic arthropathy, which is the result of bleeding into joints. The most commonly affected joints are the knees, elbows, and ankles. Joint bleeds in persons with bleeding disorders lead to both chronic and acute pain, as well as joint degeneration, swelling, and loss of range of motion. Any joint in which repeated bleeds occur is known as a target joint.

For those who suffer from arthropathy, options to correct deformities or eliminate or reduce pain include tendon lengthening, total joint replacement, arthroscopy, fusion and other treatments. Elective surgery should involve not only a surgeon but a hematologist, orthopedist, and physical therapist expert in treating bleeding disorders. In addition, joint pain can often be reduced or eliminated with the right exercise routine. Recent studies suggest starting prophylaxis at an early age to help prevent joint damage associated with frequent bleeding.

Chapter 25

Establishing an Emergency Care Plan for People with Hemophilia

According to the American College of Emergency Physicians, there are approximately 5,500 emergency departments in the United States. Renee Paper, RN, an emergency nurse, says the best way for people with bleeding disorders to use these emergency departments is to, whenever possible, stay out of them. "Diabetics don't go the emergency department for the routine infusion of insulin," says Ms. Paper, "people with bleeding disorders should not go to the emergency department for the routine infusion of factor."

In addition to her nursing career, Ms. Paper is the Program Director of the Hemophilia Foundation of Nevada. Nevertheless, one of the last things she wants to see walking into her emergency department is a person with a bleeding disorder. "There are 20,000 people with hemophilia in the country," says Ms. Paper. "Some emergency departments may not see more than one person with hemophilia over the course of a year. They may not know how to treat people with bleeding disorders."

Emergency departments are not the place for the routine management of bleeding disorders. Some homecare companies and hemophilia treatment centers (HTCs) provide nurses for home infusions, which can be very useful for infants with bleeds and people with bad venous access. Nevertheless, there will always be times when people require emergency department visits, such as when physician assessment is

---

The National Hemophilia Foundation, *NHF Community Alert*, April/May 1996; reprinted with permission.

indicated or when a homecare nurse is not an option. "Emergency departments do not provide a therapeutic environment. If and when possible, treat your bleeding disorder at home," says Ms. Paper. "Isn't that what homecare is all about?"

What about trauma? Everyone with a bleeding disorder (and/or their parents) can remember or imagine emergency situations requiring immediate action. The stories abound: a baby falls off the changing table; a toddler gets hit by a car; a child steps on a nail; gets hit by ball; a finger gets slammed in a door.

What about spontaneous bleeds? Internal bleeding doesn't always accompany a trauma. A child starts to limp, complains of a sore and swollen elbow, a toddler refuses to walk. Spontaneous bleeds can be just as frightening as those caused by trauma and they also need to be treated.

Renee Paper is the author of the pamphlet, *The Art of Negotiation: Becoming an Empowered Consumer* (available through HANDI—the information service of the National Hemophilia Foundation); she encourages families to make plans before an acute bleed, either traumatic or spontaneous, occurs. Keep sufficient factor at home and, if possible, at the child's school. Be accessible to the child's school. Infuse immediately. In most cases, Ms. Paper believes hemophilia emergencies should first be treated at home. "The emergency department is the last resort,'" she says.

How else can a family outwit a crisis? There are several steps an educated consumer can take as part of a common sense approach to living with, and treating, a chronic disease. This approach will help put the family in charge of the disease, not the other way around.

Dr. Michael Coyne is the Assistant Director of the Department of Emergency Medicine at the Berkshire Medical Center in Massachusetts, and a member of the NHF Board of Directors. He says the first thing families must do is learn as much as they can about their children's bleeding disorders. HTCs and local chapters are excellent sources of literature about bleeding disorders. Information can also be obtained through HANDI—the information service of the National Hemophilia Foundation.

Dr. Coyne concurs with Ms. Paper: don't assume every doctor is knowledgeable about bleeding disorders. Advocate for your children and be prepared, if necessary, to educate their healthcare team.

According to Dr. Coyne, the bad news is that emergency department visits—particularly in the case of trauma—may be inevitable for families with bleeding disorders. But the good news is that the extended waits and inadequate care so often experienced by families with bleeding disorders—don't have to be.

Be Proactive

Dr. Coyne echoes Ms. Paper: anticipate emergencies before they strike. According to Dr. Coyne, a good place to start is at the local hospital. Because most urban areas have more than one hospital, families should determine with which facility they are most comfortable (proximity and staff may enter into this decision). Next, they should contact the emergency department's medical and nursing directors for a "pre-emergency" appointment.

There are several materials to bring along to the meeting with the emergency department directors. Medical articles about treatment may be very useful—remember, the hospital personnel may not be knowledgeable about bleeding disorders management. Dr. Coyne's article, "Avoiding Indecision and Hesitation with Hemophilia-Related Emergencies" from the journal *Emergency Medicine Reports* (available through HANDI—the information service of the National Hemophilia Foundation) provides a wealth of information, as does the chapter on "Emergency Care" in the *Hemophilia Nursing Handbook* (can be purchased through NHF). It may be necessary to explain that children can have bleeds even though they don't exhibit any outward signs of bleeding. It may also be necessary to discuss factor: what it is and how and when it is administered.

Getting Past the Triage Barrier

Everyone who comes into the emergency department is triaged, or prioritized, based on his or her medical condition. The triage nurse is the first person to assess the patient's condition. By educating emergency care providers about bleeding disorders before a crisis ensues, a family can help ensure a child with a bleeding disorders emergency won't have a protracted wait in the emergency department.

Physicians are accustomed to running tests before they prescribe treatment. Thus, it is very important to stress that when children with bleeding disorders are brought to the emergency department and, if there is any suspicion of an acute bleed, they should be given factor **before** any diagnostic tests are administered. In an emergency situation, time is a critical element. Dr. Coyne emphasizes when a person has an acute hemorrhage, it is inappropriate to delay treatment while waiting for diagnostic test results. If invasive tests or procedures, such as lumbar puncture or joint taps, are deemed necessary, pretreatment with factor can prevent the bleeding these tests may cause.

Other treatment aspects also should be discussed. Stress the importance of having a skilled phlebotomist infuse the factor. A child in an emergency situation, especially a child with a bleeding disorder, is not the patient on whom medical students and residents should learn intravenous techniques. Similarly, the smallest caliber needle, usually one with butterfly wings, should be used. Repeated, or botched, needle sticks can cause bruising around the vein and soft tissue hematomas—conditions that may further traumatize the child, create more bleeding, and make future attempts at intravenous access problematic.

In addition to providing medical literature about bleeding disorders, families may find it useful to bring a letter from the child's primary care physician confirming the bleeding disorder diagnosis and outlining basic management principles.

Dr. Coyne emphasizes emergency medical and nursing directors will generally welcome a pre-emergency visit and appreciate the opportunity to learn about bleeding disorders and their optimal management. Renee Paper puts it this way, "the more knowledge your providers have about your child's condition, the better they will be able to manage it."

If families don't feel comfortable approaching the local emergency department staff directly, they can recruit an ally. The child's primary care physician, nurse coordinator, or local HTC physician, can be invited to the meeting. These experts can help families establish a protocol for urgent triage and care of traumatic and spontaneous bleeds. If a protocol is in place before an emergency occurs, the chances for a positive outcome are enhanced.

Learning from the Past

Of course, not all visits to the emergency department are quick, relatively painless, and productive. Stories abound involving protracted waits, repeated sticks, and medical staff who didn't believe a bleed they couldn't see. Again, Dr. Coyne urges setting up a meeting with the emergency department director, this time to analyze what went wrong. Was an inexperienced phlebotomist assigned to the child? Had the child's hematologist or primary care physician been unavailable or not contacted? Was triage delayed? Was the diagnosis given insufficient consideration? Dr. Coyne emphasizes emergency staff want to do the right thing, and says, "every error or bad outcome needs to be evaluated so it won't happen again."

Traumatic and spontaneous bleeds may be an inevitable corollary to hemophilia and related bleeding disorders, but a bad experience at an emergency department doesn't have to be.

Chapter 26

Gene Therapy Research: Seeking a Cure for Hemophilia and Other Bleeding Disorders

Gene therapy, a long awaited cure for many diseases, is progressing at a slower pace than researchers had optimistically estimated ... but it is progressing.

In September 1990, the first federally approved gene therapy protocol was initiated for the treatment of adenosine deaminase deficiency, a rare immune disorder. Following approval of this treatment protocol, the mood within the medical community was upbeat, and pioneers of the fledgling gene therapy considered federal approval an "enthusiastic vote of confidence." Researchers for many other diseases, including liver failure, several forms of cancer, familial hypercholesterolemia, hemophilia, and other bleeding disorders, kept a close watch on the progress of adenosine deaminase deficiency treatment, while awaiting National Institutes of Health (NIH) and Food and Drug Administration (FDA) approval for initiation of more widespread gene therapy treatment protocols.

In the early 1990s, still coasting on the high tide of enthusiasm, Dr. Claude Lenfant, Director of the National Heart, Lung, and Blood Institute of NIH, addressed the bleeding disorders community and said, "The time may not be far off when genetic therapy for hemophilia becomes the accepted mode of treatment." Many people felt confident gene therapy would cure hemophilia, and this cure would be available before the end of the decade.

The National Hemophilia Foundation, *NHF Community Alert*, June 1996; reprinted with permission.

At that time, the call of "before the end of the decade" resonated with many members of the bleeding disorders community and continues to do so. However, with the decade now two thirds over, perhaps it is time to take stock of the state of gene therapy and re-evaluate its progress.

How Does It Work?

To date, gene therapy for bleeding disorders has been focused on factors IX and VIII. The theory behind hemophilia gene therapy is relatively straightforward. A healthy version of the defective factor VIII or IX gene (depending on which disease—hemophilia A or B—a person has) is inserted into a person with hemophilia. Once the healthy gene is inserted, it becomes part of the person's genetic make-up, enabling him or her to manufacture factor. If a successful gene transfer is made, it would cure hemophilia. However, as Drs. Helen Blau and Matthew Springer of Stanford University said in a recent *New England Journal of Medicine* article, "Although easily comprehended in principle, gene therapy is not so simple in practice."

Healthy genes are introduced, or delivered, into the target cells of the patient's body by way of a transporting medium or "vector" that brings the gene into targeted human cells. So far, the most successful vectors produced have been viruses.

In hemophilia research, two main viral vectors have been tried. The first group of vectors are retroviruses. Although the AIDS virus is also a retrovirus, it is not from the family of viruses modified for gene therapy. Scientifically altered, replication-deficient, recombinant retrovirus vectors have been shown to transport healthy genes to the cell's genome (the part that contains the DNA). The cells' DNA should become permanently altered for the life of the cell.

One problem with retrovirus vectors is that they are only capable of carrying genes into actively dividing cells, which are in limited number. Therefore, even when gene therapy is successful, factor levels may be very low. Current retroviral vector research is focused, in part, on trying to modify retrovirus vectors so they can carry the genes into nondividing cells.

A second type of vector under study is scientifically altered adenovirus vectors. Nonaltered adenoviruses are responsible for respiratory illnesses and conjunctivitis. The main advantage of adenovirus vectors is their ability to carry their gene load into nondividing cells. When adenovirus gene therapy is successful, initial factor levels can be high. However, the disadvantage of adenoviral gene transfer is the host experiences a complex immune response that ultimately results in a loss of gene expression.

Other viruses also are being investigated. One, the adeno-associated virus, may be useful for gene therapy. Its major advantage is its ability to integrate healthy genes at a specific site in the target cell's genome.

Does It Work?

Findings from the first experiments involving gene therapy in hemophilia were published in 1993 by Gerrard and colleagues. After inserting human factor IX genes into mice, the results were minimal (small quantities of human factor IX were detected in the mice's bloodstream for one week) yet encouraging and paved the way for the next wave of research: dogs.

In 1993, Dr. Mark Kay of the University of Washington and colleagues inserted healthy factor IX dog genes into hemophilic dogs using an adenovirus vector. After treatment, the dogs were able to make factor IX for more than five months. These results, which the researchers themselves called "complete albeit transient," were greeted with cautious optimism by the scientific community. An editorial in the journal *Science* (where the results were published) praised the results and then tempered the praise by stating, "Although it offers considerable promise, this method isn't ready for the clinic yet."

In that same year, a group of researchers in China reported they inserted cells containing healthy human factor IX genes into two brothers with hemophilia B. The transfer was accomplished via retroviral vector. According to the researchers (Lu and colleagues) only one of the boys responded to the treatment. His factor levels rose from 2.9% to 6.3%, and he no longer required factor treatment. It should be noted, however, that there have been no follow-up reports to substantiate this encouraging preliminary report.

The June 1996 issue of the journal *Blood* presents work from Connelly and colleagues showing encouraging developments in hemophilia A gene therapy. In this study, a single intravenous injection of an adenovirus vector containing a portion of the human factor XIII gene was injected into mice. This resulted in therapeutic factor levels detectable for more than five months.

Future Prospects

Most of the gene therapy research conducted in the United States is funded, in part, by NIH. A recent article in *Science* reported NIH spends approximately $200 million a year funding gene therapy research for a variety of diseases. Private industry, another major supporter of gene therapy research, spends more or less the same amount. So what does this $400 million a year have to show for itself?

A special NIH committee established to answer that question reported recently in *Science* that "clinical efficacy has not been *definitely* demonstrated at this time in any gene therapy protocol, despite anecdotal claims of successful therapy." The NIH committee pointed an accusatory finger at vectors, calling both adenoviral and retroviral vectors "inefficient." The news, however, is not all negative. The commiittee confirmed the value of clinical research and emphasized the necessity of improving the quality of basic gene therapy research. Furthermore, the NIH committee emphasized the current level of funding for this research is appropriate, and they identified hemophilia as one of the most "straightforward" applications of gene therapy. Previously, NHF paved the way for $10.4 million of NIH funds to be allocated to eight hemophilia gene therapy researchers.

With NIH taking a closer look at the research it funds and groups such as the bleeding disorders community expectantly anticipating the long-awaited announcement of a cure, the onus is on gene therapy researchers to continue improving the quality of research. Through its Judith Graham Pool Fellowships, NHF can help ensure that ongoing research, as well as the next generation of research, responds to the bleeding disorders community's needs in gene therapy and other areas. It is hoped that through appropriate funding and dedicated scientific commitment, the hemophilias and von Willebrand disease, along with the other gene-affected diseases, will ultimately be cured.

Chapter 27

Von Willebrand Disease

Facts about Von Willebrand Disease

Although less widely known than hemophilia, von Willebrand disease (vWD) is actually the most common inherited bleeding disorder. It affects women and men in equal numbers. People with vWD take longer to stop bleeding due to defects or deficiencies in a clotting factor called von Willebrand factor (vWF). In most cases, the problem arises from low levels of vWF in the bloodstream. In other cases, there may be enough vWF, but it does not work properly.

The abnormal gene in vWD is located on a chromosome called an autosomal chromosome or an autosome, rather than a sex-linked (X) chromosome. Therefore, both men and women may pass the vWD gene to their offspring. A parent with von Willebrand disease has a 50% chance of passing the disease onto each of his or her children, whether or not they are male or female. vWD also can be the result of a spontaneous, new genetic mutation in the child. Individuals whose vWD is the result of such a mutation also may pass the disease on to their children.

Not everyone who has vWD shows symptoms. For those who do, typical signs include nosebleeds, easy bruising, heavy menstrual flow, and excessive or unusual bleeding from the mouth or gums.

Sometimes bleeding is caused by injury. At other times there is no obvious cause. Gastrointestinal or urinary tract bleeding also may occur in persons with vWD. It is rare for persons with vWD to have joint or muscle bleeds.

In most cases, vWD is a mild disorder with few, if any, symptoms. This is why many people do not realize they may have this disease until another family member is diagnosed. Sometimes bleeding after a serious injury or surgery may suggest a clotting disorder is present. The type and severity of symptoms a person with vWD may have are related to the amount and quality of vWF in the blood. Persons with little or no vWF are likely to have more frequent and/or severe bleeding problems that require treatment than those with milder deficiencies of vWF.

Symptoms of vWD

Some typical vWD symptoms are recurrent nosebleeds, easy bruising, heavy menstrual flow, or excessive, unusual bleeding from the mouth or gums. Bleeding may not necessarily be caused by injury, that is, it may be spontaneous. On the other hand, many people with vWD may bleed heavily or for a long time after surgery or injury. Gastrointestinal or urinary tract bleeding may also be a problem. It is more rare for people with vWD to bleed into the joints or muscles, common sources of bleeding in people with hemophilia A and B (factor VIII and factor IX deficiencies). The type and severity of symptoms may vary among different family members affected by vWD. The type of vWD cannot change. This idea is an old misconception. A person's symptoms, however, may change throughout his/her life.

VWD is most commonly a mild disorder. It may be discovered or identified at any age and may be associated with few, if any, symptoms. Affected individuals may not be identified until another family member is diagnosed or until they have a serious injury or surgery. The kind and number of symptoms or problems a person with vWD has are related to the amount of von Willebrand factor (vWF) in his/her blood. If a person has little or no vWF, he/she is considered to be "severe," and is likely to have more frequent and/or severe bleeding problems. These could include frequent nosebleeds or heavy menstrual periods that require treatment to limit the bleeding. Individuals with severe vWD will need treatment before and after having any type of surgical procedure.

Treatments for vWD

People with von Willebrand disease now have a range of treatment choices depending on whether their illness is mild or severe. A drug sprayed into the nose, Stimate, is the newest form of treatment. Bleeding is usually controlled in individuals with mild von Willebrand disease by using this nasal spray to boost their own factor VIII and vWD levels. Persons with more severe vWD may require infusions of a von Willebrand factor-containing blood product such as Humate P.

vWD: Issues and Complications

Living with von Willebrand Disease

With the current knowledge of vWD and by taking advantage of the treatments, care and services available through the hemophilia treatment center (HTC), physician, and hemophilia chapter a person can live a healthy, normal life. The process of coming to terms with the diagnosis of vWD, like any chronic illness, is different for each person. For many, it involves fears and losses, as well as mastery and gains. Talking with others—friends, health-care professionals, and other people with vWD—can help a person sort out feelings and reactions, and find support.

vWD and Physical Activity

It is important that people with vWD engage in regular exercise and physical activity to keep their joints and muscles strong and their health good. Being in good physical condition can actually reduce the number of bleeding problems a person experiences. It is often recommended that people diagnosed with vWD avoid physical activities that might cause severe bruising, such as contact sports, or those with high accident rates, such as skiing. Such activities, however, may be safe for people with mild vWD. A physician can make recommendations based upon his/her evaluation of the severity and type of vWD.

Risks of HIV/AIDS and Hepatitis

Anyone who used blood products (such as clotting concentrates or cryoprecipitate) prior to 1985 is at risk for HIV infection. In late 1984, the NHF urged the use of heat treated factor for all patients. Since 1985, products like Humate P have been specially treated and are free of HIV. Read the NHF publications, *HIV Disease in People With Hemophilia: Your Questions Answered, The Basics of HIV Disease: Questions and Answers,* and *What Women Should Know: HIV Infection, AIDS, and Hemophilia* for more information about getting an HIV test. Individuals should discuss their blood product history with their doctor.

People with vWD should be tested for Hepatitis B and vaccinated if blood tests show no evidence of previous exposure or infection. While a vaccine is not available for Hepatitis C, a physician will probably order a blood test to look for evidence of this illness, and if present, monitor liver function.

Issues for Women with vWD

It is very likely that the menstrual flow in a woman with vWD will be heavier and last longer than that of other women. Because of this heavier flow, a woman may tend to become anemic (not enough iron in the red blood cells). It is important that a woman with vWD be checked regularly for anemia. A doctor may prescribe birth control pills in an effort to control menstrual bleeding. The hormones in these pills cause an increase in vWF and factor VIII levels.

Pregnancy and childbirth can be handled successfully. The woman with vWD should see an obstetrician as soon as she suspects she is pregnant. The obstetrician can work with the HTC in providing the best prenatal care for the woman and her baby.

Delivering a baby at term should not be a problem for the woman with vWD. This is because over the nine months of pregnancy, every woman's vWF, including Factor VIII and von Willebrand factor, increases. For the woman with vWD, this means better protection from a bleeding problem at the time of delivery. However, after delivery, these clotting factor levels decrease, and women with vWD may develop post-partum (after-delivery) bleeding. If this occurs, it can be successfully treated with DDAVP or Humate P.

If a woman with von Willebrand Disease has a miscarriage or abortion early in pregnancy, before the natural increase in clotting factors occurs, she might have bleeding problems. If a woman with vWD thinks or knows she is miscarrying, or is choosing to terminate her pregnancy, she should seek immediate vWD treatment. Rarely, women with severe or moderately severe vWD may require a hysterectomy (surgical removal of the uterus) to control serious uterine bleeding that does not respond to other treatments.

It should be noted that some women with type IIA or IIB vWD may not experience an increase in clotting factor during pregnancy, thus, knowing the type of vWD is important.

Children in families with a known history of vWD should be checked to see if they have a bleeding problem. The hemophilia treatment center can order the appropriate diagnostic tests.

Newborn Testing

Since stress may elevate vWD levels, testing newborns for vWD may be difficult unless they have a type II variant. If tests are abnormally elevated, repeat testing in several days may be necessary to rule out the presence of vWD.

Chapter 28

Factor VII and Factor XI Deficiencies

Factor VII Deficiency

What Is It?

This factor deficiency has had several names, including proconvertin and serum prothrombin conversion accelerator (SPCA) deficiency. Often, people with factor VII deficiency are diagnosed as newborns because of bleeding into the brain as a result of birth trauma. The incidence of factor VII deficiency is 1 in 500,000.

Women with factor VII deficiency can experience heavy menstrual bleeding, spontaneous nosebleeds, gum bleeding, bleeding from injuries in small blood vessels, or bleeding deep within the skin, as well as bleeding into the stomach, intestine, and urinary tract. They also may experience bleeding into joints. Bleeding severity after an injury or surgery can vary greatly for people with factor VII deficiency.

Treatment Options

To date, factor VII concentrate is sold only in Europe. Because this product is not yet licensed for use in the United States it can be obtained in this country only with special permission. Other treatment choices are prothrombin complex concentrates that contain adequate

---

©1997[?] The National Hemophilia Foundation, 116 W. 32nd Steet, New York, NY 10001 (212) 328-3755; reprinted with permission. Visit the National Hemophilia Foundation on-line at www.hemophilia.org.

levels of factor VII. Recombinant factor VIIa, an activated form, is currently available only for experimental use.

Factor XI Deficiency (Hemophilia C)

What Is It?

After von Willebrand disease, this is the most common bleeding disorder affecting females. The incidence of factor XI deficiency is 1 in 100,000, though it occurs more frequently among members of some ethnic groups. Its incidence is about 1 in 10,000 among Ashkenazi Jews. There are at least three different known genetic changes associated with factor XI deficiency; these vary in their effect on bleeding. Your doctor can explain exactly what type of factor XI deficiency you have and how this will affect your care and treatment.

Factor XI deficiency is usually diagnosed after injury-related bleeding, and symptoms tend to be mild. Nearly 50% of people with factor XI deficiency report no bleeding problems.

Individuals with factor XI deficiency may experience bruising, nosebleeds, or blood in their urine. Some women have prolonged bleeding after childbirth. Spontaneous bleeding is uncommon, even in people with severe factor XI deficiency. Joint bleeding is uncommon, but delayed bleeding (bleeding long after an injury has occurred) can be a problem.

Treatment Options

No commercial concentrate of factor XI is available in the United States. Accordingly, the treatment of choice for factor XI deficiency is plasma.

Chapter 29

Thrombocytopenia

Thrombocytopenia is a condition in which the number of platelets found in the blood is abnormally low. Platelets, also called thrombocytes, are the blood cells that help stop bleeding. A person with this condition bleeds longer than is normal.

Platelets are made in the bone marrow and then released into the bloodstream, where they normally circulate for about 10 days. The normal, average platelet count in human blood is 300,000 per microliter. If the platelet count is less than 100,000 per microliter of blood, a diagnosis of thrombocytopenia is made.

Thrombocytopenia has various causes: it can result from decreased platelet production or increased platelet destruction. The spleen normally destroys old red blood cells but can become overactive and attack platelets, too.

Conditions that cause thrombocytopenia are usually acquired rather than inherited. Thrombocytopenia affects children and adults of both sexes. Treatment for thrombocytopenia is based on the type and cause.

Types

There are two types of thrombocytopenia—idiopathic and secondary.

An unnumbered, undated fact sheet produced by the National Heart, Lung, and Blood Institute (NHLBI) Information Center, P. O. Box 30105, Bethesda, MD 20824-0105. (301) 251-1222. Fax (301) 251-1223.

In **idiopathic thrombocytopenia**, the cause of the condition is not known. The most common idiopathic form is called idiopathic thrombocytopenic purpura (ITP). There are two forms of ITP—acute and chronic. Acute ITP occurs most often in childhood and affects girls and boys equally. It is most common in children 2 to 6 years old. Most cases occur after an upper respiratory or viral infection. Acute ITP is rare in adults.

ITP that lasts longer than 6 months is called chronic. People of any age can develop chronic ITP, but it is most frequently seen in adults age 20 to 40. Women are affected about three times more often than men. Patients with chronic ITP tend to go back and forth between remission and relapse over long periods. During remission, the symptoms go away; they return again when the chronic ITP relapses, or returns.

Secondary thrombocytopenia is caused by an underlying disease or other factor that decreases platelet production or leads to destruction of platelets. Some of these causes are:

- some medications—most commonly estrogens, quinidine, quinine, heparin, thiazides, and gold compounds;

- large amounts of alcohol consumed quickly ("binge drinking");

- bacterial infections, such as septicemia (also called blood poisoning, produced by the spread of bacteria or their toxins);

- viral infections, such as human immunodeficiency virus (HIV);

- immune disorders, such as systemic lupus erythematosus (SLE) and rheumatoid arthritis;

- blood diseases, including aplastic anemia, megaloblastic anemia, and preleukemic syndromes;

- malignant diseases, including such cancers as leukemia, lymphoma, and myeloproliferative disorders; and

- radiation therapy and chemotherapy given to treat many cancers.

Severe thrombocytopenia also occurs with other disorders, such as thrombotic thrombocytopenic purpura (TTP) and hemolytic uremic syndrome (HUS). In these life-threatening disorders, loose strands of fibrin (an insoluble protein formed when blood clots) are deposited in blood vessels. This uses up platelets and harms red blood cells.

TTP often affects more than one organ and is almost always fatal if not treated. HUS usually affects the kidneys, and fibrin clots in the vessels of other organs are rare. HUS tends to occur in young children, pregnant women, or women who have recently given birth. In children, HUS usually occurs after an infection, such as an episode of diarrhea caused by the bacterium, *E. coli*. Sometimes, HUS occurs in older children, as well as in women who take oral contraceptives.

Thrombocytopenia also is caused by rare hereditary disorders. These include Wiskott-Aldrich syndrome, Bernard-Soulier syndrome, May-Hegglin anomaly, and thrombocytopenia-absent radius syndrome (TAR).

Signs and Symptoms

The symptoms of thrombocytopenia are similar, regardless of its cause. These symptoms include easy or too much bruising (ecchymosis); purple patches on the skin and mucous membranes (purpura); a red, dot-like rash (petechiae) usually on the lower legs; nosebleeds; blood in vomit or stools; or a very heavy menstrual flow.

Sometimes, abnormal bleeding occurs during surgery, dental work, or trauma. Bleeding caused by thrombocytopenia is usually brief and light to moderate in amount. By contrast, bleeding from disorders due to defective clotting tends to last a long time and to be moderate to heavy in amount. In thrombocytopenia, life-threatening symptoms, such as a hemorrhage (too much bleeding) in the brain or digestive tract, are rare. In neonatal thrombocytopenia, intracranial bleeding may lead to mental retardation or death.

Diagnosis

The doctor diagnoses thrombocytopenia by taking a thorough medical history, performing a physical examination, and testing blood samples. The doctor will ask about any drugs that are being taken because medications are a very common cause of thrombocytopenia. A platelet count is taken from the blood sample—this measures the number of platelets in the blood. Normal laboratory values for a platelet count are 150,000 to 450,000 per microliter. A platelet count below 100,000 per microliter indicates thrombocytopenia.

The next step after identifying the thrombocytopenia is to find the cause. This is done by more blood tests—among these are evaluations of bleeding time, prothrombin time (PT), partial thromboplastin time (PTT), clot retraction time, and fibrinogen level.

The doctor also will look for other symptoms. For example, the doctor will check for fever or joint aches, which may indicate that thrombocytopenia is caused by an immune disorder such as SLE or an infection.

Sometimes, an aspiration and biopsy is done. In this procedure, a needle is used to remove a small amount of marrow from the bone. The marrow is then examined in the laboratory to make sure it contains normal platelet-forming cells and does not show signs of metastatic cancer that has spread to the bone marrow or leukemia, which is a cancer of the blood cells themselves.

Treatment

The treatment and prognosis of thrombocytopenia depend on the condition's cause and the number of platelets in the blood.

Sometimes, no treatment is needed—the platelet count goes back to normal. Children with acute ITP usually recover without treatment in 3 to 6 months. Ten to 15 percent of adults also recover from ITP on their own.

However, adults with very low platelet counts (fewer than 30,000 platelets per microliter of blood) usually need some treatment. The first step is often steroid therapy. Pills of the drug prednisone are taken. The pills are taken for at least 2 weeks and as long as 3 months. This therapy alone cures about 25 percent of adults with ITP.

If the condition persists, then the spleen may need to be removed. The surgery is called a splenectomy. It is effective for most patients.

However, if the platelet count is still very low, more medications may be given. These drugs will suppress the immune system and include intravenous vincristine, intravenous gamma globulin, and danaxol pills.

Sometimes a doctor tells a patient with chronic thrombocytopenia to take special measures to avoid harming their platelet function. These measures may include not taking certain drugs and being careful not to be injured. The drugs are those that affect platelet function, such as aspirin, penicillin, and tricyclic antidepressants. The prevention of injuries can include wearing helmets and protective padding when exercising and not playing contact sports, such as football and basketball.

Occasionally, transfusions of platelets are given. The transfusion has concentrated platelets in a plasma base. Plasma makes up about 55 percent of blood and is a yellowish fluid that contains blood-clotting factors, antibodies, and minerals. The transfusions control or prevent bleeding by temporarily increasing the number of platelets in the blood and help only in certain situations, such as with internal bleeding or to prepare for surgery. People with ITP rarely need such transfusions.

In secondary thrombocytopenia, the condition causing the low platelet count must be treated. The following are some examples:

- *Medications or alcohol.* The medication or alcohol is stopped, and usually the platelet count quickly returns to normal. Sometimes steroid treatment is needed when the condition has been caused by gold compounds.

- *Infections.* The infection is cured, and the platelet count returns to normal. With HIV-infected patients, the drugs used to cure the infection may also worsen immune system function. So infections in those with HIV are usually left untreated, unless the platelet count falls below 30,000 per microliter.

- *Immune disorders such as SLE.* The immune disease is treated along with the thrombocytopenia.

- *Blood or malignant diseases.* The treatment and prognosis depend on the underlying disease.

- *Radiation and chemotherapy treatments for cancer.* The platelet count usually returns to normal after these treatments are over. Occasionally, platelet transfusions are needed as the patient is being treated. The prognosis depends on the cancer.

For thrombotic thrombocytopenic purpura (TTP), treatment can involve steroid therapy, plasma exchange, aspirin, and other drugs. About 70 percent of patients recover, but 10 percent of them get sick again.

Treatment for hemolytic uremic syndrome can include transfusion, kidney dialysis, steroids, and heparin. (Dialysis is a procedure that removes waste products from the blood, usually by a machine.) Eighty to 95 percent of children with HUS need a form of supportive therapy, such as dialysis, which is followed by their spontaneous recovery. The treatment does not work well for adults, and the death rate from HUS is much higher for adults than children.

Treatments for hereditary thrombocytopenia vary. May-Hegglin anomaly and Bernard-Soulier syndrome are sometimes treated with platelet transfusions during surgery or trauma, particularly if there is excess bleeding. Wiskott-Aldrich syndrome is treated by removing the spleen. With thrombocytopenia-absent radius syndrome, infants who survive their first year have a good prognosis and will need no further treatment. Steroids do not help with these forms.

The protein that controls the production of platelets from cells in the bone marrow has recently been isolated. Results of preclinical testing appear promising, and it should be valuable in the treatment of thrombocytopenia when available for clinical use.

Seeking Help

Many types of thrombocytopenia can be treated by an internist or family doctor. However, sometimes a blood specialist (hematologist) is consulted as well. Hematologists are doctors who have received extra training in blood diseases. These doctors can be found in most cities. Most medical centers have hematology divisions in their medicine departments, and patients who need evaluation, treatment, or information often can be referred to a hematologist by their regular doctor.

For More Information

More information on specific forms of thrombocytopenia or related conditions is available from the following organizations.

Leukemia, lymphoma, myeloproliferative disorders, and radiation or chemotherapy treatment for cancer:

National Cancer Institute
(800) 4-CANCER

Rare forms of thrombocytopenia:

National Organization for Rare Disorders
P.O. Box 8923
New Fairfield, CT 06812
(203) 746-6518

Thrombocytopenia-absent radius syndrome:

Thrombocytopenia-Absent Radius Syndrome Association (TARSA)
312 Sherwood Drive
R.D. #1
Linwood, NJ 08221
(609) 927-0418

Idiopathic thrombocytopenic purpura and hemolytic uremic syndrome:

American Autoimmune-Related Diseases Association
15475 Gratiot Avenue
Detroit, MI 48205
(313) 371-8600

National Heart, Lung, and Blood Institute

This information in this chapter was provided as a public service of the National Heart, Lung, and Blood Institute (NHLBI). The NHLBI supports and conducts research related to the causes, prevention, diagnosis, and treatment of heart, vascular, lung, and blood diseases. This information is not meant to substitute for individual medical diagnosis or treatment. Only a physician, with knowledge of the patient's current condition and medical history, can provide appropriate advice. For recorded information on heart health call: 1-800-575-WELL.

Part Five

Circulatory Disorders

Chapter 30

Thrombophlebitis

Thrombosis is the formation of a blood clot that partly or completely blocks a blood vessel. Phlebitis is the inflammation of a vein usually caused by infection or injury. This inflammation can cause the blood flow through the veins to be bumpy and disturbed. Thrombophlebitis occurs when a vein becomes obstructed with a blood clot and inflamed.

Symptoms

The symptoms of thrombophlebitis are pain, redness, tenderness, itching, a hard cordlike swelling along the length of the affected vein, and sometimes (if infection is present) fever.

If a portion of a thrombus breaks away and travels to the lungs, it is called a pulmonary embolism. A person with a pulmonary embolism may experience chest pain, shortness of breath, cough, blood-streaked sputum, loss of consciousness, or sudden death. Quick diagnosis is the key to reducing negative consequences of a pulmonary embolism.

Causes

Thrombophlebitis is a response to either infection or injury. Many conditions can make a person more likely to develop thrombophlebitis,

---

An undated fact sheet produced by the National Heart, Lung, and Blood Institute.

including the use of oral contraceptives, long periods of immobility or confinement, varicose veins, heart attack, hip fracture, cancer, and obesity. Rarely, medical procedures involving the piercing of a vein with tubes or needles can cause irritation leading to phlebitis. Women also tend to be slightly more susceptible than men to developing thrombophlebitis.

Diagnosis

Diagnosis of thrombophlebitis is different for veins close to the skin's surface (surface thrombus) than for veins buried deep within the body (deep vein thrombus).

Diagnosis of a surface thrombus is based on symptoms, including pain, rash, and swelling. Diagnosis of a deep vein thrombus is more difficult, often using a Doppler ultrasound blood flow detector test that employs sound waves to provide a picture of blood flow changes or a radionuclide venography test (a special X-ray using injected dye) if the patient also is being scanned for a pulmonary embolism.

If these tests are inconclusive, contrast venography is used for diagnosis. This procedure involves a variation of an X-ray that visualizes blood clots obstructing blood flow if they are present. This test is expensive, time-consuming, and painful; therefore, it is only used when other tests are inconclusive.

Treatment

The type of treatment used to cure thrombophlebitis depends on the location, severity, and cause of the blood clot.

If thrombophlebitis occurs with an infection, then the infection usually will be treated first using antibiotics. An untreated infection could result in blood poisoning. If infection is not present, then thrombophlebitis usually resolves on its own within a week and treatment will be aimed at reducing any pain. Aspirin or other anti-inflammatory medications are often used. Zinc oxide ointment can be used to reduce itching.

All patients with thrombophlebitis are advised to rest, elevate the affected area, apply hot compresses, and wrap the affected area with an elastic bandage. However, care must be used in wrapping the extremity with uniform tightness so as not to have an area of undue restriction that could exacerbate the present thrombophlebitis or, worse, create a new area of thrombophlebitis.

Serious complications in persons with thrombophlebitis in the veins just under the skin are rare. If a thrombus occurs in a deep vein, the valves of the veins may be damaged, leading to swelling of the legs. This results from blood leaking back through the valve into the lower legs.

In either a surface thrombus or a deep vein thrombus, there is a possibility of a portion of the blood clot breaking loose, traveling through the bloodstream, and getting stuck in the lungs causing a pulmonary embolism.

A deep vein thrombus is usually treated in the hospital. Blood thinners are administered through an intravenous tube. If blood thinners are not successful in breaking down the thrombus, a small filter can be inserted with a catheter or by surgery into the vein that carries blood back to the heart (the inferior vena cave). This filter prevents the thrombus from traveling to the lungs.

Treatment of a pulmonary embolism may include a blood-thinning or clot-dissolving medication or surgical removal of the clot.

Seeking Help

The sooner thrombophlebitis is treated, the better. People who have any abnormal symptoms, especially infection or injury, should see a doctor immediately.

Chapter 31

Buerger's Disease (Thromboangiitis Obliterans)

Abstract

Thromboangiitis obliterans (Buerger's disease) is an inflammatory obliterative, nonatherosclerotic, vascular disease that affects the small- and medium-sized arteries, veins, and nerves. It is causally related to tobacco use, although the exact mechanism is unknown. Its clinical presentation is manifested by distal arterial ischemia and superficial thrombophlebitis. Thromboangiitis obliterans usually becomes quiescent if the patient is able to stop smoking cigarettes. However, if smoking continues, amputation commonly results.

Introduction

Thromboangiitis obliterans (Buerger's disease) is an inflammatory obliterative, nonatherosclerotic vascular disease that most commonly affects the small- and medium-sized arteries, veins, and nerves. In the acute phase, a highly inflammatory thrombus forms, and although there is some inflammation in the blood vessel wall itself, the inflammatory changes are not nearly as prominent as in other forms of vasculitis. Although thromboangiitis obliterans is a form of vasculitis it is rarely discussed in writings about vasculitis. In the American College of Rheumatology 1990 criteria for the classification of vasculitis, thromboangiitis obliterans is not discussed at all [1]. It is not clear

"Thromboangiitis obliterans," *Current Opinion in Rheumatology* 1994, 6:44-49, ©1994 Current Science; reprinted with permission.

whether this is because thromboangiitis obliterans is so uncommon or because of the failure to recognize thromboangiitis obliterans as a true form of vasculitis. Also, in a recent review of immunologic aspects of cardiovascular disease, thromboangiitis obliterans is not discussed, whereas most other forms of vasculitis are discussed in detail [2].

Thromboangiitis obliterans was first described by von Winiwarter in 1879 [3]. In 1908, Buerger provided a detailed and accurate description of the pathology of thromboangiitis obliterans in 11 amputated limbs [4]. Thromboangiitis obliterans is usually considered a disease of predominantly male, heavy cigarette smokers. Recently, the clinical spectrum of thromboangiitis obliterans has changed [5].

The exact incidence of thromboangiitis obliterans is not known. It varies in different geographic regions and appears to be highest in populations that have the largest percentage of cigarette smokers. In a report from the Mayo Clinic [6], a progressive decline was noted in the clinical diagnosis of thromboangiitis obliterans from 1947 to 1986. In 1947, there were 121 cases per 116,232 registrants (0.1%) compared with 28 cases per 221,000 registrants (0.01%) in 1986. The reason for this 10-fold decline may be the application of more strict criteria for the diagnosis of thromboangiitis obliterans or a progressive decline in the percentage of individuals who smoke cigarettes in the United States, or both. Other societies such as Japan, Eastern Europe, southeastern Asia, India, and Israel have not shown a similar decline in incidence of thromboangiitis obliterans [7,8].

Etiology

The exact etiology of thromboangiitis obliterans is unknown. Pathologically, thromboangiitis obliterans is a vasculitis [9]. There is an extremely strong association with tobacco use, suggesting that many of the patients who develop thromboangiitis obliterans may be allergic to tobacco. In India, most individuals who develop thromboangiitis obliterans are of poor socioeconomic status and smoke bidis (homemade cigarettes with raw tobacco); this may account for the higher incidence of thromboangiitis obliterans in the Indian population. Some investigators have suggested purified tobacco glycoprotein as a cause of increased vascular reactivity in cigarette smokers. Papa and Adar [10] and Papa *et al.* [11] studied 13 patients with definite thromboangiitis obliterans for cellular and humoral sensitivity to tobacco glycoprotein. They compared the patients with smokers and nonsmokers without thromboangiitis obliterans and found no difference in the humoral response. Patients with thromboangiitis obliterans and healthy smokers had the same cellular response to tobacco glycoprotein antigen, whereas nonsmokers did not respond at all. Therefore, these investigators as well as others believe that although tobacco use may be an important etiologic factor in patients who develop thromboangiitis obliterans, it is not the only factor. There may be other important etiologic factors in the pathogenesis of thromboangiitis obliterans.

The results of several studies suggest that there may be a genetic predisposition to the development of thromboangiitis obliterans. Considerable differences were found in the HLA haplotypes among different populations. In the United Kingdom, McLaughlin et al. [12] showed a preponderance of HLA-A9 and HLA-B5 antigen, whereas other HLA haplotypes were noted to be increased in thromboangiitis obliterans patients from Japan, Austria, and Israel [10].

Other investigators have suggested that autoimmune mechanisms may be important in thromboangiitis obliterans. Adar et al. [13] demonstrated that patients with thromboangiitis obliterans exhibit increased cellular sensitivity to types I and III collagen, which are constituents of human arteries. They also detected significant levels of anticollagen antibodies in thromboangiitis obliterans patients [11].

It was suggested in a recent report that there is no difference in the fibrinolytic system between patients suffering from Buerger's disease and control patients [14]. However, in Buerger's disease, the level of urokinase-plasminogen activator was twofold higher, and free plasminogen activator inhibitor 1 was 40% lower in patients with thromboangiitis obliterans compared with healthy volunteers. After venous occlusions, although tissue plasminogen activator antigen increased in both groups, increases were much more pronounced in the control patients. The authors suggest that in Buerger's disease, there is endothelial derangement that could be characterized by increased urokinase-plasminogen activator release and decreased plasminogen activator inhibitor 1 release.

Increased levels of antiphospholipid antibodies in a pregnant patient with Buerger's disease have been described [15]. However, it is possible that this patient did not have thromboangiitis obliterans because both thromboangiitis obliterans and antiphospholipid antibody syndrome can cause similar signs, symptoms, and arteriographic appearances.

There is no clear etiologic mechanism that is operative in patients with thromboangiitis obliterans. Tobacco use seems to play a central role in all patients who have thromboangiitis obliterans. Other etiologic factors may be important as well, such as genetic predisposition and possibly, autoimmune mechanisms.

Clinical Aspects

Thromboangiitis obliterans usually occurs in young smokers. Ischemia begins distally, involving the small- and medium-sized arteries and veins. Occasionally, large-artery involvement may be present, but it is uncommon.

At the Cleveland Clinic Foundation, 112 patients with Buerger's disease were evaluated between 1970 and 1987 [5]. The mean age of this population was 42 years (range, 20 to 75 years). Whereas in other series the male-to-female ratio was reported to be 9 to 1, in our series it was about 3 to 1 [5]. It appears that Buerger's disease occurs more commonly in women in societies in which there is a greater percentage of women who smoke. In populations in which few women smoke (e.g., Japan and India), a very strong male-to-female preponderance remains.

Table 31.1. Presenting signs and symptoms of thromboangiitis obliterans (from Olin *et al.* [5]; with permission).

Symptoms	Patients, n(%)
Intermittent claudication	70(63)
Rest pain	91(81)
Ischemic ulcers	85(76)
Upper extremity	24(28)
Lower extremity	39(46)
Both	22(26)
Thrombophlebitis	43(38)
Raynaud's phenomenon	49(44)
Sensory findings	77(69)
Abnormal Allen's test results	71(63)
Abnormal pulses	
Brachial	0
Radial	22(20)
Ulnar	46(41)
Popliteal	25(22)
Dorsalis pedis	87(78)
Posterior tibial	73(65)

The presenting clinical signs and symptoms in our series of patients are shown in Table 31.1. Intermittent claudication often occurs initially in the arch of the foot, and as the disease progresses more proximally, calf claudication may occur. A large percentage of patients present with ischemic rest pain or ischemic ulcerations. In patients with lower-extremity ulcerations in whom Buerger's disease is a consideration, an Allen's test should be performed to assess circulation in the hands and fingers. Abnormal Allen's test results in a young smoker with lower extremity ulcerations suggest the diagnosis of thromboangiitis obliterans because small-vessel involvement in both the upper and lower extremities is demonstrated. It is important to recognize that an absent radial artery pulse may occur in only 20% of individuals, and an absent ulnar artery pulse may occur in 41% of individuals with thromboangiitis obliterans. However, 63% of all individuals with thromboangiitis obliterans will have abnormal Allen's test results, which illustrates the distal nature of the disease involvement. One may encounter normally palpable radial and ulnar pulses, but the circulation distal to these arteries in the wrist may be significantly impaired.

The sensory findings in patients with thromboangiitis obliterans may be due to severe ischemic neuropathy. However, there is another explanation for the inordinately high percentage of patients who have sensory abnormalities. In thromboangiitis obliterans, there is fibrous tissue encasement of the artery, vein, and nerve. Encasement of small neurofibers may account for sensory abnormalities.

Differential Diagnosis

Diseases that can mimic thromboangiitis obliterans must be excluded. The most important and common of these diseases are atherosclerosis and emboli. All patients suspected of having thromboangiitis obliterans should undergo an echocardiogram to rule out cardiac thrombi and an arteriogram to rule out proximal atherosclerosis. Other diseases that should be included in the differential diagnosis of thromboangiitis obliterans are systemic lupus erythematosus, rheumatoid arthritis, scleroderma, polyarteritis nodosa, antiphospholipid antibody syndrome, giant-cell or Takayasu's arteritis, leukocytoclastic vasculitis, various blood dyscrasias such as polycythemia vera, ergotamine abuse, occupational hazards such as the frequent use of vibratory tools, hypothenar hammer syndrome, Ehlers-Danlos syndrome, pseudoxanthoma elasticum, calciphylaxis, and thrombosed aneurysms.

Arteriographic findings in patients with thromboangiitis obliterans are suggestive but not pathognomonic of the disease. There is involvement of the small- and medium-sized blood vessels. The most commonly involved vessels are the digital arteries of the fingers and toes as well as those of the palmar, plantar, tibial, peroneal, radial, and ulnar arteries. The arteriographic appearance is noted for its segmentally occlusive lesions. Affected arteries may have normal segments. More severe disease occurs distally. An increase in collateral vessels often occurs around areas of occlusion. The collaterals may take on a corkscrew appearance. Most importantly, the proximal arteries are normal; there is no evidence for underlying atherosclerosis or emboli.

Pathology

It is not common to obtain pathologic specimens during the acute phase of thromboangiitis obliterans. Reluctance to obtain biopsy specimens of these vessels is due to the fact that the distal extremity is usually ischemic and fear that biopsy will lead to new ulcerations. Therefore, most pathologic specimens come from amputated limbs in which the disease is generally chronic. Nonetheless, available data suggest that there are three phases of disease in thromboangiitis obliterans. The acute phase is characterized by a pan vasculitis with involvement of the intima, media, and adventitia. There is a highly cellular thrombus with lymphocytes, neutrophils, giant cells, and often microabscess formation. There may be endothelial-cell and fibroblast proliferation in the vessel wall and in the thrombus, but fibrinoid necrosis is absent. Segments of normal-appearing artery are often interspersed with segments showing acute, inflammatory reactions. In the subacute phase, there is much less cellularity and microabscess formation, and recanalization of the thrombus is apparent. There may be evidence of perivascular fibrosis and "vascularization" of the blood vessel wall. One also may begin to see the development of collateral and anastomotic vessels. In the late phase of the disease, there is often organized and recanalized thrombus and perivascular and perineural fibrosis. This represents an end-stage lesion that is not pathognomonic of thromboangiitis obliterans; it may occur in other vascular diseases.

Occasionally, thromboangiitis obliterans has been noted in the coronary arteries. Mautner *et al.* [16] analyzed the morphology of coronary plaque composition in a patient with Buerger's disease. The predominant component of the arterial narrowing was cellular (65%)

and dense fibrous tissue (30%). Extracellular lipid, foam cells, and calcified tissue made up less than 5% of the arterial narrowing.

It is not necessary to have a pathologic specimen to diagnose thromboangiitis obliterans. The diagnosis can be made on clinical grounds if the scenario is compatible and if there is no proximal source of emboli or atherosclerosis. However, if there are unusual features such as older age or unusual disease distribution, a pathologic specimen is necessary to make this diagnosis [17].

Therapy

The most important aspects of the treatment of thromboangiitis obliterans are shown in Table 31.2. It is imperative that the patient discontinue smoking or using tobacco in any form. In the active phases of the disease, even smokeless tobacco or passive smoking can be enough to keep the disease active. In patients who are able to discontinue cigarette smoking, amputations are extremely uncommon [5]. Of the 37 patients in our series who discontinued smoking, two (5%) underwent amputation. Both patients had critical limb ischemia with frank gangrene when they stopped smoking. If there was no tissue loss at the time the patient discontinued cigarette smoking, amputation did not occur [5].

Table 31.2. Therapy for thromboangiitis obliterans.

Cessation of smoking or tobacco use in any form
Treatment of local ischemic ulcerations
    Foot care
        Lubricate skin with lanolin-based cream
        Place lamb's wool between toes
        Avoid trauma, i.e., heel protectors, bed cradle
    Trial of calcium channel blockers and/or pentoxifylline
    Iloprost (not currently available in the United States)
    Sympathectomy
Treat cellulitis with antibiotics
Treat superficial phlebitis with nonsteroidal anti-inflammatory drugs
Amputate limb when all else fails

Other forms of therapy are merely palliative. In one report, the authors demonstrated that iloprost was more effective than aspirin in patients with critical limb ischemia due to thromboangiitis obliterans [18]. Fifteen of 68 patients (85%) treated with iloprost showed healing of ischemic ulcerations and/or relief of ischemic rest pain compared with 11 of 65 patients (17%) treated with aspirin (P< 0.05).

Usually, surgical revascularization is not an option in Buerger's disease. Because vascular involvement is distal, appropriate sites for bypass graft insertion are generally not present. In the few patients who have undergone arterial bypass, long-term results are poor. Thrombolytic therapy with low-dose intra-arterial streptokinase was attempted in 11 patients [19]. The catheter tip was advanced toward the occluding thrombus but not into the thrombus. Ten thousand units of streptokinase were given as a bolus, followed by 5000 U/hr for 24 hours. The overall success rate with amputation being avoided or altered was 58.3%. Although results are encouraging, in our experience, thrombolytic therapy generally has not been effective.

Conclusions

Thromboangiitis obliterans is a distal occlusive vascular disease that affects both arteries and veins. It is causally related to tobacco use in some, as of yet, undefined way. In individuals who are able to discontinue smoking or using tobacco, the outcome of the disease is almost always favorable. However, in patients who continue to use tobacco, amputation is common.

—by Jeffrey W. Olin, DO

Jeffrey W. Olin, DO, Department of Vascular Medicine, The Cleveland Clinic Foundation, 9500 Euclid Avenue, Cleveland, OH 44195, USA

References

1. Hunder GG, Arend WP, Bloch DA, Calabrese LH, Fauci AS, Fries JF, Leavitt RY, Lie JT, Lightfoot RW, Masi AT, *et al.*: The American College of Rheumatology 1990 Criteria for the Classification of Vasculitis. *Arthritis Rheum* 1990, 33:1065-1114.

2. Ledford DK: Immunologic Aspects of Cardiovascular Disease. *JAMA* 1992, 268:2923-2929.

3.   Von Winiwarter F: Ueber Eine Eigenthumliche Form von Endarteritis und Endophlebitis mit Gangran des Fusses. *Arch Klin Chir* 1879, 23:202-206.

4.   Buerger L: Thrombo-Angiitis Obliterans: A Study of the Vascular Lesion Leading to Pre-Senile Spontaneous Gangrene. *Am J Med Sci* 1908, 136:567-580.

5.   Olin JW, Young JR, Graor RA, Ruschhupt WF, Bartholomew JR: The Changing Clinical Spectrum of Thromboangiitis Obliterans (Buerger's Disease). *Circulation* 1990, 82 (suppl IV):IV-3-IV-8.

6.   Lie JT: The Rise and Fall and Resurgence of Thromboangiitis Obliterans (Buerger's Disease). *Acta Pathol Jpn* 1989, 39:153-158.

7.   Grove WJ, Stansby GP: Buerger's Disease in Cigarette Smoking in Bangladesh. *Ann R Coll Surg Engl* 1992, 74:115-118. Thirty-nine patients with Buerger's disease were reported on over a 2-month period. Their clinical presentation and smoking habits are presented in detail.

8.   Gindal RM: Buerger's Disease in Cigarette Smoking in Bangladesh [Letter]. *Ann R Coll Surg Engl* 1992, 74:436-437.

9.   Lie JT: Diagnostic Histopathology of Major Systemic and Pulmonary Vasculitic Syndromes. *Rheum Clin North Am* 1990, 16:269-292.

10. Papa MZ, Adar R: A Critical Look at Thromboangiitis Obliterans (Buerger's Disease). *Perspect Vasc Surg* 1992, 5:1-21. The world's literature regarding the etiology, clinical features, angiographic features, histologic features, and diagnostic criteria for thromboangiitis obliterans are reviewed in this important article.

11. Papa M, Bass A, Adar R, Halperin Z, Schneiderman J, Becker CG, Brautbar H, Mozes E: Autoimmune Mechanisms in Thromboangiitis Obliterans (Buerger's Disease): The Role of Tobacco Antigen and the Major Histocompatibility Complex. *Surgery* 1992, 111:527-531. Patients with Buerger's disease and healthy smokers had the same rate of cellular response to tobacco glycoprotein, whereas nonsmokers did not respond at

all. It was suggested that if tobacco glycoprotein has an immunologic role in the pathogenesis of thromboangiitis obliterans, an additional factor must also be operative. Buerger's disease patients had a higher frequency of HLA-DR4 and a significantly lower frequency of HLA-DRw6 antigen than did both the control group and the group of patients who smoked but did not have Buerger's disease.

12. McLaughlin GA, Helsby CR, Evans CC, Chapman DM: Association of HLA-A9 and HLA-B5 With Buerger's Disease. *BMJ* 1976, 2:1165-1166.

13. Adar R, Papa MZ, Halperin Z, Mozes M, Shoshan S, Softer B, Zinger H, Dayan M, Mozes E: Cellular Sensitivity to Collagen and Thromboangiitis Obliterans. *N Engl J Med* 1983, 308:1113-1116.

14. Chaudhury NA, Pietraszek MH, Hachiya T, Baba S, Sakaguchi S, Takada Y, Takada A: Plasminogen Activators and Plasminogen Activator Inhibitor 1 Before and After Venous Occlusion of the Upper Limb and Thromboangiitis Obliterans (Buerger's Disease). *Thromb Res* 1992, 6:321-329. Endothelial dysfunction in patients with Buerger's disease is reflected by elevated levels of urokinase, enhanced plasminogen activator release, and depressed levels of plasminogen activator inhibitor 1.

15. Casellas M, Perez A, Cabero L: Buerger's Disease and Antiphospholipid Antibodies in Pregnancy. *Ann Rheum Dis* 1993, 52:247-248. A case of elevated levels of antiphospholipid antibodies is described in a patient with "Buerger's disease" who was pregnant.

16. Mautner GC, Mautner SL, Lin F, Roggin M, Roberts WC: Amounts of Coronary Arterial Luminal Narrowing and Composition of Material Causing the Narrowing in Buerger's Disease. *Am J Cardiol* 1993, 71:486-490. The coronary arteries of a 37-year-old man were studied postmortem. The composition of the arterial lesion is described in great detail. Cellular and fibrous tissue made up approximately 95% of the lesion in this patient with Buerger's disease.

17. Olin JW, Lie JT: Thromboangiitis Obliterans (Buerger's Disease). In *Current Management of Hypertension and Vascular*

Diseases. Edited by Cook JP, Frohlich ED. St. Louis: BC Decker, Mosby Yearbook; 1992:265-271. The diagnosis and treatment of thromboangiitis obliterans is reviewed in detail.

18. Fiessinger JN, Schafer M: Trial of Iloprost vs. Aspirin Treatment for Critical Limb Ischaemia of Thromboangiitis Obliterans. *Lancet* 1990, 335:555-557.

19. Hussein E, El Dorri A: Intra-Arterial Streptokinase as Adjuvant Therapy for Complicated Buerger's Disease: Early Trials. *Int Surg* 1993, 78:54-58. Eleven cases of thromboangiitis obliterans treated with thrombolytic therapy are described.

Chapter 32

Raynaud's Phenomenon

What Is Raynaud's Phenomenon?

Raynaud's phenomenon is a disorder that affects the blood vessels in the fingers, toes, ears, and nose. This disorder is characterized by episodic attacks, called vasospastic attacks, that cause the blood vessels in the digits (fingers and toes) to constrict (narrow). Although estimates vary, recent surveys show that Raynaud's phenomenon may affect 5 to 10 percent of the general population in the United States. Women are more likely than men to have the disorder. Raynaud's phenomenon appears to be more common in people who live in colder climates. However, people with the disorder who live in milder climates may have more attacks durinq periods of colder weather.

What Happens During an Attack?

For most people, an attack is usually triggered by exposure to cold or emotional stress. In general, attacks affect the fingers or toes but may affect the nose, lips, or ear lobes.

Reduced Blood Supply to the Extremities

When a person is exposed to cold, the body's normal response is to slow the loss of heat and preserve its core temperature. To maintain

Fact Sheet AR-125, National Institute of Arthritis and Musculoskeletal and Skin Diseases (NIAMS), AMT 6/96, June 1996.

this temperature, the blood vessels that control blood flow to the skin surface move blood from arteries near the surface to veins deeper in the body. For people who have Raynaud's phenomenon, this normal body response is intensified by the sudden spasmodic contractions of the small blood vessels (arterioles) that supply blood to the fingers and toes. The arteries of the fingers and toes may also collapse. As a result, the blood supply to the extremities is greatly decreased, causing a reaction that includes skin discoloration and other changes.

Changes in Skin Color and Sensation

Once the attack begins, a person may experience three phases of skin color changes (white, blue, and red) in the fingers or toes. The order of the changes of color is not the same for all people, and not everyone has all three colors. Pallor (whiteness) may occur in response to spasm of the arterioles and the resulting collapse of the digital arteries. Cyanosis (blueness) may appear because the fingers or toes are not getting enough oxygen-rich blood. The fingers or toes may also feel cold and numb. Finally, as the arterioles dilate (relax) and blood returns to the digits, rubor (redness) may occur. As the attack ends, throbbing and tingling may occur in the fingers and toes. An attack can last from less than a minute to several hours.

How Is Raynaud's Phenomenon Classified?

Doctors classify Raynaud's phenomenon as either the primary or the secondary form. In medical literature, "primary Raynaud's phenomenon" may also be called Raynaud's disease, idiopathic Raynaud's phenomenon, or primary Raynaud's syndrome. The terms idiopathic and primary both mean that the cause is unknown.

Primary Raynaud's Phenomenon

Most people who have Raynaud's phenomenon have the primary form (the milder version). A person who has primary Raynaud's phenomenon has no underlying disease or associated medical problems. More women than men are affected, and approximately 75 percent of all cases are diagnosed in women who are between 15 and 40 years old.

People who have only vasospastic attacks for several years, without involvement of other body systems or organs, rarely have or will develop a secondary disease (that is, a connective tissue disorder such as scleroderma) later. Several researchers who studied people who appeared to have primary Raynaud's phenomenon over long periods of time found that less than 9 percent of these people developed a secondary disease.

Secondary Raynaud's Phenomenon

Although secondary Raynaud's phenomenon is much less common than the primary form, it is often a more complex and serious disorder. Secondary means that patients have an underlying disease or condition that causes Raynaud's phenomenon. Connective tissue diseases are the most common cause of secondary Raynaud's phenomenon. Some of these diseases reduce blood flow to the digits by causing blood vessel walls to thicken and the vessels to constrict too easily. Raynaud's phenomenon is seen in approximately 85 to 95 percent of patients with scleroderma and mixed connective tissue disease, and it is present in about one-third of patients with systemic lupus erythematosus. For most people with lupus, Raynaud's phenomenon acts like the primary form of the disorder. Raynaud's phenomenon also can occur in patients who have other connective tissue diseases, including Sjögren's syndrome, dermatomyositis, and polymyositis.

Possible causes of secondary Raynaud's phenomenon, other than connective tissue diseases, are carpal tunnel syndrome and obstructive arterial disease (blood vessel disease). Some drugs, including beta-blockers (used to treat high blood pressure), ergotamine preparations (used for migraine headaches), certain agents used in cancer chemotherapy, and drugs that cause vasoconstriction such as some over-the-counter cold medications and narcotics are linked to Raynaud's phenomenon.

People in certain occupations may be more vulnerable to secondary Raynaud's phenomenon. Some workers in the plastics industry (who are exposed to vinyl chloride) develop a scleroderma-like illness, of which Raynaud's phenomenon can be a part. Workers who operate vibrating tools can develop a type of Raynaud's phenomenon called vibration-induced white finger. In addition, people whose fingers are subject to repeated stress, such as typing or playing the piano, are more vulnerable to the disorder.

People with secondary Raynaud's phenomenon often experience associated medical problems. The more serious problems are skin ulcers (sores) or gangrene (tissue death) in the fingers or toes. Painful ulcers and gangrene are fairly common and can be difficult to treat. In addition, a person may experience heartburn or difficulty in swallowing. These two problems are caused by weakness in the muscle of the esophagus (the tube that takes food and liquids from the mouth to the stomach) that can occur in people with connective tissue diseases.

How Does a Doctor Diagnose Raynaud's Phenomenon?

If a doctor suspects Raynaud's phenomenon, he or she will ask the patient for a detailed medical history. The doctor will then examine the patient to rule out other medical problems. The patient might have a vasospastic attack during the office visit, which makes it easier for the doctor to diagnose Raynaud's phenomenon. Most doctors find it fairly easy to diagnose Raynaud's phenomenon but more difficult to identify the form of the disorder. (See *Diagnostic Criteria for Raynaud's Phenomenon*, below, for the criteria doctors use to diagnose primary or secondary Raynaud's phenomenon.)

Nailfold capillaroscopy (study of capillaries under a microscope) can help the doctor distinguish between primary and secondary Raynaud's phenomenon. During this test, the doctor puts a drop of oil on the patient's nailfolds, the skin at the base of the fingernail. The doctor then examines the nailfolds under a microscope to look for abnormalities of the tiny blood vessels called capillaries. If the capillaries are enlarged or deformed, the patient may have a connective tissue disease.

The doctor may also order two particular blood tests, an antinuclear antibody test (ANA) and an erythrocyte sedimentation rate (ESR). The ANA test determines whether the body is producing special proteins (antibodies) often found in people who have connective tissue diseases or other autoimmune disorders. The ESR test is a measure of inflammation in the body and tests how fast red blood cells settle out of unclotted blood. Inflammation in the body causes an elevated ESR.

Diagnostic Criteria for Raynaud's Phenomenon

Primary Raynaud's Phenomenon

- Periodic vasospastic attacks of pallor or cyanosis (some doctors include the additional criterion of the presence of these attacks for at least two years)

- Normal nailfold capillary pattern

- Negative antinuclear antibody test

- Normal erythrocyte sedimentation rate

- Absence of pitting scars or ulcers of the skin, or gangrene (tissue death) in the fingers or toes

Secondary Raynaud's Phenomenon

- Periodic vasospastic attacks of pallor and cyanosis
- Abnormal nailfold capillary pattern
- Positive antinuclear antibody test
- Abnormal erythrocyte sedimentation rate
- Presence of pitting scars or ulcers of the skin, or gangrene in the fingers or toes

What Is the Treatment for Raynaud's Phenomenon?

The aims of treatment are to reduce the number and severity of attacks and to prevent tissue damage and loss in the fingers and toes. Most doctors are conservative in treating patients with primary and secondary Raynaud's phenomenon; that is, they recommend nondrug treatments and self-help measures first. Doctors may prescribe medications for some patients, usually those with secondary Raynaud's phenomenon. In addition, patients are treated for any underlying disease or condition that causes secondary Raynaud's phenomenon.

Nondrug Treatments and Self-Help Measures

Several nondrug treatments and self-help measures can decrease the severity of Raynaud's attacks and promote overall well-being.

- *Take Action During an Attack.* An attack should not be ignored. Its length and severity can be lessened by a few simple actions. The first and most important action is to warm the hands or feet. In cold weather, people should go indoors. Running warm water over the fingers or toes or soaking them in a bowl of warm water will warm them. Taking time to relax will further help to end the attack. If a stressful situation triggers the attack, a person can help stop the attack by getting out of the stressful situation and relaxing. People who are trained in biofeedback can use this technique along with warming the hands or feet in water to help lessen the attack.

- *Keep Warm.* It is important not only to keep the extremities warm but also to avoid chilling any part of the body. In cold weather, people with Raynaud's phenomenon must pay particular attention to dressing. Several layers of loose clothing, socks, hats, and gloves or mittens are recommended. A hat is important because a great deal of body heat is lost through the scalp. Feet should be kept dry and warm. Some people find it helpful to wear mittens and socks to bed during winter. Chemical warmers, such as small heating pouches that can be placed in pockets, mittens, boots, or shoes, can give added protection during long periods outdoors. People who have secondary Raynaud's phenomenon should talk to their doctors before exercising outdoors in cold weather.

People with Raynaud's phenomenon should also be aware that air conditioning can trigger attacks. Turning down the air conditioning or wearing a sweater may help prevent attacks. Some people find it helpful to use insulated drinking glasses and to put on gloves before handling frozen or refrigerated foods.

- *Quit Smoking.* The nicotine in cigarettes causes the skin temperature to drop, which may lead to an attack.

- *Control Stress.* Because stress and emotional upsets may trigger an attack, particularly for people who have primary Raynaud's phenomenon, learning to recognize and avoid stressful situations may help control the number of attacks. Many people have found that relaxation or biofeedback training can help decrease the number and severity of attacks. Biofeedback training teaches people to bring the temperature of their fingers under voluntary control. Local hospitals and other community organizations, such as schools, often offer programs in stress management.

- *Exercise.* Many doctors encourage patients who have Raynaud's phenomenon, particularly the primary form, to exercise regularly. Most people find that exercise promotes overall well-being, increases energy level, helps control weight, and promotes restful sleep. Patients with Raynaud's phenomenon should talk to their doctors before starting an exercise program.

- *See a Doctor.* People with Raynaud's phenomenon should see their doctors if they are worried or frightened about attacks or if they have questions about caring for themselves. They should always see their doctors if attacks occur only on one side of the body (one hand or one foot) and any time an attack results in sores or ulcers on the fingers or toes.

Treatment with Medications

People with secondary Raynaud's phenomenon are more likely than those with the primary form to be treated with medications. Many doctors believe that the most effective and safest drugs are calcium-channel blockers, which relax smooth muscle and dilate the small blood vessels. These drugs decrease the frequency and severity of attacks in about two-thirds of patients who have primary and secondary Raynaud's phenomenon. These drugs also can help heal skin ulcers on the fingers or toes.

Other patients have found relief with drugs called alpha blockers that counteract the actions of norepinephrine, a hormone that constricts blood vessels. Some doctors prescribe a nonspecific vasodilator (drug that relaxes blood vessels), such as nitroglycerine paste, which is applied to the fingers, to help heal skin ulcers. Patients should keep in mind that the treatment for Raynaud's phenomenon is not always successful. Often, patients with the secondary form will not respond as well to treatment as those with the primary form of the disorder.

Patients may find that one drug works better than another. Some people may experience side effects that require stopping the medication. For other people, a drug may become less effective over time. Women of childbearing age should know that the medications used to treat Raynaud's phenomenon may affect the growing fetus. Therefore, women who are pregnant or are trying to become pregnant should avoid taking these medications if possible.

Self-Help Reminders

- Take action during an attack
- Keep warm
- Don't smoke
- Control stress
- Exercise regularly
- See a doctor if questions or concerns develop

What Research Is Being Conducted to Help People Who Have Raynaud's Phenomenon?

Researchers are studying the use of other drugs to treat Raynaud's phenomenon; for example, oral and intravenous prostaglandins, such as iloprost. Other investigators are studying the molecular mechanisms behind Raynaud's phenomenon and the anatomy of blood vessels. Several medical centers in the United States are studying the use of biofeedback to control attacks. Researchers studying scleroderma and other connective tissue diseases are also investigating Raynaud's phenomenon in relation to these diseases.

Raynaud's Phenomenon Glossary

Antibodies. Special proteins (produced by the body's immune system) that help fight and destroy viruses, bacteria, and other foreign substances that invade the body.

Antinuclear antibody. Abnormal antibodies that are often present in people who have connective tissue diseases or other autoimmune disorders. These antibodies target material in the nucleus (the "command center") of healthy cells instead of fighting specific disease-causing agents.

Antinuclear antibody test (ANA). A blood test done to find out if the body is producing antinuclear antibodies.

Arteries. Large blood vessels that carry blood and oxygen from the heart to all parts of the body.

Arterioles. Small blood vessels that branch off from arteries and connect to capillaries.

Biofeedback. A technique designed to help a person gain control over involuntary (independent of the will) body functions, such as heart rate, blood pressure, or skin temperature.

Capillaries. Tiny blood vessels that carry blood between arterioles (the smallest arteries) and venules (the smallest veins). Capillaries form networks throughout the body's organs and tissues. They open and close in response to the organs' needs for oxygen and nutrients.

Connective tissue. The tissue that supports body structures and holds parts together. Some parts of the body, such as tendons and cartilage, are made up of connective tissue. Connective tissue is also the basic substance of bone and blood vessels.

Connective tissue disease. A group of diseases that affect the body's connective tissues, including tissue in the joints, blood vessels, heart, skin, and other supporting structures. Some of these diseases are caused by a malfunctioning of the immune system. Connective tissue diseases are fairly common and include systemic lupus erythematosus, rheumatoid arthritis, scleroderma, polymyositis, and dermatomyositis.

Cyanosis. Bluish, grayish, or dark purple discoloration of the skin that occurs when blood cannot circulate freely and gives up all its oxygen.

Erythrocyte sedimentation rate (ESR). A blood test that determines how fast erythrocytes (red blood cells) settle out of unclotted blood and is used to detect inflammation in the body. Connective tissue diseases can change blood proteins, which changes how quickly red blood cells settle out of unclotted blood to the bottom of a test tube. Higher ESRs (indicating more rapid settling of red blood cells and the presence of inflammation) are found in all of the connective tissue diseases.

Gangrene. A condition that occurs when tissue dies. Tissue death is usually caused by a loss of blood supply. Gangrene may affect a small area, such as a finger or toe, or a large portion of a limb.

Ischemic lesion. A sore or other skin abnormality caused by an insufficient supply of blood to the tissue.

Nailfold capillaroscopy. A test used to identify the primary or secondary form of Raynaud's phenomenon. The examiner places a drop of oil on the nailfold (the skin at the cuticle or base of the nail) and uses a hand-held magnifying glass or microscope to look at the capillaries in the nailfold. Certain changes in theses capillaries can be characteristic of connective tissue diseases.

Smooth muscle. The muscles of the body that are not under a person's conscious control. Smooth muscle is found mainly in the internal organs, including the digestive tract, respiratory passages, urinary bladder, and walls of blood vessels.

Spasm. An involuntary, sudden muscle contraction. In Raynaud's phenomenon, involuntary contraction of the smooth muscle in the blood vessels decreases the flow of blood to the fingers or toes (which leads to color changes in the skin).

Vasodilator. An agent, usually a drug, that widens blood vessels and allows more blood to reach the tissues.

Vasospasm or Vasoconstriction. A sudden muscle contraction that narrows the blood vessels, reducing blood flow to a part of the body.

The NIAMS gratefully acknowledges the assistance of Phillip J. Clements, M.D., of the University of Califomia, Los Angeles; Jay D. Coffman, M.D., of the Boston University Medical Center; and Frederick M. Wigley, M.D., of The Johns Hopkins University School of Medicine in the preparation and review of this fact sheet.

Chapter 33

Varicose Vein Treatments

Fast Facts

- Varicose veins are bulging veins that become enlarged when they fail to circulate the blood properly.

- Spider veins are the smaller thread-like or "starburst" vessels appearing on the surface of the skin.

- Doctors use a variety of methods to treat venous disease. Problem veins may be surgically removed or injected with a solution.

- Varicose veins and spider veins may recur following treatment by any known method. New varicose and spider also may appear.

- Question doctors carefully about the cosmetic side effects and health risks for each type of treatment.

- Be wary of claims promising "major breakthroughs," "permanent results," "unique treatments," "painless," or "absolutely safe" treatments.

Thousands of people every year consider getting treatment for varicose veins and spider veins. Advertisements for treating venous disease often tout "unique," "permanent," "painless," or "absolutely safe" methods—making it difficult to decide on the best treatment. If you are considering this procedure, the following information may help.

Federal Trade Commission, January 1994, #F030421.

Remember, though, this cannot substitute for a consultation with a properly trained physician.

What are varicose veins?

Veins can become enlarged with pools of blood when they fail to circulate the blood properly. These visible and bulging veins, called varicose veins, are often associated with symptoms such as tired, heavy, or aching limbs. In severe cases, varicose veins can rupture, or open sores (called "ulcers") can form on the skin. Varicose veins are most common in the legs and thighs.

What are spider veins?

Small "spider veins" also can appear on the skin's surface. These may look like short, fine lines, "starburst" clusters, or a web-like maze. Spider veins are most common in the thighs, ankles, and feet. They may also appear on the face.

Who gets varicose and spider veins?

Varicose and spider veins can occur in men or women of any age but most frequently affect women of childbearing years and older. Family history of the problem and aging increase one's tendency to develop varicose and spider veins.

What causes varicose and spider veins?

The causes of varicose and spider veins are not entirely understood. In some instances, the absence or weakness of valves in the veins, which prevent the backward flow of blood away from the heart, may cause the poor circulation. In other cases, weaknesses in the vein walls may cause the pooling of the blood. Less commonly, varicose veins are caused by such diseases as phlebitis or congenital abnormalities of the veins. Venous disease is generally progressive and cannot be prevented entirely. However, in some cases, wearing support hosiery and maintaining normal weight and regular exercise may be beneficial.

Is treatment always necessary?

No. Varicose and spider veins may be primarily a cosmetic problem. Severe cases of varicose veins, especially those involving ulcers, typically require treatment. Check with a doctor if you are uncertain.

What procedures are available to treat varicose and spider veins?

Varicose veins are frequently treated by eliminating the "bad" veins. This forces the blood to flow through the remaining healthy veins. Various methods can be used to eliminate the problem veins, including, most commonly, surgery or sclerotherapy. Less commonly, laser or electro-cautery treatments have been used to treat the smallest spider veins, especially on the face.

Surgery to treat varicose veins, commonly referred to as "stripping," is usually done under local or partial anesthesia, such as an "epidural." Here, the problematic veins are "stripped" out by passing a flexible device through the vein and removing it through an incision near the groin. Smaller tributaries of these veins also are stripped with this device or removed through a series of small incisions. Those veins that connect to the deeper veins are then tied off. This stripping method has been used since the 1950s.

Spider veins cannot be removed through surgery. Sometimes, they disappear when the larger varicose veins feeding the spider veins are removed. Remaining spider veins also can be treated with "sclerotherapy."

"Sclerotherapy" uses a fine needle to inject a solution directly into the vein. This solution irritates the lining of the vein, causing it to swell and the blood to clot. The vein turns into scar tissue that fades from view. Some doctors treat both varicose and spider veins with sclerotherapy. Today, the substances most commonly used in the United States are hypertonic saline or Sotradecol (sodium tetradecyl sulfate). Polidocanol (aethoxyskerol) is undergoing FDA testing but has not yet been approved in the U.S. for sclerotherapy.

During sclerotherapy, after the solution is injected, the vein's surrounding tissue is generally wrapped in compression bandages for several days, causing the vein walls to stick together. Patients whose legs have been treated are put on walking regimens, which forces the blood to flow into other veins and prevents blood clots. This method and variations of it have been used since the 1920s. In most cases, more than one treatment session will be required.

Do these procedures hurt?

For all of these procedures, the amount of pain an individual feels will vary, depending on the person's general tolerance for pain, how extensive the treatments are, which parts of the body are treated, whether complications arise, and other factors. Because surgery is performed under anesthesia, you will not feel pain during the procedure. After the anesthesia wears off, you will likely experience pain near the incisions.

For sclerotherapy, the degree of pain will also depend on the size of the needle used and which solution is injected. Most people find hypertonic saline to be the most painful solution and experience a burning and cramping sensation for several minutes when it is injected. Some doctors mix a mild local anesthetic in with the saline solution to minimize the pain.

What types of doctors provide treatments for varicose and spider veins?

Doctors providing surgical treatment include general and vascular surgeons. Sclerotherapy is often performed by dermatologists. Some general, vascular, and plastic surgeons also perform sclerotherapy treatments. You may want to consult more than one doctor before deciding on a method of treatment. Be sure to ask doctors about their experience in performing the procedure you want.

What are the side effects of these treatments?

Carefully question doctors about the safety and side effects for each type of treatment. Thoroughly review any "informed consent" forms your doctor gives you explaining the risks of a procedure.

For surgical removal of veins, the side effects are those for any surgery performed under anesthesia, including nausea, vomiting, and the risk of wound infection. Surgery also results in scarring where small incisions are made and may occasionally cause blood clots.

For sclerotherapy, the side effects can depend on the substance used for the injection. People with allergies may want to be cautious. For example, Sotradecol may cause allergic reactions, occasionally severe. Hypertonic saline solution is unlikely to cause allergic reactions. Either substance may burn the skin (if the needle is not properly inserted) or permanently mark or "stain" the skin. (These brownish marks are caused by the scattering of blood cells throughout the tissue after the vein has been injected and may fade over time). Occasionally, sclerotherapy can lead to blood clots.

Laser and electro-cautery treatments can cause scarring and changes in the color of the skin.

How long do results last?

Many factors will affect the rate at which treated veins recur. These include the diagnosis, the method used and its suitability for treating a particular condition, and the skill of the physician. Sometimes the body forms a new vein in place of the one removed by a surgeon. An injected vein that was not completely destroyed by sclerotherapy may reopen, or a new vein may appear in the same location as a previous one. Many studies have found that varicose veins are more likely to recur following sclerotherapy than following surgery. However, no treatment method has been scientifically established as free from recurrences. For all types of procedures, recurrence rates increase with time. Also, because venous disease is typically progressive, no treatment can prevent the appearance of new varicose or spider veins in the future.

Is one treatment better than another?

The method you select for treating venous disease should be based on your physician's diagnosis, the size of the veins to be treated, your treatment history, your age, your history of allergies, and your ability to tolerate surgery and anesthesia, among other factors. As noted above, small spider veins cannot be surgically removed and can only be treated with sclerotherapy. On the other hand, larger varicose veins may, according to many studies, be more likely to recur if treated with sclerotherapy.

Be wary of claims touting "major breakthroughs," "permanent results," "unique treatments," "brand-new," "painless," or "absolutely safe" methods. Always ask for specific documentation for claims made about particular recurrence rates or fewer health risks or cosmetic side effects.

How expensive is the procedure?

Sclerotherapy can cost anywhere from a few hundred dollars to several thousand dollars, depending on the number of injections and treatment sessions required and the area of the country where the procedure is performed.

Surgery can cost approximately $600 – $2,000 per leg for the surgeon's fee, plus charges for anesthesia and hospitalization. Most vein surgery can be performed on an out-patient basis. Costs can vary depending on how many veins must be removed and the area of the country where the procedure is performed.

301

You may want to check to see if the procedure is covered under your medical insurance. Many policies do not cover costs for elective cosmetic surgery.

For More Information

If you need to resolve a problem with a doctor regarding treatment for varicose veins, you may want to contact your county medical society, state medical board, or local consumer protection agency.

You also may want to report any concerns about advertising claims to the Federal Trade Commission (FTC). Write: Correspondence Branch, Federal Trade Commission, Washington, DC 20580. Although the FTC does not generally intervene in individual disputes, the information you provide may indicate a pattern of possible law violations requiring action by the Commission or referral to state authorities.

For a free brochure on **Cosmetic Surgery**, write: Public Reference, Federal Trade Commission, Washington, DC 20580; 202-326-2222. You also may request **Best Sellers**, which lists all of the FTC's consumer publications.

Chapter 34

Venous Ulcers

Leg Ulcers

Veins are the problem more than half the time. They can be painful and make walking difficult. They look raw, weep fluid and frequently become infected.

Leg and foot ulcers affect approximately 500,000 Americans. Although they're most common in people older than 60, the ulcers can also occur in younger adults.

Fortunately, most ulcers respond to conservative care. Yet a severe ulcer can take weeks or months to heal, only to recur. And some ulcers never heal.

Here's a look at the most common type of leg ulcer and how it's managed, including the newest developments in research.

Poor Venous Circulation Can Cause an Ulcer

The venous system is made up of superficial and deep veins. Smaller veins connect the superficial and deep systems at many locations throughout your legs and feet. All three systems have one-way valves.

Normal venous pressure and the contraction of your leg muscles return blood to your heart. One-way valves in the veins keep blood from flowing backward.

Reprinted from August 1995 *Mayo Clinic Health Letter* with permission of Mayo Foundation for Medical Education and Research, Rochester, Minnesota 55905. For subscription information, call 1-800-333-9038.

More than half of all leg ulcers occur when venous circulation becomes impaired. Poor venous blood flow may develop from inflammation (vasculitis) or inflammation with obstruction by a blood clot within a vein (thrombophlebitis). Weakening in venous walls caused by heredity, age, obesity or pregnancy can also impair venous circulation. Weakened venous walls are a main cause of varicose veins.

How Venous Ulcers Develop

When inflammation in the deep veins and their valves occurs, venous pressure increases. Elevated pressure stretches venous walls and their valves, preventing the valves from closing tightly.

Blood flows backward and pools in small connecting veins near your feet. This can lead to a dull ache in your legs that grows worse with prolonged standing and is relieved by raising your legs.

Increased venous pressure allows fluid to leak out of tiny blood vessels (capillaries), resulting in edema. Blood components may also leak into the surface layer of your skin, impairing exchange of nutrients between blood and tissues. As a result, your skin is more vulnerable to injury and slow healing.

Even the slightest trauma to your skin, such as friction from tight elastic in your socks, a bump, an insect bite or a scratch, may lead to an ulcer. Varicose veins also commonly cause venous ulcers.

Location and Appearance Are Clues to Diagnosis

Venous ulcers typically develop near your anklebone, where gravity causes blood to pool in greatest amounts. They almost never occur above your knee or on your sole.

Most venous ulcers are irregularly shaped. Continuous leakage of fluid from capillaries causes a weeping and raw appearance. In addition to edema, the skin surrounding a venous ulcer may be dry, itchy and inflamed.

When the location and appearance aren't enough to diagnose the ulcer as venous, your doctor may use noninvasive tests. Doppler ultrasound uses high-frequency sound waves to evaluate venous blood flow and determine whether valves work effectively.

In plethysmography (ple-thiz-MOG-rah-fe), a type of pump placed around your calf is used to evaluate venous blood flow before, during and after exercise. If venous circulation is impaired, blood volume during exercise drops an abnormally small amount and returns more quickly than expected.

Treatment Ranges from Conservative to Aggressive

Years ago, having a leg ulcer meant hospitalization or strict bed rest at home. Now, treating leg ulcers generally involves these conservative approaches:

Dressings. Wet dressings promote healing by absorbing weeping fluids and preventing tissues from drying out. They also reduce the risk of infection by keeping the ulcer clean and protected from bacteria.

During initial healing, gauze dressings moistened with a saline solution are changed daily. If an ulcer is free from infection, your doctor may apply an adhesive film or absorbent gel or foam instead of a gauze dressing.

Elastic wraps. An elastic compressive wrap improves venous blood flow while the ulcer heals. A wrap is gentler on the ulcer than therapeutic compressive stockings during healing.

Once the ulcer is healed, wearing support stockings during the day can help prevent a recurrent venous ulcer (see "Reduce Your Risk").

For a severe ulcer, your doctor may add these more aggressive approaches:

Mechanical pumps. A sleeve attached to a small pump fits over your lower leg. Intermittent compression of the sleeve promotes venous blood flow by forcing blood and fluids out of swollen leg tissues. Your doctor may prescribe use of the pump a few hours each day in addition to wearing elastic stockings or a wrap.

Skin grafting. For a large ulcer, taking skin from your back or leg and placing it over the ulcer may be preferable to prolonged, conservative care.

Surgery. For enlarged varicose veins, you may need to have a damaged section of vein removed (vein stripping). Bypass surgery or repair of leaky valves is rarely needed for venous ulcers.

What May Lie Ahead

Although most ulcers heal with conservative care, chronic recurrent ulcers continue to challenge doctors and frustrate those who have them. Better treatments may eventually come from methods that take advantage of your skin's natural ability to heal.

One treatment uses growth factors contained in human blood platelets. When applied to an ulcer, growth factors stimulate formation of new skin tissue over the ulcer. In combination with other approaches, growth factor therapy seems to enhance healing of chronic venous ulcers.

Other treatments involve grafting human skin grown in the laboratory over chronic venous ulcers to promote and speed healing. Growth factor therapy and cultured skin treatments are currently under review by the Food and Drug Administration.

Reduce Your Risk

Follow these steps to prevent new or recurrent ulcers:

Wear support stockings. Gentle compression promotes venous circulation. You can buy the knee-high stockings at most medical supply stores or drugstores. Wear them when standing or sifting for long periods.

Ask your doctor or other health-care professional for advice on the amount of compression you need for your condition.

To prevent severe recurrent ulcers, your doctor may prescribe specially designed stockings that provide greater compression at your ankles.

Walk daily. Contraction of your leg muscles during activity helps pump blood back to your heart.

Change your position frequently. During long car trips, stop to take a walk every couple of hours.

On flights, stand up and stretch periodically. Walk through the cabin about once every hour. Flex your ankles or press your feet against the seat in front of you.

Elevate your legs. Place your legs at least 12 inches above the level of your heart when sitting or lying down. Do this for 10 to 15 minutes three or four times daily.

Control your weight. Being overweight puts pressure on your veins, stretching venous walls and valves.

Chapter 35

Aneurysms

Just before Christmas in 1964, officials of the Houston Methodist Hospital in Texas stood at the entrance awaiting the arrival of famous visitors: the Duke and Duchess of Windsor. But the former king of England and his commoner wife were coming to Houston for more than a visit. The duke was scheduled to undergo surgery during the holidays.

Four years earlier, British physicians had detected a small pulsating mass in the duke's abdomen. They diagnosed the mass as an abdominal aneurysm, a balloon-like dilation of the wall of the aorta, the large, sturdy blood vessel that comes out of the heart and branches into other arteries that carry oxygen and nutrients to all parts of the body. Such aneurysms can rupture spontaneously, with dire consequences.

The duke's medical advisers had monitored the aneurysm closely as it slowly grew larger each year. When the aneurysm suddenly grew dangerously large, they sent him to a renowned heart surgeon, Methodist's Michael E. DeBakey, M.D., a specialist in aneurysm repair. At that time, DeBakey did about a thousand such procedures each year, sometimes as many as six a day.

In an operation lasting little more than an hour, DeBakey cut out the swollen part of the aorta—normally less than an inch in diameter at this point in the body, but now the size of a large grapefruit—and replaced it with a 4-inch length of knitted Dacron tubing. The Duke of Windsor recovered without incident and lived until 1972, when he died of throat cancer at age 78.

FDA Consumer, October 1992, 26(8):36-39.

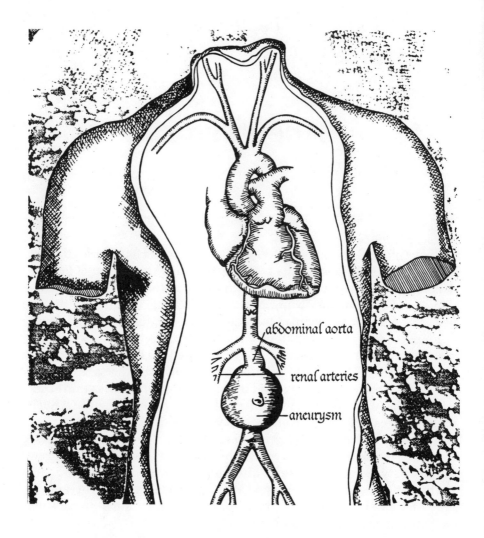

Figure 35.1. *The abdominal aorta, below the renal arteries, is the most common place for an aneurysm, a ballooning of an artery resulting from weakening of the artery wall. The Duke of Windsor in 1964 underwent successful surgery in the United States for an abdominal aortic aneurysm. If such aneurysms rupture, death can result.*

Aortic Aneurysms

Although aneurysms may develop in the wall of any blood vessel in the body, they almost always form in an artery, such as the aorta. Aortic aneurysms that develop in the chest area, where the aorta branches off from the heart, are called thoracic aneurysms. Aneurysms that develop in the part of the aorta that extends through the abdominal area, as in the Duke of Windsor's case, are called abdominal aneurysms. About 90 percent of aortic aneurysms are abdominal.

Abdominal aneurysms are four times more common in men than in women, and are most prevalent in whites aged 50 to 80. Ruptured aortic aneurysms are the ninth leading killer of American men over 55.

When an aneurysm hemorrhages, blood pours into body cavities. Tissues beyond the rupture are deprived of blood and cannot function properly, causing shock and death if not treated promptly. The larger the aneurysm, the greater the risk of rupture. A person with an abdominal aortic aneurysm that measures over 2½ inches in diameter (over 6 centimeters) faces a 50 percent chance of dying within one year: 75 percent within two years; and over 90 percent within five years.

About a quarter of those with abdominal aneurysms experience pain in the abdomen or lower back that may be mistaken for a kidney stone attack or a ruptured vertebral disk. But in most cases, there are no warning symptoms.

The doctor may see or feel a throbbing, tender mass in the middle or lower abdomen during a routine physical, or may discover the aneurysm by chance when ultrasound imaging is done for some other reason.

Since abdominal aneurysms less than 2 inches (5 centimeters) in diameter rarely rupture, physicians usually prescribe blood pressure-lowering drugs, such as beta blockers, to reduce the pounding of blood against arterial walls. Patients with small aneurysms are monitored regularly with full exams and imaging techniques.

When the aneurysm is large or when there are many, surgeons can replace all or most of the aorta with Dacron tubing. Jere W. Lord Jr., M.D., retired professor of surgery, New York University, calls this "probably the most difficult operation a surgeon is required to perform on a human patient."

Thoracic aneurysms may also be symptomless, and are sometimes discovered unexpectedly on a routine chest x-ray. If symptoms do occur, they include pain in the shoulders, lower back, neck, or abdomen. A dry, brassy cough that doesn't respond to cough medication is another warning signal. The swelling aneurysm may press on the nerve that opens and shuts the vocal cords, causing hoarseness, even loss of voice.

When blood works its way through a tear in the aorta's innermost wall and separates the layers of the artery wall, creating a second channel, a dangerous complication known as a dissecting aortic aneurysm results. The most common symptom is an excruciating tearing or ripping pain in the chest, often mistaken for a heart attack. Unless the aorta is repaired immediately, most people with a dissect-

Table 35.2. Tests to Diagnose Aneurysms.

Angiogram	an x-ray examination of arteries, veins or heart chambers, which is obtained by injecting a radiopaque (contrasting) dye into the bloodstream to make these structures more visible.
Computed tomography (CT) scan	special x-rays used with a computer to provide cross-sectional images or "slices" of body tissues.
Magnetic resonance imaging (MRI)	diagnostic technique that uses the response of atoms to a strong magnetic field to produce cross-sectional images of soft tissues, such as veins and arteries.
Spinal tap	puncture of the spinal cavity with a needle to extract the spinal fluid for diagnostic purposes.
Ultrasound	use of high-frequency sound waves to produce an image or photograph of an organ or tissues. Echocardiography—a diagnostic procedure that uses ultrasound waves to visualize structures within the heart.
X-ray	a photograph obtained by bombarding a target in a vacuum tube with high-velocity electrons, enabling them to penetrate solid matter and act on photographic film.

ing aneurysm die. About 60 percent of thoracic aneurysms dissect; abdominal aneurysms rarely do. Dissecting aneurysms are more common in blacks than whites.

Atherosclerosis, or hardening of the arteries, which weakens artery walls, is a factor in 95 percent of aortic aneurysms. High blood pressure may speed up damage to vessel walls. Aortic aneurysms may also result from congenital defects, heredity, injuries, diabetes, and syphilis.

More than half of patients with one aortic aneurysm will develop another, so physicians use a variety of tests, not available in the Duke of Windsor's time, to monitor patients: computed tomography (CT) scans, ultrasound, echocardiography, or magnetic resonance imaging (MRI).

People who have Marfan's syndrome, a connective tissue disorder, tend to be particularly vulnerable to aortic aneurysms because of weak arterial walls. About 10 percent of patients with aortic aneurysms have Marfan's syndrome.

Berry Aneurysms

Aneurysms that balloon out to look like berries may form in congenitally weak spots in a ring of arteries at the base of the brain known as the circle of Willis. All the brain's major arteries open into this ring, which then circulates blood to the areas of the brain that control movement, sight, feeling, and thinking. The circle of Willis guarantees the brain a continual supply of blood in the event that one of these arteries, such as the carotid, is blocked.

Berry aneurysms have been aptly described as time bombs, because they are liable to burst at any time, resulting in hemorrhagic strokes that affect 30,000 Americans each year. One-third of such ruptures occur during sleep. About half of the people with ruptured berry aneurysms die immediately. Many of the survivors die later from recurring hemorrhage or suffer irreversible brain damage. Ruptured berry aneurysms are most common in people 40 to 60 years old, and in slightly more women than men.

Before berry aneurysms rupture, some people get warning signs. Small amounts of blood may leak from the aneurysm for hours or days, causing headaches, nausea and neck stiffness. Angiograms can locate a suspected unruptured aneurysm.

Unfortunately, in more than 90 percent of cases there are no symptoms until the aneurysm bursts. Rupture results in an excruciating headache, often accompanied by nausea and vomiting. Loss of consciousness that follows may be temporary or may proceed to coma and death. Other symptoms may include personality changes, blurred vision, paralysis on one side of the body, speech impairment, seizures, and difficulty walking or talking, depending on where the rupture occurred and the amount of bleeding.

In some cases, the ruptured artery stops bleeding by itself because swollen brain tissues in the area press against the rupture or a clot forms and plugs the rupture. When a burst aneurysm is suspected, the best diagnostic tool is the computed tomography (CT) scan, which locates the clot and indicates the amount of blood spillage in the brain in 80 percent of cases. A spinal tap (lumbar puncture) will confirm the presence of blood in the cerebrospinal fluid, the watery cushion that protects the brain and spinal cord from shock. Angiograms are usually necessary to show how large and where the rupture is located, and can pinpoint other aneurysms as well.

Neurosurgeons can open the skull and repair the aneurysm, in most cases, by placing a metal clamp at its base. Ideally, this should be done within 48 hours after hemorrhage, because the rupture can start to bleed again at any time. However, when surgery is performed by experienced hands within one to two weeks after hemorrhage on patients in good neurological condition, mortality rate is 5 percent or less. Another danger with subarachnoid hemorrhage—so-called because the blood seeps into the fluid-filled area around the brain called the subarachnoid space—is that an artery near the ruptured aneurysm may constrict or go into spasm, causing another stroke. Nimodipine (Nimotop), a calcium channel-blocking agent, has bee shown to decrease the severity of neurologic damage from spasm in people who have suffered a subarachnoid hemorrhage.

When a patient is very ill, surgery is postponed to allow brain swelling to go down, usually a matter of weeks. Besides bed rest, the patient awaiting surgery may be treated with drugs to reduce severe high blood pressure, corticosteroids to reduce swelling, and analgesics to relieve headache.

Unruptured aneurysms that cause pain or other symptoms by pressing on nerves in the brain should be surgically removed. If they are detected, unruptured aneurysms that cause no symptoms should also be removed if they are more than two-fifths of an inch (10 millimeters) in diameter. Sometimes the tendency to have such aneurysms is inherited.

Medical management of people with a family history of aneurysms is controversial. "If your mother and your sister and your aunt all had aneurysms, and you are one of the worried well, you might want to have some tests," says neurologist Alexander W. Dromerick Jr., M.D., Princeton University researcher and fellow of the Hospital of the University of Pennsylvania. "MRIs are being used to screen asymptomatic relatives, but nobody is quite sure how accurate they are. An MRI will pick up large aneurysms, and some of the smaller ones, but will miss some. A CT scan will pick up evidence of bleeding, but not usually an unruptured aneurysm. What we call the 'gold standard,' the test against which all other tests are measured, is the angiogram. But there's a 1 to 2 percent chance of TIAs [transient ischemic attacks, or ministrokes], stroke and death with an angiogram, and no physician wants to expose an asymptomatic patient to this risk without good reason."

About 20 percent of people initially diagnosed with one berry aneurysm are found to have at least one more. (Berry aneurysms are found in up to 4 percent of routine adult autopsies.) As in other types of aneurysms, atherosclerosis and high blood pressure, which exerts pressure on weakened areas, cause these areas to stretch like a balloon and eventually rupture. Heavy cigarette smoking and cocaine use have also been implicated in aneurysm rupture.

Peripheral Artery Aneurysms

The third most frequent type of aneurysm occurs in the large arteries that run down the leg and in back of the knee (the femoral and popliteal arteries). They chiefly affect men and usually result from atherosclerosis, only occasionally from congenital weakness of arterial walls, injuries, or bacterial infections. They can be felt as throbbing masses in the groin and behind the knee.

Behind-the-knee aneurysms rarely burst, but they may grow so large that they interfere with circulation in the lower leg. Clots may also develop suddenly in the aneurysm, cutting off the supply of blood to the lower leg and foot, possibly leading to and necessitating amputation. Such complications can usually be prevented by replacing the affected part of the artery by a (saphenous) leg vein, as in bypass surgery.

Diagnosis may be confirmed by angiograms, which give a picture of the arteries, or ultrasound, which can determine the size of the arteries. The physician will also look for abdominal aortic aneurysms in these patients, because very often patients have both.

Aneurysms in the groin rupture more frequently than those in the knee, but otherwise are subject to the same kinds of complications. Risk factors for the development of peripheral aneurysms are high blood pressure, high blood cholesterol levels, diabetes, obesity, lack of regular exercise, and the chief culprit, smoking. Since these same risk factors are implicated in heart disease and stroke, lifestyle changes to keep blood vessels healthy will have other health benefits, as well.

—by Evelyn Zamula

Evelyn Zamula is a freelance writer in Potomac, Md.

Chapter 36

Stroke: Brain Attack

Introduction

If you're like most Americans, you plan for your future. When you choose a college, you balance long-range career goals against short-range factors such as size, location, and cost of the school. When you take a job, you examine its pension plan. When you buy a home, you consider its location and condition so that your investment grows. Today, more and more Americans are protecting their most important asset—their health. Are you?

Stroke ranks as the third leading killer in the United States. A stroke can be devastating to individuals and their families, robbing them of their independence. It is the most common cause of adult disability. Each year more than 500,000 Americans have a stroke, with about 145,000 dying from stroke-related causes. Officials at the National Institute of Neurological Disorders and Stroke (NINDS) are committed to reducing that burden through biomedical research.

What Is a Stroke?

A stroke, or "brain attack," occurs when blood circulation to the brain fails. Brain cells can die from decreased blood flow and the resulting lack of oxygen. There are two broad categories of stroke: those

National Institute of Neurological Disorders and Stroke, from http://www.ninds.nih.gov/healinfo/disorder/stroke/strokepr.htm; last updated October 28, 1997.

caused by a blockage of blood flow and those caused by bleeding. While not usually fatal, a blockage of a blood vessel in the brain or neck is the most frequent cause of stroke and is responsible for about 80 percent of strokes. These blockages stem from three conditions: the formation of a clot within a blood vessel of the brain or neck, called thrombosis; the movement of a clot from another part of the body such as the heart to the neck or brain, called embolism; or a severe narrowing of an artery in or leading to the brain, called stenosis. Bleeding into the brain or the spaces surrounding the brain causes the second type of stroke, called hemorrhagic stroke.

Two key steps you can take will lower your risk of death or disability from stroke: know stroke's warning signs and control stroke's risk factors. Scientific research conducted by the NINDS has identified warning signs and a large number of risk factors.

What Are Warning Signs of a Stroke?

Warning signs are clues your body sends that your brain is not receiving enough oxygen. If you observe one or more of these signs of a stroke or "brain attack," don't wait, call a doctor or 911 right away!

- Sudden weakness or numbness of the face, arm, or leg on one side of the body.
- Sudden dimness or loss of vision, particularly in one eye.
- Sudden difficulty speaking or trouble understanding speech.
- Sudden severe headache with no known cause.
- Unexplained dizziness, unsteadiness or sudden falls, especially with any of the other signs.

Other danger signs that may occur include double vision, drowsiness, and nausea or vomiting. Sometimes the warning signs may last only a few moments and then disappear. These brief episodes, known as transient ischemic attacks or TIAs, are sometimes called "mini-strokes." Although brief, they identify an underlying serious condition that isn't going away without medical help. Unfortunately, since they clear up, many people ignore them. Don't. Heeding them can save your life.

What Are Risk Factors for a Stroke?

A risk factor is a condition or behavior that occurs more frequently in those who have, or are at greater risk of getting, a disease than in those who don't. Having a risk factor for stroke doesn't mean you'll have a stroke. On the other hand, not having a risk factor doesn't mean you'll avoid a stroke. But your risk of stroke grows as the number and severity of risk factors increases.

Stroke occurs in all age groups, in both sexes, and in all races in every country. It can even occur before birth, when the fetus is still in the womb. In African-Americans, the death rate from stroke is almost twice that of the white population. Scientists have found more and more severe risk factors in some minority groups and continue to look for patterns of stroke in these groups.

What Are the Treatable Risk Factors?

Some of the most important treatable risk factors for stroke are:

- *High blood pressure.* Also called hypertension, this is by far the most potent risk factor for stroke. If your blood pressure is high, you and your doctor need to work out an individual strategy to bring it down to the normal range. Some ways that work: Maintain proper weight. Avoid drugs known to raise blood pressure. Cut down on salt. Eat fruits and vegetables to increase potassium in your diet. Exercise more. Your doctor may prescribe medicines that help lower blood pressure. Controlling blood pressure will also help you avoid heart disease, diabetes, and kidney failure.

- *Cigarette smoking.* Cigarette smoking has been linked to the buildup of fatty substances in the carotid artery, the main neck artery supplying blood to the brain. Blockage of this artery is the leading cause of stroke in Americans. Also, nicotine raises blood pressure; carbon monoxide reduces the amount of oxygen your blood can carry to the brain; and cigarette smoke makes your blood thicker and more likely to clot. Your doctor can recommend programs and medications that may help you quit smoking. By quitting, at any age, you also reduce your risk of lung disease, heart disease, and a number of cancers including lung cancer.

- *Heart disease.* Common heart disorders such as coronary artery disease, valve defects, irregular heart beat, and enlargement of one of the heart's chambers can result in blood clots that may break loose and block vessels in or leading to the brain. The most common blood vessel disease, caused by the buildup of fatty deposits in the arteries, is called atherosclerosis. Your doctor will treat your heart disease and may also prescribe medication, such as aspirin, to help prevent the formation of clots. Your doctor may recommend surgery to clean out a clogged neck artery if you match a particular profile. If you are over 50, NINDS scientists believe you and your doctor should make a decision about aspirin therapy. A doctor can evaluate your risk factors and help you decide if you will benefit from aspirin or other blood-thinning therapy.

- *Warning signs or history of stroke.* If you experience a TIA, get help at once. Many communities encourage those with stroke's warning signs to dial 911 for emergency medical assistance. If you have had a stroke in the past, it's important to reduce your risk of a second stroke. Your brain helps you recover from a stroke by drawing on backup systems that now do double duty. That means a second stroke can be twice as bad.

- *Diabetes.* You may think this disorder affects only the body's ability to use sugar, or glucose. But it also causes destructive changes in the blood vessels throughout the body, including the brain. Also, if blood glucose levels are high at the time of a stroke, then brain damage is usually more severe and extensive than when blood glucose is well-controlled. Treating diabetes can delay the onset of complications that increase the risk of stroke.

Do You Know Your Stroke Risk?

Some of the most important risk factors for stroke can be determined during a physical exam at your doctor's office. If you are over 55 years old, a worksheet in a pamphlet available from the NINDS can help you estimate your risk of stroke and show the benefit of risk-factor control. The worksheet was developed from NINDS-supported work in the well-known Framingham Study. Working with your doctor, you can develop a strategy to lower your risk to average or even below average for your age. Many risk factors for stroke can be managed, some very successfully. Although risk is never zero at any age, by starting early and controlling your risk factors you can lower your risk of death or disability from stroke. With good control, the risk of stroke in most age groups can be kept below that for accidental injury or death.

To obtain a copy of the worksheet, write requesting the pamphlet *Brain Basics: Preventing Stroke* from the NINDS Office of Scientific and Health Reports.

National Institute of Neurological Disorders and Stroke
Office of Scientific and Health Reports
P.O. Box 5801
Bethesda, MD 20824

Americans have shown that stroke is preventable and treatable. A better understanding of the causes of stroke has helped Americans make lifestyle changes that have cut the stroke death rate nearly in half in the last two decades. More than a million stroke survivors suffer little or no long-lasting disability from their strokes. Another two million, however, live with the crippling and lifelong disabilities of paralysis, loss of speech, and poor memory. Scientists at the NINDS predict that, with continued attention to reducing the risks of stroke and by using currently available therapies and developing new ones, Americans should be able to prevent 80 percent of all strokes by the end of the decade.

Chapter 37

Fainting

Passing out is usually scary but not always serious: You felt fine. Then with little warning, you found yourself lying on the floor with a circle of concerned faces peering down at you.

One in three people faints at least once in a lifetime, most often after age 65. Although frightening and maybe a bit embarrassing, fainting generally isn't a reason to panic.

When the Lights Go Out

Fainting, also called syncope (SING-kuh-pe), occurs when not enough oxygen-rich blood reaches your brain. Without adequate oxygen, brain metabolism slows, causing you to lose consciousness briefly.

You may have no warning. But usually you feel nauseated or lightheaded, become sweaty and pale, then experience a graying out of your vision.

Within about a minute of lying flat, sufficient blood flow to your brain is restored and you regain consciousness.

A Symptom with Many Causes

About 25 percent of adults faint because of a heart condition (see "When Fainting Signals Something Serious"). In as many as 35 percent of people, the reason is unknown.

Reprinted from January 1996 *Mayo Clinic Health Letter* with permission of Mayo Foundation for Medical Education and Research, Rochester, Minnesota 55905. For subscription information, call 1-800-333-9038.

In other cases, fainting may be due to a drop in blood pressure related to these factors:

Standing Too Quickly. When you stand, your sympathetic nervous system triggers release of the hormone adrenaline. This leads to an increase in your heart rate and blood pressure, preserving adequate blood flow to your brain.

With age, this cardiovascular response can slow. Standing too quickly may cause blood to pool in your legs, leading to a sudden drop in blood pressure.

Medications. High blood pressure drugs and antiarrhythmics that slow heart rate are typically associated with fainting.

These drugs can make you more susceptible to blood pressure changes. They also can keep your heart from beating fast enough to meet higher demands caused by a change in position or activity.

Anxiety. Emotional stress or sudden severe pain can trigger interplay between your neurologic and cardiovascular systems that results in stimulation of your vagus nerve. This signals your heart to slow and your arteries to dilate. When the changes occur too quickly, blood pressure drops suddenly.

Activity. Adequate sodium helps maintain blood pressure. Sodium lost through excessive sweat during strenuous activity, especially in heat and humidity, can lead to a drop in blood pressure.

Ways to Prevent Fainting

A few simple steps may keep you from fainting:

Lower Your Head. If you feel as though you're going to faint, lie down. Raise your legs above the level of your head to increase blood flow to your brain. If you can't lie down, sit or bend forward with your head between your knees. Wait until the lightheadedness or nausea has subsided before trying to stand.

Stand Slowly. This gives your blood pressure and heart rate more time to adjust to an upright position.

Check Medications. If a new drug or change in prescription causes occasional lightheadedness, talk with your doctor. You may need an adjustment in your dosage.

If you take several medications, don't take them all at the same time unless your doctor advises otherwise. The combined effect may over whelm your body's ability to maintain homeostasis.

Pace Yourself. When working or exercising in heat and humidity, take frequent breaks and drink plenty of liquids.

Don't Minimize Fainting

If you have a chronic health condition such as cardiovascular disease, high blood pressure or diabetes coupled with recurrent fainting, have your doctor evaluate the problem. Contact your doctor about even a single fainting episode if you're more than 40 years old.

When Fainting Signals Something Serious

Serious causes of fainting typically involve problems with your heart or the blood vessels leading to your brain. An irregular rhythm, the most common heart condition, reduces blood pumped from your heart. Severe narrowing of your aortic valve (aortic stenosis) or accumulation of plaque in your carotid arteries may cause fainting by limiting blood flow to your brain.

See your doctor right away if fainting occurs without warning, when you turn your head or extend your neck, or when accompanied by:

- Irregular heartbeat
- Chest pain
- Shortness of breath
- Blurred vision
- Confusion
- Trouble talking

Chapter 38

Hypotension

Hypotension is a drop in blood pressure. It results in symptoms such as fainting and lightheadedness, since blood flow to the brain decreases. There are two main forms:

- *Orthostatic hypotension* refers to a drop in blood pressure usually due to changes in posture. Orthostatic hypotension is experienced most commonly upon standing upright after lying down or sitting.

- *Postprandial hypotension* refers to a drop in blood pressure following a meal. Although postprandial hypotension can occur with posture change, it is distinct in that it is meal-induced.

In both cases, the drop in blood pressure is almost always greater than or equal to 20/10 mm Hg. (Example: Normal blood pressure is 120/80 mm Hg. Hypotension may cause a drop to 100/70 mm Hg and may be associated with symptoms.)

Hypotension is common in the elderly and affects more people with advancing age. Recent research suggests postprandial hypotension may be more common in the elderly than orthostatic hypotension.

Symptoms

Hypotension can lead to the following symptoms:

An undated fact sheet produced by the National Heart, Lung, and Blood Institute.

- syncope (fainting)
- lightheadedness
- dizziness
- confusion
- weakness
- nausea
- vision that is spotted or blurred
- angina (chest pain)
- difficulties in walking
- frequent falls

Causes

Orthostatic Hypotension

A number of different disorders can cause orthostatic hypotension. These disorders affect the body's ability to maintain normal blood pressure. Here are some terms related to hypotension:

- *Autonomic neuropathies* are diseases that affect the peripheral nervous system, which consists of nerves outside the brain and spinal cord.

- *Baroreceptor dysfunction* means the pressure-sensitive nerve endings that control blood pressure do not work properly.

- *Endocrinologic disorders* are problems with glands (and/or the hormones these glands secrete) of the endocrine system such as the thyroid and pancreas.

- *Vascular insufficiency* is a term used to describe inadequate blood flow in the blood vessels.

- *Hypovolemic disorders* indicate low blood volume.

Drugs can also cause orthostatic hypotension. The most common drugs known to contribute to orthostatic hypotension are tricyclic antidepressants, diuretics, antihypertensives, vasodilators, clonidine, and marijuana.

Postprandial Hypotension

The causes of postprandial hypotension are not fully understood. Research suggests that, with the process of aging, blood pressure regulation may be negatively affected or that specific diseases may impair the ability of the body to maintain normal blood pressure. Additional studies are necessary to determine whether these theories are in fact true.

Diagnosis

Hypotension can be determined by blood pressure measurement. Blood pressure should be measured while standing, sitting, and lying down as well as before and after meals in order to observe blood pressure changes.

Other diagnostic procedures are often necessary to determine the underlying cause of hypotension if the reason for it is unknown. These tests will vary according to each patient's symptoms.

Treatment

In *orthostatic hypotension* the goals of treatment are (1) to make sure that there is an adequate flow of blood to the brain in the upright position (when standing or sitting), (2) to avoid situations that cause blood pressure to drop when upright, and (3) to reduce symptoms. Common drugs used to treat orthostatic hypotension include fludrocortisone and α_1-adrenergic agonists.

Treatment will vary according to the patient since the best way to treat hypotension is to treat the underlying cause.

In *postprandial hypotension*, treatment is aimed at reducing symptoms. Be aware that the risks of syncope (fainting) and falling are greatest 15 to 90 minutes following a meal. Also, ask your doctor if you are taking any medications that lower blood pressure or blood volume. You may be able to stop taking them.

To lessen symptoms, you may be advised by your doctor to do the following:

- Take any hypotension medicine prescribed by your doctor *between* meals rather than during meals.

- Eat frequent small meals rather than three large meals a day.

- Avoid alcohol before and after meals (if you drink, it is better to do so during meals).

- Drink lots of fluids.

- Increase caffeine intake (although this recommendation is controversial).

- Avoid sitting or standing for long periods after meals.

Prognosis

The outlook for patients with hypotension depends on the underlying cause of their condition. Usually hypotension can be controlled so that daily activities can take place without difficulty.

Seeking Help

If you are experiencing any symptoms of hypotension, you should see a doctor at once.

For Related Information

For more information on the diseases that can cause hypotension, contact:

National Institute of Neurological Disorders and Stroke (NINDS)
Building 31, Room 8A06
31 Center Drive, MSC 2540
Bethesda, MD 20892-2540
 (301) 496-5751

National Institute of Diabetes and Digestive and Kidney Disorders
(NIDDK)
Building 31, Room 9A04
31 Center Drive, MSC 2560
Bethesda, MD 20892-2560
 (301) 496-3583

Chapter 39

Hypertension

It's Important to Know about High Blood Pressure

High blood pressure, also called hypertension, is a risk factor for heart and kidney diseases and stroke. This means that having high blood pressure increases your chance (or risk) of getting heart or kidney disease, or of having a stroke. This is serious business: Heart disease is the number one killer in the United States, and stroke is the third most common cause of death.

About one in every four American adults has high blood pressure. High blood pressure is especially dangerous because it often gives no warning signs or symptoms. Fortunately, though, you can find out if you have high blood pressure by having your blood pressure checked regularly. If it is high, you can take steps to lower it. Just as important, if your blood pressure is normal, you can learn how to keep it from becoming high. This text will tell you how.

The National High Blood Pressure Education Program

The National Heart, Lung, and Blood Institute—part of the National Institutes of Health—sponsors a nationwide education program to help people avoid the ill effects of high blood pressure, and to help prevent high blood pressure altogether.

The National High Blood Pressure Education Program (NHBPEP), coordinated by the National Heart, Lung, and Blood Institute

NIH Publication No. 94-3281, May 1994.

(NHLBI), works to reduce death and disability related to high blood pressure. The program also promotes prevention of this important public health problem. This nationwide network is composed of many organizations and gives information to health professionals, patients, family members, and the public about the dangers of this serious problem.

The progress made to date has been impressive. The NHBPEP has helped to improve blood pressure control, contributing to a 50 percent decrease in deaths from coronary heart disease and a 57 percent decrease in deaths from stroke over the last 20 years. Many Americans are alive today because they are controlling their high blood pressure.

What Is Blood Pressure—And What Happens When It Is High?

Since blood is carried from the heart to all of your body's tissues and organs in vessels called arteries, blood pressure is the force of the blood pushing against the walls of those arteries. In fact, each time the heart beats (about 60-70 times a minute at rest), it pumps out blood into the arteries. Your blood pressure is at its greatest when the heart contracts and is pumping the blood. This is called systolic pressure. When the heart is at rest, in between beats, your blood pressure falls. This is the diastolic pressure.

Blood pressure is always given as these two numbers, systolic and diastolic pressures. Both are important. Usually they are written one above or before the other, such as 120/80 mm Hg, with the top number the systolic, and the bottom the diastolic.

Different actions make your blood pressure go up or down. For example, if you run for a bus, your blood pressure goes up. When you sleep at night, your blood pressure goes down. These changes in blood pressure are normal. Some people have blood pressure that stays up all or most of the time. Their blood pushes against the walls of their arteries with higher-than-normal force. If untreated this can lead to serious medical problems like these:

- *Arteriosclerosis ("hardening of the arteries")*. High blood pressure harms the arteries by making them thick and stiff. This speeds the build up of cholesterol and fats in the blood vessels like rust in a pipe, which prevents the blood from flowing through the body, and in time can lead to a heart attack or stroke.

- *Heart attack*. Blood carries oxygen to the body. When the arteries that bring blood to the heart muscle become blocked, the heart cannot get enough oxygen. Reduced blood flow can cause chest pain (angina). Eventually, the flow may be stopped completely, causing a heart attack.

- *Enlarged heart.* High blood pressure causes the heart to work harder. Over time, this causes the heart to thicken and stretch. Eventually the heart fails to function normally causing fluids to back up into the lungs. Controlling high blood pressure can prevent this from happening.

- *Kidney damage.* The kidney acts as a filter to rid the body of wastes. Over a number of years, high blood pressure can narrow and thicken the blood vessels of the kidney. The kidney filters less fluid and waste builds up in the blood. The kidneys may fail altogether. When this happens, medical treatment (dialysis) or a kidney transplant may be needed.

- *Stroke.* High blood pressure can harm the arteries, causing them to narrow faster. So, less blood can get to the brain. If a blood clot blocks one of the narrowed arteries, a stroke (thrombotic stroke) may occur. A stroke can also occur when very high pressure causes a break in a weakened blood vessel in the brain (hemorrhagic stroke).

Who's Likely to Develop High Blood Pressure?

Anyone can develop high blood pressure, but some people are more likely to develop it than others. For example, high blood pressure is more common—it develops earlier and is more severe—in African-Americans than in whites. In the early and middle adult years, men have high blood pressure more often than women. But as men and women age, the reverse is true. More women after menopause have high blood pressure than men of the same age. And the number of both men and women with high blood pressure increases rapidly in older age groups. More than half of all Americans over age 65 have high blood pressure. And older African-American women who live in the Southeast are more likely to have high blood pressure than those in other regions of the United States. In fact, the southeastern states have some of the highest rates of death from stroke. High blood pressure is the key risk factor for stroke. Other risk factors include cigarette smoking and overweight. These 11 states—Alabama, Arkansas, Georgia, Indiana, Kentucky, Louisiana, Mississippi, North Carolina,

South Carolina, Tennessee, and Virginia—have such high rates of stroke among persons of all races and in both sexes that they are called the "Stroke Belt States."

Finally, heredity can make some families more likely than others to get high blood pressure. If your parents or grandparents had high blood pressure, your risk may be increased. While it is mainly a disease of adults, high blood pressure can occur in children as well. Even if everyone is healthy, be sure you and your family get your blood pressure checked. Remember high blood pressure has no signs or symptoms.

How Is Blood Pressure Checked?

Having your blood pressure checked is quick easy, and painless. Your blood pressure is measured with an instrument called a sphygmomanometer (sfig'-mo-ma-nom-e-ter).

It works like this: A blood pressure cuff is wrapped around your upper arm and inflated to stop the blood flow in your artery for a few seconds. A valve is opened and air is then released from the cuff and the sounds of your blood rushing through an artery are heard through a stethoscope. The first sound heard and registered on the gauge or mercury column is called the systolic blood pressure. It represents the maximum pressure in the artery produced as the heart contracts and the blood begins to flow. The last sound heard as more air is released from the cuff is the diastolic blood pressure. It represents the lowest pressure that remains within the artery when the heart is at rest.

What Do the Numbers Mean?

Blood pressure is always expressed in two numbers that represent the systolic and diastolic pressures. These numbers are measurements of millimeters (mm) of mercury (Hg). The measurement is written one above or before the other, with the systolic number on the top and the diastolic number on the bottom. For example, a blood pressure measurement of 120/80 mm Hg is expressed verbally as "120 over 80." Table 39.1 shows categories for blood pressure levels in adults.

If your blood pressure is less than 140/90 mm Hg it is considered normal. However, a blood pressure below 120/80 mm Hg is even better for your heart and blood vessels. People used to think that low blood pressure (for example, 105/65 mm Hg in an adult) was unhealthy. Except for rare cases, this is not true. High blood pressure or "hypertension" is classified by stages and is more serious as the numbers get higher.

Table 39.1. Categories for Blood Pressure Levels in Adults (Age 18 Years and Older).

Category	Blood Pressure Level (mm Hg)	
	Systolic	Diastolic
Normal	<130	<85
High normal	130-139	85-89
Hypertension*		
Stage 1	140-159	90-99
Stage 2	160-179	100-109
Stage 3	180-209	110-119
Stage 4	210 or higher	120 or higher

*Note: "Hypertension" is the medical term for high blood pressure. These categories are from the National High Blood Pressure Education Program, JNCV report.

What Causes High Blood Pressure?

For most people, there is no single known cause of high blood pressure. This type of high blood pressure is called "primary" or "essential" hypertension. This type of blood pressure can't be cured, although in most cases it can be controlled. That's why it's so important for everyone to take steps to reduce their chances of developing high blood pressure.

In a few people, high blood pressure can be traced to a known cause like tumors of the adrenal gland, chronic kidney disease, hormone abnormalities, use of birth control pills, or pregnancy. This is called "secondary hypertension." Secondary hypertension is usually cured if its cause passes or is corrected.

How Can You Prevent High Blood Pressure?

Everyone—regardless of race, age, sex, or heredity—can help lower their chance of developing high blood pressure. Here's how:

1. Maintain a healthy weight, lose weight if you are overweight,
2. Be more physically active,
3. Choose foods lower in salt and sodium, and
4. If you drink alcoholic beverages, do so in moderation.

These rules are also recommended for treating high blood pressure, although medicine is often added as part of the treatment. It is far better to keep your blood pressure from getting high in the first place.

Another important measure for your health is to not smoke: While cigarette smoking is not directly related to high blood pressure, it increases your risk of heart attack and stroke.

Let's look more closely at the four rules to prevent high blood pressure and for keeping a healthy heart:

1. Maintain a Healthy Weight; Lose Weight If You Are Overweight

As your body weight increases, your blood pressure rises. In fact, being overweight can make you two to six times more likely to develop high blood pressure than if you are at your desirable weight. Keeping your weight in the desirable range is not only important to prevent high blood pressure but also for your overall health and well being.

It's not just how much you weigh that's important: It also matters where your body stores extra fat. Your shape is inherited from your parents just like the color of your eyes or hair. Some people tend to gain weight around their belly; others, around the hips and thighs. "Apple-shaped" people who have a pot belly (that is, extra fat at the waist) appear to have higher health risks than "pear-shaped" people with heavy hips and thighs.

No matter where the extra weight is, you can reduce your risk of high blood pressure by losing weight. Even small amounts of weight loss can make a big difference in helping to prevent high blood pressure. Losing weight, if you are overweight and already have high blood pressure, can also help lower your pressure.

To lose weight, you need to eat fewer calories than you burn. But don't go on a crash diet to see how quickly you can lose those pounds. The healthiest and longest-lasting weight loss happens when you do it slowly, losing ½ to 1 pound a week. By cutting back by 500 calories a day by eating less and being more physically active, you can lose about 1 pound (which equals 3,500 calories) in a week.

Losing weight and keeping it off involves a new way of eating and increasing physical activity for life. Here's how to eat and get on your way to a lower weight:

- **Choose foods low in calories and fat.** Naturally, choosing low-calorie foods cuts calories. But did you know that choosing foods low in fat also cuts calories? Fat is a concentrated source of calories, so eating fewer fatty foods will reduce calorie intake. Some examples of fatty foods to cut down on are: butter, margarine, regular salad dressings, fatty meats, skin of poultry, whole-milk dairy foods like cheese, fried foods, and many cookies, cakes, pastries and snacks.

  Try these low fat foods: baked, broiled, or poached chicken and turkey (without the skin); fish; lean cuts of meat (like round or sirloin); skim or 1% milk or evaporated skim milk; lower-fat, low-sodium cheeses; fresh, frozen, or canned fruit; fresh, frozen, or canned (no salt added) vegetables (without cream or cheese sauces); plain rice and pasta; English muffins, bagels, sandwich breads and rolls, soft tortillas; cold (ready-to-eat) cereals lower in sodium; cooked hot cereals (not instant because it is higher in sodium). Note: When choosing cheeses, breads, and cereals, use the food label to choose those lower in fat and sodium.

- **Choose foods high in starch and fiber.** Foods high in starch and fiber are excellent substitutes for foods high in fat. They are lower in calories than foods high in fat. These foods are also good sources of vitamins and minerals.

  Foods high in starch and/or fiber: fruits, vegetables, whole-grain cereals, pasta and rice, whole-grain breads, dry peas and beans. Note: Use the food label to choose breads and cereals lower in sodium.

- **Limit serving sizes.** To lose weight, it's not just the type of foods you eat that's important, but also the amount. To take in fewer calories, you need to limit your portion sizes. Try especially to take smaller helpings of high calorie foods like high fat meats and cheeses. And try not to go back for seconds.

  Here's a good tip to help you control or change your eating habits: Keep track of what you eat, when you eat, and why, by writing it down. Note whether you snack on high fat foods in front of the television, or if you skip breakfast and then eat a large

A SAMPLE WALKING PROGRAM

	Warm up	Target zone exercising*	Cool down time	Total
Week 1				
Session A	Walk normally 5 min.	Then walk briskly 5 min.	Then walk normally 5 min.	15 min.
Session B	Repeat above pattern			
Session C	Repeat above pattern			

Continue with at least three exercise sessions during each week of the program. If you find a particular week's pattern tiring, repeat it before going on to the next pattern. You do not have to complete the walking program in 12 weeks.

Week 2	Walk 5 min.	Walk briskly 7 min.	Walk 5 min.	17 min.
Week 3	Walk 5 min.	Walk briskly 9 min.	Walk 5 min.	19 min.
Week 4	Walk 5 min.	Walk briskly 11 min.	Walk 5 min.	21 min.
Week 5	Walk 5 min.	Walk briskly 13 min.	Walk 5 min.	23 min.
Week 6	Walk 5 min.	Walk briskly 15 min.	Walk 5 min.	25 min.
Week 7	Walk 5 min.	Walk briskly 18 min.	Walk 5 min.	28 min.
Week 8	Walk 5 min.	Walk briskly 20 min.	Walk 5 min.	30 min.
Week 9	Walk 5 min.	Walk briskly 23 min.	Walk 5 min.	33 min.
Week 10	Walk 5 min.	Walk briskly 26 min.	Walk 5 min.	36 min.
Week 11	Walk 5 min.	Walk briskly 28 min.	Walk 5 min.	38 min.
Week 12	Walk 5 min.	Walk briskly 30 min.	Walk 5 min.	40 min.

Week 13 on:

Check your pulse periodically to see if you are exercising within your target zone. As you get more in shape, try exercising within the upper range of your target zone. Gradually increase your brisk walking time to 30 to 60 minutes, three or four times a week. Remember that your goal is to get the benefits you are seeking and enjoy your activity.

* Here's how to check if you are within your target heart rate zone:

1) Right after you stop exercising, take your pulse: Place the tips of your first two fingers lightly over one of the blood vessels on your neck, just to the left or right of your Adam's apple. Or try the pulse spot inside your wrist just below the base of your thumb.

2) Count your pulse for 10 seconds and multiply the number by 6.

3) Compare the number to the right grouping below: Look for the age grouping that is closest to your age and read the line across. For example, if you are 43, the closest age on the chart is 45; the target zone is 88-131 beats per minute.

AGE	Target HR Zone
20 years	100-150 beats per minute
25 years	98-146 beats per minute
30 years	95-142 beats per minute
35 years	93-138 beats per minute
40 years	90-135 beats per minute
45 years	88-131 beats per minute
50 years	85-127 beats per minute
55 years	83-123 beats per minute
60 years	80-120 beats per minute
65 years	78-116 beats per minute
70 years	75-113 beats per minute

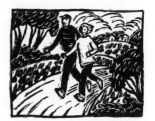

SOURCE: *Exercise and Your Heart*, National Heart, Lung, and Blood Institute and the American Heart Association, NIH Publication No. 93-1677.

Figure 39.2. A Sample Walking Program.

lunch. Once you see your habits, you can set goals for yourself: Cut back on TV snacks and, when you do snack, have fresh fruit, unsalted air-popped popcorn, or unsalted pretzels. If there's no time for breakfast at home, take a low fat muffin, bagel (skip the cream cheese), or cereal with you to eat at work. Changing your behavior will help you change your weight for the better.

- **Increase physical activity.** There's more to weight loss than just eating less. Another important ingredient is increasing physical activity, which burns calories. Cutting down on fat and calories combined with regular physical activity can help you lose more weight and keep it off longer than either way by itself.

2. Be More Physically Active

Besides losing weight, there are other reasons to be more active: Being physically active can reduce your risk for heart disease, help lower your total cholesterol level and raise HDL-cholesterol (the "good" cholesterol that does not build up in the arteries), and help lower high blood pressure. And people who are physically active have a lower risk of getting high blood pressure—20 to 50 percent lower-than people who are not active.

You don't have to be a marathon runner to benefit from physical activity. Even light activities, if done daily, can help lower your risk of heart disease. So you can fit physical activity into your daily routine in small but important ways: take a walk at lunch time or after dinner; use the stairs instead of the elevator; get off the bus one or two stops early and walk the rest of the way; park farther away from the store or office; ride a bike; work in the yard or garden; go dancing.

More vigorous exercise has added benefits. It helps improve the fitness of the heart and lungs. And that in turn protects you more against heart disease. Activities like swimming, brisk walking, running, and jumping rope are called "aerobic." This means that the body uses oxygen to make the energy it needs for the activity. Aerobic activities can condition your heart and lungs if done at the right intensity for at least 30 minutes, three to four times a week. But if you don't have 30 minutes for a break, try to find two 15-minute periods or even three 10-minute periods. Try to do some type of aerobic activity in the course of a week.

MEAT, POULTRY, FISH, AND SHELLFISH

Fresh meat (including lean cuts of beef, pork, lamb and veal),poultry, finfish, cooked, 3 oz	Less than 90
Shellfish, 3 oz	100-325
Tuna, canned, 3 oz	300
*Sausage,2 oz	515
*Bologna, 2 oz	535
*Frankfurter, 1-1/2 oz	560
Boiled ham, 2 oz	750
Lean ham, 3 oz	1,025

EGGS

Egg white, 1	55
*Whole egg, 1	65
Egg substitute, 1/4 cup =1 egg	80-120

DAIRY PRODUCTS

Milk

*Whole milk, 1 cup	120
Skim or 1% milk, 1 cup	125
Buttermilk (salt added), 1 cup	260

Cheese

*Natural cheese:	
*Swiss cheese, 1 oz	75
*Cheddar cheese, 1 oz	175
*Blue cheese, 1 oz	395
Low fat cheese, 1 oz	150
*Process cheese and cheese spreads, 1 oz	340-450
Lower sodium and fat versions	Read the label
*Cottage cheese (regular), 1/2 cup	455
Cottage cheese (low fat), 1/2 cup	460

Yogurt

*Yogurt, whole milk, plain, 8 oz	105
Yogurt, fruited or flavored, low fat or nonfat, 8 oz	120-150
Yogurt, nonfat or low fat, plain, 8 oz	160-175

VEGETABLES

Fresh or frozen vegetables, or no salt added canned (cooked without salt), 1/2 cup	Less than 70
Vegetables, canned, no sauce, 1/2 cup	55-470
*Vegetables, canned or frozen with sauce, 1/2 cup	Read the label
Tomato juice, canned, 3/4 cup	660

BREADS, CEREALS, RICE, PASTA, DRY PEAS AND BEANS

Breads and crackers

Bread, 1 slice	110-175
English muffin, 1/2	130
Bagel, 1/2	190
Cracker, saltine type, 5 squares	195
*Baking powder biscuit, 1	305

Cereals

Ready-to-eat

Shredded wheat, 3/4 cup	Less than 5
Puffed wheat and rice cereals, 1-1/2 to 1-2/3 cup	Less than 5
Granola-type cereals, 1/2 cup	5-25
Ring and nugget cereals, 1 cup	170-310
Flaked cereals, 2/3 to 1 cup	170-360

Cooked

Cooked cereal (unsalted), 1/2 cup	Less than 5
Instant cooked cereal, 1 packet = 3/4 cup	180

Pasta and rice

Cooked rice and pasta, (unsalted), 1/2 cup	Less than 10
*Flavored rice mix, cooked, 1/2 cup	250-390

Peas and beans

Peanut butter, unsalted, 2 tbsp	Less than 5
Peanut butter, 2 tbsp	150
Dry beans, home cooked, (unsalted), or no salt added canned, 1/2 cup	Less than 5
Dry beans, plain, canned, 1/2 cup	350-590
*Dry beans, canned with added fat or meat, 1/2 cup	425-630

FRUITS

Fruits (fresh, frozen, canned), 1/2 cup	Less than 10

FATS AND OILS

Oil, 1 tbsp	0
*Butter, unsalted, 1 tsp	1
*Butter, salted, 1 tsp	25
Margarine, unsalted, 1 tsp	Less than 5
Margarine, salted, 1 tsp	50
Imitation mayonnaise, 1 tbsp	75
*Mayonnaise, 1 tbsp	80
Prepared salad dressings, low calorie, 2 tbsp	50-310
*Prepared salad dressings, 2 tbsp	210-440

SNACKS

Popcorn, chips, and nuts

Unsalted nuts, 1/4 cup	Less than 5
Salted nuts, 1/4 cup	185
*Unsalted potato chips and corn chips, 1 cup	Less than 5
*Salted potato chips and corn chips, 1 cup	170-285
Unsalted popcorn, 2-1/2 cups	Less than 10
Salted popcorn, 2-1/2 cups	330

Candy

Jelly beans, 10 large	5
*Milk chocolate bar, 1 oz. bar	25

Frozen desserts

*Ice cream, 1/2 cup	35-50
Frozen yogurt, low fat or nonfat, 1/2 cup	40-55
Ice milk, 1/2 cup	55-60

CONDIMENTS

Mustard, chili sauce, hot sauce, 1 tsp	35-65
Catsup, steak sauce, 1 tbsp	100-230
Salsa, tartar sauce, 2 tbsp	200-315
Salt, 1/6 tsp	390
Pickles, 5 slices	280-460
Soy sauce, lower sodium, 1 tbsp	600
Soy sauce, 1 tbsp	1030

CONVENIENCE FOODS

**Canned and dehydrated soups, 1 cup	600-1,300
**Lower sodium versions	Read label
***Canned and frozen main dishes, 8 oz	500-1,570
***Lower sodium versions	Read label

*Choices are higher in saturated fat, cholesterol, or both.

**Creamy soups are higher in saturated fat and cholesterol.

***Limit main dishes that have ingredients higher in saturated fat, cholesterol, or both.

Source: Adapted from Home and Garden Bulletin 253-7, United States Department of Agriculture, July 1993.

Figure 39.3. Sodium in Foods (in milligrams).

Most people don't need to see a doctor before they start exercising, since a gradual, sensible exercise program has few health risks. But if you have a health problem like high blood pressure; if you have pains or pressure in the chest or shoulder area; if you tend to feel dizzy or faint; if you get very breathless after a mild workout; or are middle-age or older and have not been active, and you are planning a vigorous exercise program, you should check with your doctor first. Otherwise, get out, get active, and get fit-and help prevent high blood pressure. The sample walking program described in Figure 39.2 can help you get started.

3. *Choose Foods Lower in Salt and Sodium*

Americans eat more salt (sodium chloride) and other forms of sodium than they need. And guess what? They also have higher rates of high blood pressure than people in other countries who eat less salt. Often, if people with high blood pressure cut back on salt and sodium, their blood pressure falls. Cutting back on salt and sodium also prevents blood pressure from rising. Some people like African-Americans and the elderly are more affected by sodium than others. Since there's really no practical way to predict exactly who will be affected by sodium, it makes sense to limit intake of salt and sodium to help prevent high blood pressure. All Americans, especially people with high blood pressure, should eat no more than about 6 gams of salt a day, which equals about 2,400 milligrams of sodium. That's about 1 teaspoon of table salt. But remember to keep track of ALL salt eaten—including that in processed foods and added during cooking or at the table. Americans eat 4,000 to 6,000 milligrams of sodium a day, so most people need to cut back on salt and sodium. See Figure 39.3 for the range of sodium in some types of foods.

You can teach your taste buds to enjoy less salty foods. Here are a few tips:

- Check food labels for the amount of sodium in foods. Choose those lower in sodium most of the time. Look for products that say "sodium free," "very low sodium," "low sodium," "light in sodium," "reduced or less sodium," or "unsalted," especially on cans, boxes, bottles, and bags.

- Buy fresh, plain frozen, or canned with "no salt added" vegetables. Use fresh poultry, fish and lean meat, rather than canned or processed types.

- Use herbs, spices, and salt-free seasoning blends in cooking and at the table instead of salt. Try these foods with the suggested flavorings, spices, and herbs:

  Meat, Poultry, and Fish
  Beef. Bay leaf, marjoram, nutmeg, onion, pepper, sage, thyme
  Lamb. Curry powder, garlic, rosemary, mint
  Pork. Garlic, onion, sage, pepper, oregano
  Veal. Bay leaf, curry powder, ginger, marjoram, oregano
  Chicken. Ginger, marjoram, oregano, paprika, poultry seasoning, rosemary, sage, tarragon, thyme
  Fish. Curry powder, dill, dry mustard, lemon juice, marjoram, paprika, pepper

  Vegetables
  Carrots. Cinnamon, cloves, marjoram, nutmeg, rosemary, sage
  Corn. Cumin, curry powder, onion, paprika, parsley
  Green beans. Dill, curry powder, lemon juice, marjoram, oregano, tarragon, thyme
  Greens. Onion, pepper
  Potatoes. Dill, garlic, onion, paprika, parsley, sage
  Summer squash. Cloves, curry powder, marjoram, nutmeg, rosemary, sage
  Winter squash. Cinnamon, ginger, nutmeg, onion
  Tomatoes. Basil, bay leaf, dill, marjoram, onion, oregano, parsley, pepper

- Cook rice, pasta, and hot cereals without salt. Cut back on instant or flavored rice, pasta, and cereal mixes because they usually have added salt.

- Choose "convenience" foods that are lower in sodium. Cut back on frozen dinners, mixed dishes like pizza, packaged mixes, canned soups or broths, and salad dressings which often have a lot of sodium.

- When available, buy low- or reduced-sodium, or "no-salt-added" versions of foods like these: Canned soup, dried soup mixes, bouillon; Canned vegetables and vegetable juices; Cheeses, lower in fat; Margarine; Condiments like catsup, soy sauce;

Crackers and baked goods; Processed lean meats; Snack foods like chips, pretzels, nuts

- Rinse canned foods like tuna to remove some sodium.

4. If You Drink Alcoholic Beverages, Do So in Moderation

Drinking too much alcohol can raise your blood pressure. It may also lead to the development of high blood pressure. So to help prevent high blood pressure, if you drink alcohol, limit how much you drink to no more than 2 drinks a day. The "Dietary Guidelines for Americans" recommend that for overall health women should limit their alcohol to no more than 1 drink a day.

This is what counts as a drink:

- 1½ ounces of 80-proof or 1 ounce of 100-proof whiskey,
- 5 ounces of wine, or
- 12 ounces of beer (regular or light).

You may have heard that some alcohol is good for your heart health. Some news reports suggest that people who consume a drink or two a day have lower blood pressure and live longer than those who consume no alcohol or those who consume excessive amounts of alcohol. Others note that wine raises the "good" blood cholesterol that prevents the build up of fats in the arteries. While these news stories may be correct they don't tell the whole story: Too much alcohol contributes to a host of other health problems, such as motor vehicle accidents, diseases of the liver and pancreas, damage to the brain and heart, an increased risk of many cancers, and fetal alcohol syndrome. Alcohol is also high in calories. So you should limit how much you drink.

What Else Might Prevent High Blood Pressure?

Other things also may help prevent blood pressure. Here's a roundup of what's being said about them—and whether it's true or false.

Dietary Supplements: Potassium, Calcium, Magnesium, Fish Oils

- **Potassium.** Eating foods rich in potassium appears to protect some people from developing high blood pressure. You probably can get enough potassium from your diet, so a supplement isn't

341

necessary. Many fruits, vegetables, dairy foods, and fish are good sources of potassium. These include: catfish; lean pork; lean veal; cod; flounder; trout; milk; yogurt; dry peas and beans; green beans; apricots; peaches; bananas; prunes and prune juice; orange juice; lima beans; stewed tomatoes; spinach; plantain; sweet potatoes; pumpkin; potatoes; and winter squash.

- **Calcium.** Populations with low calcium intakes have high rates of high blood pressure. However, it has not been proven that taking calcium tablets will prevent high blood pressure. But it is important to be sure to get at least the recommended amount of calcium—800 milligrams per day for adults (pregnant and breast-feeding women need more)—from the foods you eat. Dairy foods like, low fat selections of milk, yogurt, and cheese are good sources of calcium. Low fat and nonfat dairy products have even more calcium than the high fat types.

- **Magnesium.** A diet low in magnesium may make your blood pressure rise. But doctors don't recommend taking extra magnesium to help prevent high blood pressure—the amount you get in a healthy diet is enough. Magnesium is found in whole grains, green leafy vegetables, nuts, seeds, and dry peas and beans.

- **Fish oils.** A type of fat called "omega-3 fatty acids" is found in fatty fish like mackerel and salmon. Large amounts of fish oils may help reduce high blood pressure, but their role in prevention is unclear. But taking fish oil pills is not recommended because high doses can cause unpleasant side effects. The pills are also high in fat and calories. Of course, most fish if not fried or made with added fat are low in saturated fat and calories and can be eaten often.

Other Factors

- **Fats, Carbohydrates, and Protein.** Varying the amount and type of fats, carbohydrates, and protein in the diet has little, if any, effect on blood pressure. But for overall heart health, it is crucial to limit the amount of fat in your diet, especially the saturated fat found in foods like fatty meats and whole milk dairy foods. Saturated fats raise your blood cholesterol level, and a high blood cholesterol level is another risk factor for heart disease. Foods high in fat are also high in calories. Remember, foods high in complex carbohydrate (starch and fiber) are low in fat and calories—so eating these foods in moderate amounts instead of high fat foods can help you to lose weight if you are overweight or to prevent you from gaining weight.

- **Caffeine.** The caffeine in drinks like coffee, tea, and sodas may cause blood pressure to go up, but only temporarily. In a short time your blood pressure will go back down. Unless you are sensitive to caffeine and your blood pressure does not go down, you do not have to limit caffeine to prevent developing high blood pressure.

- **Garlic or Onions.** Increased amounts of garlic and onions have not been found to affect blood pressure. Of course, they are tasty substitutes for salty seasonings and can be used often.

- **Stress Management.** Stress can make blood pressure go up for a while and, over time, may contribute to the cause of high blood pressure. So it's natural to think that stress management techniques like biofeedback meditation, and relaxation would help prevent high blood pressure. But this doesn't seem to be the case: the few studies that have looked at this have not shown that stress management helps to prevent high blood pressure. Of course, stress management techniques are helpful if they help you feel better or stick to a weight-loss and/or exercise program.

Here's a Recap

After going through all the things that may affect blood pressure, it's worth noting again the things that are sure to help you prevent high blood pressure:

1. Maintaining a healthy weight—losing weight if you are overweight,
2. Being more physically active,
3. Choosing foods low in salt and sodium, and
4. If you drink alcoholic beverages, doing so in moderation.

By following these guidelines, you can help reduce or prevent high blood pressure for life—and, in turn, lower your risk for heart disease and stroke.

Want to Know More?

For more information on either high blood pressure or weight and physical activity, contact:

National Heart, Lung, and Blood Institute Information Center
P.O. Box 30105
Bethesda, MD 20824-0105
(301) 251-1222

Chapter 40

High Blood Cholesterol and Atherosclerosis

Cholesterol and Heart Disease

True or False?

Are you cholesterol smart? Test your knowledge about high blood cholesterol with the following statements. Answer each true or false. The answers are given below.

1. High blood cholesterol is one of the risk factors for heart disease that you can do something about.

2. To lower your blood cholesterol level you must stop eating meat altogether.

3. Any blood cholesterol level below 240 mg/dL is desirable for adults.

4. Fish oil supplements are recommended to lower blood cholesterol.

5. To lower your blood cholesterol level you should eat less saturated fat, total fat, and cholesterol, and lose weight if you are overweight.

6. Saturated fats raise your blood cholesterol level more than anything else in your diet.

This chapter includes text from NIH Publication Nos. 95-3794 (May 1995), 96-2696 (August 1996), and 95-3045 (September 1995).

7. All vegetable oils help lower blood cholesterol levels.

8. Lowering blood cholesterol levels can help people who have already had a heart attack.

9. All children need to have their blood cholesterol levels checked.

10. Women don't need to worry about high blood cholesterol and heart disease.

11. Reading food labels can help you eat the heart healthy way.

Answers

1. **True.** High blood cholesterol is one of the risk factors for heart disease that a person can do something about. High blood pressure, cigarette smoking, diabetes, overweight, and physical inactivity are the others.

2. **False.** Although some red meat is high in saturated fat and cholesterol, which can raise your blood cholesterol, you do not need to stop eating it or any other single food. Red meat is an important source of protein, iron, and other vitamins and minerals. You should, however, cut back on the amount of saturated fat and cholesterol that you eat. One way to do this is by choosing lean cuts of meat with the fat trimmed. Another way is to watch your portion sizes and eat no more than 6 ounces of meat a day. Six ounces is about the size of two decks of playing cards.

3. **False.** A total blood cholesterol level of under 200 mg/dL is desirable and usually puts you at a lower risk for heart disease. A blood cholesterol level of 240 mg/dL is high and increases your risk of heart disease. If your cholesterol level is high, your doctor will want to check your level of LDL-cholesterol ("bad" cholesterol). A HIGH level of LDL-cholesterol increases your risk of heart disease, as does a LOW level of HDL-cholesterol ("good" cholesterol). An HDL-cholesterol level below 35 mg/dL is considered a risk factor for heart disease. A total cholesterol level of 200-239 mg/dL is considered borderline-high and usually increases your risk for heart disease. All adults 20 years of age or older should have their blood cholesterol level checked at least once every 5 years.

4. **False.** Fish oils are a source of omega-3 fatty acids, which are a type of polyunsaturated fat. Fish oil supplements generally

do not reduce blood cholesterol levels. Also, the effect of the long-term use of fish oil supplements is not known. However, fish is a good food choice because it is low in saturated fat.

5. **True.** Eating less fat, especially saturated fat, and cholesterol can lower your blood cholesterol level. Generally your blood cholesterol level should begin to drop a few weeks after you start on a cholesterol-lowering diet. How much your level drops depends on the amounts of saturated fat and cholesterol you used to eat, how high your blood cholesterol is, how much weight you lose if you are overweight, and how your body responds to the changes you make. Over time, you may reduce your blood cholesterol level by 10-50 mg/dL or even more.

6. **True.** Saturated fats raise your blood cholesterol level more than anything else. So, the best way to reduce your cholesterol level is to cut back on the amount of saturated fats that you eat. These fats are found in largest amounts in animal products such as butter, cheese, whole milk, ice cream, cream, and fatty meats. They are also found in some vegetable oils—coconut, palm, and palm kernel oils.

7. **False.** Most vegetable oils—canola, corn, olive, safflower soybean, and sunflower oils—contain mostly monounsaturated and polyunsaturated fats, which help lower blood cholesterol when used in place of saturated fats. However, a few vegetable oils—coconut, palm, and palm kernel oils—contain more saturated fat than unsaturated fat. A special kind of fat, called "trans fat," is formed when vegetable oil is hardened to become margarine or shortening, through a process called "hydrogenation." The harder the margarine or shortening, the more likely it is to contain more trans fat. Choose margarine containing liquid vegetable oil as the first ingredient. Just be sure to limit the total amount of any fats or oils, since even those that are unsaturated are rich sources of calories.

8. **True.** People who have had one heart attack are at much higher risk for a second attack. Reducing blood cholesterol levels can greatly slow down (and, in some people, even reverse) the buildup of cholesterol and fat in the wall of the coronary arteries and significantly reduce the chances of a second heart attack. If you have had a heart attack or have

347

coronary heart disease, your LDL level should be around 100 mg/dL which is even lower than the recommended level of less than 130 mg/dL for the general population.

9. **False.** Children from "high risk" families, in which a parent has high blood cholesterol (240 mg/dL or above) or in which a parent or grandparent has had heart disease at an early age (at 55 years or younger), should have their cholesterol levels tested. If a child from such a family has a cholesterol level that is high, it should be lowered under medical supervision, primarily with diet, to reduce the risk of developing heart disease as an adult. For most children, who are not from high-risk families, the best way to reduce the risk of adult heart disease is to follow a low saturated fat, low cholesterol eating pattern. All children over the age of 2 years and all adults should adopt a heart healthy eating pattern as a principal way of reducing coronary heart disease.

10. **False.** Blood cholesterol levels in both men and women begin to go up around age 20. Women before menopause have levels that are lower than men of the same age. After menopause, a woman's LDL-cholesterol level goes up—and so her risk for heart disease increases. For both men and women, heart disease is the number one cause of death.

11. **True.** Food labels have been changed. Look on the nutrition label for the amount of saturated fat, total fat, cholesterol, and total calories in a serving of the product. Use this information to compare similar products. Also look for the list of ingredients. Here, the ingredient in the greatest amount is first and the ingredient in the least amount is last. So to choose foods low in saturated fat or total fat, go easy on products that list fats or oil first, or that list many fat and oil ingredients.

Facts about Blood Cholesterol and Atherosclerosis

Why Blood Cholesterol Matters

Blood cholesterol plays an important part in deciding a person's chance or risk of getting coronary heart disease (CHD). The higher your blood cholesterol level, the greater your risk. That's why high blood cholesterol is called a risk factor for heart disease. Did you know that heart disease is the number one killer of men and of women in the United States? About a half million people die each year from heart attacks caused by CHD. Altogether 1.25 million heart attacks occur each year in the United States.

Even if your blood cholesterol level is close to the desirable range, you can lower it and reduce your risk of getting heart disease. Eating in a heart-healthy way, being physically active, and losing weight if you are overweight are things everyone can do to help lower their levels. This text will show you how. But first, a few things you ought to know...

The Blood Cholesterol—Heart Disease Connection

When you have too much cholesterol in your blood, the excess builds up on the walls of the arteries that carry blood to the heart. This buildup is called "atherosclerosis" or "hardening of the arteries." It narrows the arteries and can slow down or block blood flow to the heart. With less blood, the heart gets less oxygen. With not enough oxygen to the heart, there may be chest pain ("angina" or "angina pectoris"), heart attack ("myocardial infarction"), or even death. Cholesterol buildup is the most common cause of heart disease, and it happens so slowly that you are not even aware of it. The higher your blood cholesterol, the greater your chance of this buildup.

Other Risk Factors for Heart Disease

A high blood cholesterol level is not the only thing that increases your chance of getting heart disease. Here is a list of known risk factors:

Factors You Can Do Something About

- Cigarette smoking
- High blood cholesterol (high total and LDL-cholesterol)
- Low HDL-cholesterol
- High blood pressure
- Diabetes
- Obesity/overweight
- Physical inactivity

Factors You Cannot Control

- Age: 45 years or older for men; 55 years or older for women
- Family history of early heart disease (heart attack or sudden death): father or brother stricken before the age of 55; mother or sister stricken before the age of 65

The more risk factors you have, the greater your chance of heart disease. Fortunately, most of these risk factors are things you can do something about.

Who Can Benefit From Lowering Blood Cholesterol?

Almost everyone can benefit from lowering his or her blood cholesterol. Lowering cholesterol slows the fatty buildup in the arteries, and in some cases can help reduce the buildup already there. And, if you have two or more other risk factors for heart disease or already have heart disease, you have a great deal to gain from lowering your high blood cholesterol. In this case, lowering your level may greatly reduce your risk of any more heart problems.

Many Americans have had success in lowering their blood cholesterol levels. From 1978 to 1990, the average blood cholesterol level in the U.S. dropped from 213 mg/dL to 205 mg/dL.

Cholesterol—In Your Blood, In Your Diet

Cholesterol is a waxy substance found in all parts of your body. It helps make cell membranes, some hormones, and vitamin D. Cholesterol comes from two sources: your body and the foods you eat. Blood cholesterol is made in your liver. Your liver makes all the cholesterol your body needs. Dietary cholesterol comes from animal foods like meats, whole milk dairy foods, egg yolks, poultry, and fish. Eating too much dietary cholesterol can make your blood cholesterol go up. Foods from plants, like vegetables, fruits, grains, and cereals, do not have any dietary cholesterol.

LDL- and HDL-Cholesterol:
The Bad and The Good

Just like oil and water, cholesterol and blood do not mix. So, for cholesterol to travel through your blood, it is coated with a layer of protein to make a "lipoprotein." Two lipoproteins you may have heard about are low density lipoprotein (LDL) and high density lipoprotein (HDL). LDL-cholesterol carries most of the cholesterol in the blood. Remember, when too much LDL-cholesterol is in the blood, it can lead to cholesterol buildup in the arteries. That is why LDL-cholesterol is called the "bad" cholesterol. HDL-cholesterol helps remove cholesterol from the blood and helps prevent the fatty buildup. So HDL-cholesterol is called the "good" cholesterol.

Things That Affect Blood Cholesterol

Your blood cholesterol level is influenced by many factors. These include:

What You Eat. High intake of saturated fat, dietary cholesterol, and excess calories leading to overweight can increase blood cholesterol levels. Americans eat an average of 12 percent of their calories from saturated fat, and 34 percent of their calories from total fat. These intakes are higher than what is recommended for the health of your heart. The average daily intake of dietary cholesterol is 220-260 mg for women and 360 mg for men.

Overweight. Being overweight can make your LDL-cholesterol level go up and your HDL-cholesterol level go down.

Physical Activity. Increased physical activity lowers LDL-cholesterol and raises HDL-cholesterol levels.

Heredity. Your genes partly influence how your body makes and handles cholesterol.

Age and Sex. Blood cholesterol levels in both men and women begin to go up around age 20. Women before menopause have levels that are lower than men of the same age. After menopause, a woman's LDL-cholesterol level goes up—and so her risk for heart disease increases.

Have Your Blood Cholesterol Checked

All adults age 20 and over should have their blood cholesterol (also called "total" blood cholesterol) checked at least once every 5 years. If an accurate HDL-cholesterol measurement is available, HDL should be checked at the same time. If you do not know your total and HDL levels, ask your doctor to measure them at your next visit.

Total and HDL-cholesterol measurements require a blood sample that is taken from your arm or finger. You do not have to fast for this test. If you have had your total and HDL-cholesterol checked, check the chart "Total Blood Cholesterol and HDL-Cholesterol Categories" to see how they measure up.

Blood cholesterol levels of under 200 mg/dL are called "desirable" and put you at lower risk for heart disease. Any cholesterol level of 200 mg/dL or more increases your risk; over half the adults in the

United States have levels of 200 mg/dL or greater. Levels between 200 and 239 mg/dL are "borderline-high." A level of 240 mg/dL or greater is "high" blood cholesterol. A person with this level has more than twice the risk of heart disease compared to someone whose cholesterol is 200 mg/dL. About one out of every five American adults has a high blood cholesterol level of 240 mg/dL or greater.

Unlike total cholesterol, the lower your HDL, the higher your risk for heart disease. An HDL level less than 35 mg/dL increases your risk for heart disease. The higher your HDL level, the better.

In certain cases, it may be necessary to have your LDL-cholesterol checked, too, because it is a better predictor of heart disease risk than your total blood cholesterol. You will need to fast. That means you can have nothing to eat or drink but water, coffee, or tea, with no cream or sugar, for 9 to 12 hours before the test.

Table 40.1. Total Blood Cholesterol and HDL-Cholesterol Categories

Total Cholesterol

Less than 200 mg/dL .... Desirable
200 to 239 mg/dL .... Borderline-High
240 mg/dL or greater .... High

HDL-Cholesterol

Less than 35 mg/dL .... Low HDL-cholesterol

Note: These categories apply to adults age 20 and above.

Table 40.2. LDL-Cholesterol Categories

Less than 130 mg/dL .... Desirable
130 to 159 mg/dL .... Borderline-High Risk
160 mg/dL and above .... High Risk

Note: These categories apply to adults age 20 and above.

If your doctor has checked your LDL level, use the chart "LDL-Cholesterol Categories" to see how it measures up.

If your LDL-cholesterol level is high or borderline-high and you have other risk factors for heart disease, your doctor will likely plan a treatment program for you. Following an eating plan low in saturated fat and cholesterol and increasing your physical activity is usually the first and main step of treatment. Some people will also need to take medicine.

Guidelines for Heart-Healthy Living

Whatever your blood cholesterol level, you can make changes to help lower it or keep it low and reduce your risk for heart disease. These are guidelines for heart-healthy living that the whole family (including children ages 2 and above) can follow:

1. Choose foods low in saturated fat.

All foods that contain fat are made up of a mixture of saturated and unsaturated fats. Saturated fat raises your blood cholesterol level more than anything else you eat. The best way to reduce blood cholesterol is to choose foods lower in saturated fat. One way to help your family do this is by choosing foods such as fruits, vegetables, and whole grains—foods naturally low in total fat and high in starch and fiber.

2. Choose foods low in total fat.

Since many foods high in total fat are also high in saturated fat, eating foods low in total fat will help your family eat less saturated fat. When you do eat fat, substitute unsaturated fat—either polyunsaturated or monounsaturated—for saturated fat. Fat is a rich source of calories, so eating foods low in fat will also help you eat fewer calories. Eating fewer calories can help you lose weight—and, if you are overweight, losing weight is an important part of lowering your blood cholesterol. (Consult your family doctor if you have a concern about your child's weight.)

3. Choose foods high in starch and fiber.

Foods high in starch and fiber are excellent substitutes for foods high in saturated fat. These foods—breads, cereals, pasta, grains, fruits, and vegetables—are low in saturated fat and cholesterol. They are also lower in calories than foods that are high in fat. But limit fatty toppings and spreads like butter and sauces made with cream and whole milk dairy products. Foods high in starch and fiber are also good sources of vitamins and minerals.

When eaten as part of a diet low in saturated fat and cholesterol, foods with soluble fiber—like oat and barley bran and dry peas and beans—may help to lower blood cholesterol.

4. Choose foods low in cholesterol.

Remember, dietary cholesterol can raise blood cholesterol, although usually not as much as saturated fat. So it's important for your family to choose foods low in dietary cholesterol.

Dietary cholesterol is found only in foods that come from animals. And even if an animal food is low in saturated fat, it may be high in cholesterol; for instance, organ meats like liver and egg yolks are low in saturated fat but high in cholesterol. Egg whites and foods from plant sources do not have cholesterol.

5. Be more physically active.

Being physically active helps improve blood cholesterol levels: it can raise HDL and lower LDL. Being more active also can help you lose weight, lower your blood pressure, improve the fitness of your heart and blood vessels, and reduce stress. And being active together is great for the entire family.

6. Maintain a healthy weight, and lose weight if you are overweight.

People who are overweight tend to have higher blood cholesterol levels than people of a healthy weight. Overweight adults with an "apple" shape—bigger (pot) belly—tend to have a higher risk for heart disease than those with a "pear" shape—bigger hips and thighs.

Whatever your body shape, when you cut the fat in your diet, you cut down on the richest source of calories. A family eating pattern high in starch and fiber instead of fat is a good way to help control weight. Do not go on crash diets that are very low in calories since they can be harmful to your health. If you are overweight, losing even a little weight can help to lower LDL-cholesterol and raise HDL-cholesterol.

The National Cholesterol Education Program Recommendations

The National Cholesterol Education Program (NCEP) recommends that all healthy Americans ages 2 and above adopt an eating pattern lower in saturated fat and cholesterol to lower their blood cholesterol. The recommended eating pattern for everyone in the family over 2 years old is:

- less than 10 percent of calories from saturated fat.
- an average of 30 percent of calories or less from total fat.
- less than 3M mg a day of dietary cholesterol.

These goals are to be averaged over several days.

What about Cholesterol Levels in Children?

Most children do not need to have their blood cholesterol checked. But, all children should be encouraged to eat in a heart-healthy way along with the rest of the family. Children who should be tested at age 2 or older include those who have any of these conditions:

- at least one parent who has been found to have high blood cholesterol (240 mg/dL or greater),or

- a family history of early heart disease (before age 55 in a parent or grandparent).

Also, if the parent's medical history is not known, the doctor may want to check the child's blood cholesterol level, especially in children with other risk factors like obesity.

Table 40.3. Total and LDL-Cholesterol Levels in children and Teenagers from Families with High Blood Cholesterol or Early Heart Disease.

	Total Cholesterol	LDL-Cholesterol
Acceptable	Less than 170 mg/dL	Less than 110 mg/dL
Borderline	170 to 199 mg/dL	110 to 129 mg/dL
High	200 mg/dL or greater	130 mg/dL or greater

Note: These blood cholesterol levels apply to children 2 to 19 years old.

How High Is a Child's "High" Blood Cholesterol?

If your child does need to have a cholesterol test, it can be part of a regular doctor's visit. Your doctor will likely measure your child's total cholesterol level first. However, if your family has a history of early heart disease, the doctor may measure the LDL-cholesterol level right from the start. Otherwise, your child's LDL-cholesterol level should be measured if his or her total cholesterol level was checked and found to be 170 mg/dL or greater. The blood cholesterol categories for children from families with high blood cholesterol or early heart disease are shown in Table 40.3.

Should You Know Your Cholesterol Ratio?

When you have your cholesterol checked, some laboratories may give you a number called a cholesterol ratio. This number is your total cholesterol or LDL level divided by your HDL level. The idea is that combining the levels into one number gives you an overall view of your risk for heart disease. But the ratio is too general: It is more important to know the value for each level separately because LDL- and HDL-cholesterol both predict your risk of heart disease.

What Are Triglycerides?

Triglycerides are the form in which fat is carried through your blood to the tissues. The bulk of your body's fat tissue is in the form of triglycerides. Your triglycerides are measured whenever your LDL-cholesterol is checked. Triglyceride levels less than 200 mg/dL are considered normal.

It is not clear whether high triglycerides alone increase your risk of heart disease. But many people with high triglycerides also have high LDL or low HDL levels, which do increase the risk of heart disease.

Will Lowering My Blood Cholesterol Help Me Live Longer?

Many studies show that lowering cholesterol levels reduces the risk of illness or death from heart disease, which kills more men and women each year than any other illness. If you have heart disease, lowering your cholesterol level will probably help you to live longer. If you don't have heart disease, the studies so far do not show that you will live longer, but you will definitely reduce your risk of illness and death from heart attack.

Is It Safe to Eat in a Heart-Healthy Way?

Eating in a way that is lower in saturated fat and cholesterol is safe and can be more nutritious than an eating plan higher in saturated fat and cholesterol. It will even meet the higher needs that women, children, and teenagers have for nutrients like calcium, iron, and zinc, and an eating pattern lower in total fat will reduce the risk for other chronic diseases, such as cancer. And an eating pattern lower in saturated fat, total fat, and cholesterol can still provide enough calories for the proper growth and development of children ages 2 and above. Children younger than 2 years have special nutrient needs for fat.

How Much Will Your Cholesterol Levels Change?

Generally your blood cholesterol level should begin to drop a few weeks after you start eating the heart-healthy way. How much it drops depends on the amount of saturated fat you used to eat, how high your high blood cholesterol is, how much weight you lose if you are overweight, and how your body responds to the changes you make. Over time, you may reduce your cholesterol level by 5 to 35 mg/dL or even more.

How to Find Out More

The National Cholesterol Education Program (NCEP) has other booklets for the public and health professionals on lowering blood cholesterol. Most are free of charge. The NCEP has booklets for adults with high blood cholesterol, age-specific booklets for children and adolescents with high blood cholesterol and their parents, and a pamphlet on physical activity and how to get started. To order publications on cholesterol, weight and physical activity or request a catalog, write to the NHLBI Information Center, P.O. Box 30105, Bethesda, MD 20824-0105.

Recommendations Regarding Public Screening for Measuring Blood Cholesterol

Summary Recommendations

Since the initiation of the National Cholesterol Education Program (NCEP) and the development of simpler, more rapid laboratory measurements of cholesterol levels, screening for blood cholesterol levels has become widespread. Public screening has the possibility of detecting large numbers of individuals with high blood cholesterol levels in addition to those detected in the physician's office. However, if screening is to provide useful results, it must provide reliable measurement and ensure adequate education and followup.

Results of research on screening programs were presented at a National Heart, Lung, and Blood Institute (NHLBI) Workshop on Public Screening for High Blood Cholesterol in October 1988. The workshop participants suggested methods that could make public screening more effective in detecting high blood cholesterol in individuals who might otherwise not be identified in the health-care system and that could ensure followup of appropriate cases and public education about cholesterol. Recommendations for cholesterol screening programs were first issued by the National Heart, Lung, and Blood Institute and the American Heart Association in 1989. This text is an update of these recommendations and contains information in new reports of the National Cholesterol Education Program, in particular, the second Adult Treatment Panel report (ATP II). One important recommendation is that measurement of high density lipoprotein (HDL)-cholesterol should be added to initial cholesterol testing. The current document updates previous screening guidelines by incorporating this new recommendation. But it also emphasizes that if HDL-cholesterol measurements are not available in the screening setting, measurement of total cholesterol levels still provides valuable information that can be utilized for cholesterol management.

The purpose of cholesterol screening is twofold: to augment the public health approach to cholesterol control and to support the clinical strategy. The first approach is designed to reduce the average blood cholesterol level in the general population, and this is accomplished by increasing public awareness of high blood cholesterol as a risk factor for coronary heart disease (CHD) as the initial step toward modification of life habits that lead to high cholesterol levels. Cholesterol screening is one important step toward increasing public awareness of high blood cholesterol. Cholesterol screening in young adults may be particularly valuable for making them aware of the need to modify life habits early in life to delay development of CHD for as long as possible in later life. The clinical approach aims to identify individuals who have elevated blood cholesterol or related disorders and who are candidates for cholesterol management in the clinical setting. If cholesterol abnormalities are detected in such individuals, they will appropriately be referred to their physicians for further evaluation.

Recommendations

Public screening must meet customary standards for recruitment of participants, reliable measurement of cholesterol level, the provision of appropriate information, staff training, and referral for further evaluation.

Public screening programs should:

- Use recruitment approaches that attract all adult segments of the community and develop special approaches to reach groups that would be underrepresented in usual detection programs. These include men, younger adults, low-income or low-education groups, and minorities.

- Adhere to all applicable requirements established under the Clinical Laboratory Improvement Amendments of 1988 (CLIA).

- Ensure precise and accurate cholesterol measurements. Public screening should meet the standards defined by the Laboratory Standardization Panel of the NCEP. Laboratory instruments to measure cholesterol should undergo prefield evaluation and should be subject to an ongoing system of quality control. As required by CLIA, a health professional must be available to fulfill the role of clinical consultant.

- Include education as part of screening by providing reliable verbal and printed information about cholesterol levels from knowledgeable staff. Simply telling a participant his or her cholesterol number is not sufficient in a screening program.

- Ensure that staff members have received training specific to their responsibilities, have access to consultation from appropriate health professionals, and have adequate supervision.

- Screening sites should be convenient, efficiently accommodate the numbers of screenees, be designed to ensure quality-control procedures, and ensure privacy.

- Provide cholesterol screening at a reasonable cost to the participant.

- Coordinate public screening with the local medical community by establishing liaisons with community health-care resources.

- Provide active referral and followup programs. The screening agency should be responsible for taking steps to increase the likelihood that referred screenees reach medical care. Followup methods such as letters or telephone calls are desirable.

Public screening programs should recommend referrals on the basis of the NCEP guidelines given below:

- Any person with a history of heart attack, chest pain indicative of angina pectoris, coronary bypass operation, coronary angioplasty, recurrent transient ischemic attacks (TIAs) or known blockage of a carotid artery, abdominal aortic aneurysm, or ischemic peripheral arterial disease should be referred to a physician for cholesterol evaluation, beginning with a complete lipoprotein profile (total, low density lipoprotein [LDL]-, and HDL-cholesterol, and triglycerides). Cholesterol screening in the public setting is not necessary or advisable.

- A total cholesterol (TC) of 200 mg/dL in an adult 20 years of age or older calls for referral to a physician for further cholesterol evaluation:

  - within 2 months if TC is 240 mg/dL or greater, or if TC is 200-239 mg/dL with two or more other CHD risk factors
  - within 1 year if TC is 200-239 mg/dL with fewer than two other CHD risk factors

- If an HDL-cholesterol measurement is available, a level below 35 mg/dL calls for referral to a physician for further testing. If an HDL test is not available, the individual should be reminded of the advisability of obtaining an HDL-cholesterol measurement. This test is especially needed if the person has other CHD risk factors.

- If the HDL-cholesterol is 35 mg/dL or higher and total cholesterol is less than 200 mg/dL, cholesterol testing should be carried out again in 5 years.

Introduction/Background

The congruence of many types of scientific evidence has led to general agreement in the medical community of the need to lower blood cholesterol to reduce the incidence of CHD. In 1985, the NCEP, a consortium of practitioners, public health professionals, voluntary health organizations, and government agencies, began a collaborative effort of professional and public education. In 1988, the Adult Treatment Panel of NCEP delineated guidelines for the detection, evaluation, and treatment of high blood cholesterol in adults. Treatment of individuals at risk cannot proceed, of course, until their cholesterol levels have been defined. Accordingly, NCEP advises adults: "Know your cholesterol number."

The second report of the Adult Treatment Panel II, released in 1993, updated recommendations for cholesterol management in adults. This report is similar to the first in outline, and it continues to identify LDL as the primary target of cholesterol-lowering therapy. However, the report contains three new features that distinguish it from the first. These include:

- Increased emphasis on CHD risk status as a guide to type and intensity of cholesterol-lowering therapy.

  - Identification of the patient with existing CHD or other atherosclerotic diseases as being at highest risk, and establishment of lower targets for LDL-cholesterol for these patients.

  - Addition of age to the list of major CHD risk factors, defined as 45 years or older in men and 55 years or older in women.

  - Recommendation of delaying the use of drug therapy in most young adult men (less than 35 years) and premenopausal women with LDL-cholesterol levels in the range of 160-220 mg/dL who are otherwise at low risk for CHD in the near future.

  - Enhanced recognition that high-risk postmenopausal women, and high-risk elderly patients who are otherwise in good health, are candidates for cholesterol-lowering therapy.

- More attention to HDL as a CHD risk factor.

  - Addition of HDL-cholesterol to initial cholesterol testing.

  - Designation of high HDL-cholesterol as a "negative" CHD risk factor.

  - Consideration of HDL-cholesterol levels in the choice of drug therapy.

- Increased emphasis on weight loss and physical activity as components of the dietary therapy of high blood cholesterol.

The second new emphasis, more attention to HDL as a CHD risk factor, has important implications for cholesterol screening. Increasing scientific evidence indicates that a low HDL-cholesterol is a major risk factor for CHD. The purpose of HDL testing is to identify individuals who may have either a low or an elevated HDL-cholesterol, in order to improve initial CHD risk assessment and to guide later therapy. If the HDL test is available, it should be added to initial total cholesterol testing, providing that accuracy is assured. Although practical circumstances may dictate that cholesterol screening be carried out without the HDL-cholesterol measurement, ATP II recommendations should be kept in mind, and screenees should be reminded of the importance of obtaining an HDL test in the future.

The NCEP advocates a dual strategy for lowering cholesterol levels in the general population. The first is the public health strategy, which encourages the general public to modify life habits with the aim of reducing CHD risk factors, including high blood cholesterol. This approach makes use of public education, governmental policy, and food industry actions to foster healthful changes in habits. The second approach is the clinical strategy, which attempts to identify high-risk individuals in the clinical setting. It is primarily a case-finding approach and is based on the premise that a large portion of the general population periodically passes through the clinical setting where the opportunity for appropriate cholesterol testing exists. Cholesterol screening outside the medical setting serves both the public health and clinical approaches. It assists in increasing the general public's awareness of the dangers of high blood cholesterol, while at the same time it facilitates the finding of new cases.

The NCEP guidelines, as well as the availability of portable chemistry analyzers that make cholesterol measurement rapid, affordable, relatively painless, and readily available, initially led to widespread screening outside the physician's office and enthusiastic public responses. Hospitals, nursing homes, health fairs, supermarkets, exercise clubs, and many nonmedical sites have provided screening for blood cholesterol. In addition, public screening has also become commercialized, with profit-oriented organizations selling these services. Recently, public screening activities appear to have declined, but there still exists a need to provide updated guidance on this subject.

In October 1988, the NHLBI sponsored a Workshop on Public Screening for High Blood Cholesterol to review and evaluate data from public cholesterol screenings and make recommendations for quality control, recruitment, referral, and education. Data were presented from NHLBI-supported community heart disease prevention demonstration projects, the Model Systems for Cholesterol Screening Program, and scientists working in the field. The workshop proposed objectives for public screening and made recommendations for achieving these objectives. This text updates the workshop guidelines in light of recent developments, including the recommendations of ATP II.

Objectives for Public Cholesterol Screening

- To detect individuals with high levels of blood cholesterol and make appropriate referrals to sources of medical care.

- To raise public consciousness and knowledge about the relation of blood cholesterol to CHD.

- To provide information about eating patterns and other approaches to achieve and maintain appropriate levels of blood cholesterol.

- To reach those who might not otherwise have their blood cholesterol measured as part of routine health care.

Research Findings and Recommendations

Recruitment of Screening Participants

An increased portion of the population know their blood cholesterol level and its relation to CHD risk. According to national surveys conducted in 1983, 1986, and 1990, the percentage of adults who reported ever having their cholesterol measured has increased from 35 to 65 percent, while the percentage who can report their own cholesterol number has increased from 3 to 37 percent. Nevertheless, the substantial proportion of people who do not yet know their cholesterol number necessitates continued detection and educational efforts.

Public screening can attract participants from all segments of the population. However, certain groups such as the elderly, women, white adults, those who are better educated or have higher incomes, and previously screened individuals are more likely to take advantage of screening opportunities. Conversely, men, younger and middle-aged adults, and those with low incomes or low levels of education may participate less frequently in public screenings. Minorities can be significantly underrepresented. The ability of public screenings to detect high-risk individuals in these underrepresented groups is currently limited without targeted efforts.

Targeted screenings at locations such as worksites and certain community locations can improve access for the groups mentioned above. Targeted screenings at multiple sites within a community can achieve a screening population representative of the whole, including high-risk groups.

As screening becomes more widely available, certain people will often return to repeat their blood cholesterol measurement. Between 25 and 40 percent of those attending a screening have had at least one previous assessment. This proportion will increase as more people are screened. Although rescreening for self-monitoring purposes may have some benefit, it can detract from work on undetected population groups and can promote reliance on screening as a surrogate for medical care.

Screening programs should utilize recruitment strategies that enhance participation by all population segments to ensure detection in those high-risk groups that are otherwise less likely to seek medical care.

Recruitment Strategies. Recruitment strategies should be constructed to take account of the following needs:

- Marketing approaches that emphasize participation of the entire adult population and that emphasize the underrepresented groups.

- Targeted screening at sites where underserved populations are found.

- Flexible hours at the screening site, including evenings and weekends, for maximum availability. Since testing for total cholesterol and HDL-cholesterol does not require fasting, flexibility in screening is further enhanced.

- Screening facilities that are accessible and affordable to all elements of the population.

- Recruitment of individuals unaware of their cholesterol level to enhance detection of new high-risk cases and to discourage substitution of screening for medical care.

Analyzer Operation and Quality Control

Many desktop analyzers are available. Accuracy and precision of blood cholesterol measurements, which are critical for the classification and referral of screening participants, depend on appropriate quality control and staff training. However, even with these standards, it is inevitable that analytic and biologic variability will lead to some misclassification of individuals. Poor staff training and quality control could worsen the problem and lead to substantial misclassification. It should be stressed that a single elevated cholesterol measurement, even under rigorous quality control, does not establish the diagnosis of high blood cholesterol, for which two or more cholesterol measurements are needed. By the same token, a single low reading may fail to identify a person who is in need of professional cholesterol management. However, most screening participants will proceed to have a further cholesterol determination in a medical setting, and a major role of screening is to begin the process of determining the individual's cholesterol level. In any case, a repeat measurement within 5 years is recommended.

The premise that measurements meeting quality-control standards are possible in field settings is supported by a growing body of data. Reliable measurement is dependent on rigorous quality control and effective training of technical personnel. Internal quality-control procedures (regular analysis of known standards) and external quality-control procedures (comparative analysis of blinded samples with a reference lab) enable laboratory standards to be met. The cost of these quality-control procedures is estimated at 10 percent of analysis cost, which is modest compared with that engendered by excessive misclassification.

For HDL measurements, field experience with desktop analyzers is still limited, and a definitive statement about the reliability of fingerstick HDL determinations cannot currently be made.

Measurement Recommendations: Blood Sampling

- Either fingerstick or venipuncture samples can be used for total cholesterol. Good collection techniques should be observed.

- Blood obtained from either fasting or nonfasting individuals can be used for total cholesterol and HDL-cholesterol analysis.

- Differences in the measured concentrations of cholesterol in serum and plasma should be considered when reporting values. Referral should be based on levels adjusted to serum cutpoints as recommended by NCEP.

- The blood sampling procedures should be standardized to the sitting position if possible, preferably for at least 5 minutes, because postural changes can alter blood cholesterol concentrations.

- Cholesterol analysis should not be carried out in an individual with concomitant illness.

Measurement Recommendations: Analytic Devices and Laboratory Quality Control

- Desktop analyzers ideally should meet the performance standards of the NCEP Laboratory Standardization Panel, i.e., total error 8.9 percent or less.

  Accuracy is defined as proximity to the true value as determined by a reference method, and the coefficient of variation is an estimate of the reproducibility (or precision) of the measurement.

- Operators should be trained and able to demonstrate competence before screening.

- Liaison with a certified clinical chemistry laboratory whose cholesterol analyses meet NCEP laboratory standards should be maintained for consultation and quality control.

Each analyzer should be evaluated and shown to demonstrate acceptable performance in the laboratory setting before field use. Individual instruments, even those from the same manufacturer, may differ in performance and calibration, and the quality of measurement for each machine should be established.

- This evaluation should include analysis of control samples that are traceable to the National Reference System for Cholesterol Measurements (NRSCM) established by the Centers for Disease Control and Prevention (CDC) and the National Bureau of Standards. Total cholesterol controls should have values that are near the decision levels of 200 mg/dL and 240 mg/dL.

- Multiple runs of these quality-control materials should be made in a laboratory during a 2-week period on 5 to 10 different days, and appropriate quality-control limits should be established for that instrument.

- Precision and accuracy should meet NCEP laboratory standards. Analyzers not meeting these standards should not be used until appropriate corrective measures have been taken and documented.

Measurement Recommendations: Field Quality Control (Internal Program)

- Screening programs should establish a continuous quality-control program that follows accepted laboratory principles and is adequate both to maintain and document performance. Control serum pools at two levels, near or bracketing the 200 and 240 mg/dL decision values, should be used. These are available from manufacturers or reference laboratories. They should be analyzed at the beginning of each screening day, after every 20 samples, and at the end of each day. If bias is outside the established control limits, the pool should be analyzed again, and if bias is still outside the established control limits, the instrument should be taken out of service until the problem has been corrected.

- Coefficient of variation and instrument bias should be calculated and logged weekly for each control pool. Instruments should receive appropriate corrective attention if these measures are outside NCEP guidelines.

Measurement Recommendations: Field Quality Control (External Program)

Screening centers may be either extensions of licensed clinical laboratories or independently licensed under CLIA.

- Screening centers that are extensions of licensed laboratories should make comparisons with the licensed laboratory on duplicate aliquots ("split" samples) drawn from a screenee or received as blinded samples sent from the licensed laboratory. One or two of these samples should be analyzed each day, and the values should be returned to the licensed laboratory. The accuracy of the licensed laboratory should be traceable to the NRSCM. This licensed laboratory must be part of a Health Care Financing Administration (HCFA)–approved proficiency testing program (e.g., College of American Pathologists proficiency surveys).

- Screening centers that are independently licensed under CLIA must participate in a HCFA-approved proficiency testing program (e.g., College of American Pathologists proficiency surveys). These screening centers are also encouraged to make comparisons with a licensed laboratory on duplicate aliquots ("split" samples) drawn from a screenee or received as blinded samples sent from the licensed laboratory. One or two of these samples should be analyzed each day, and the values should be returned to the licensed laboratory. The accuracy of the licensed laboratory should be traceable to the NRSCM.

Measurement Recommendations: Remeasurement

- Screening values of total cholesterol above 300 mg/dL or below 100 mg/dL should be remeasured at the same sitting. The same is true for HDL-cholesterol values above 100 mg/dL or below 25 mg/dL.

Measurement Recommendations: Documentation

- Protocols documenting operating and trouble-shooting procedures should be kept with the instrument.

- An operations checklist should be provided and should be used by field personnel. A log should be maintained to document instrument problems and corrective action taken.

- Overall quality assurance of the testing process should be audited, and quality-control results should be logged and reviewed regularly by supervisory personnel.

- The screening team should maintain logs identifying all participants, their results, date of specimen collection, and any problems with specimens that may affect results. A copy of the test report must be maintained by the screening center for 2 years.

- Optimally, the instrument should provide hard copy readouts to minimize transcription errors and maximize participants' privacy in receiving their cholesterol numbers.

Education of Participants

Information about total blood cholesterol, HDL-cholesterol, and CHD risk provided with cholesterol measurements can improve knowledge, attitudes, and health behaviors. Effective education requires knowledgeable, trained staff supported by print (and possibly video) materials suitable for the target audience. The staff should be able to provide intelligent answers to questions about the relation of both total cholesterol and HDL-cholesterol to CHD risk. This would extend to a meaningful knowledge about the role of diet and exercise in control of total and HDL-cholesterol levels. Background information supplied to patients should be consistent with ATP II guidelines and should not embrace extremes of dietary and exercise advice that some people have advocated.

Receipt of a total cholesterol (and HDL-cholesterol) number by a participant is not sufficient in a screening program. Screenees should be able to obtain verbal and printed information on blood cholesterol from screening center staff. It is essential for public screening programs to provide education for all screenees who attend, regardless of their personal cholesterol level.

Education Recommendations

To ensure the usefulness of the screening experience, educational materials should provide:

- Information on the relationship of total blood cholesterol (and HDL-cholesterol) and other risk factors for CHD.

- Explanations on the meaning and limitations of a single total blood cholesterol (and HDL-cholesterol) value, the causes of variability, and the need for multiple measurements to define an individual as having high blood cholesterol.

- Information on the relationship of diet to blood cholesterol and the importance of a balanced healthy eating pattern to lower blood cholesterol. This should include clear information on cholesterol-lowering dietary alternatives.

- Information on the importance of following advice to seek physician followup for confirmatory cholesterol testing. Physician evaluation is especially urgent for patients with established CHD or other atherosclerotic diseases.

- Information presented by a variety of means, including print and video materials. However, the participant should always receive print materials that delineate these messages. They should be presented in a clear and understandable format. The needs of special groups should be taken into account.

Staff Training

Staff members at public screening centers should have training appropriate to their responsibilities. Although health professionals are not required for many screening tasks, in their absence those employed should undergo training programs. These training programs and materials may come from a variety of sources; however, they should be taught by health professionals with experience in the measurement, detection, and management of high blood cholesterol.

Training Recommendations: General Training

All staff members must be made aware of the following requirements in screening programs:

- Importance of professional appearance and conduct.

- Understanding of the confidential nature of personal health information.

- Ability to deal with emergency situations such as fainting and anxiety reactions.

- Understanding of the importance of accurate information reporting and documentation of screening center activity.

Training Recommendations: Phlebotomists (Blood Drawers)

- Because errors in measurement frequently originate in poor sampling methods, technicians who collect blood should be properly trained and certified. They should have a clear understanding of sample collection methodology and the various factors that can affect cholesterol measurement such as posture, prolonged application of the tourniquet, and others.

- Technicians should understand safe techniques for infection control and prevention. This should include education on the CDC recommendations for preventing the transmission of hepatitis and human immunodeficiency virus (HIV) in health-care settings.

- Technicians should be specifically trained in dealing with participants who faint, bleed excessively, or develop other medical emergencies common to screening activities.

- Special attention should be given to hygienic aspects of the screening setting. The area of screening should be kept spotless and devoid of spilled blood; all used gloves should be immediately disposed of and out of sight.

Training Recommendations: Instrument Operators

- These operators may differ in background (e.g. nurses, technicians), but all must be appropriately trained and by CLIA requirements must have a minimum of a high school education. A minimum of 1 day's training conducted by experienced laboratory trainers should consist of classroom instruction and hands-on experience in calibrating and operating the instrument, detecting problems, and performing usual maintenance.

- Operators should have a minimum of 1 week's supervised field experience operating the instrument for cholesterol analysis before operating the instrument alone.

Training Recommendations: Staff Providing Education Information

- Screening center staff members who provide information to participants should receive training in the delivery of accurate educational messages. This should include teaching skills for clear, credible, and persuasive educational counseling. A minimum of 12 days should be devoted to educational counselor training. It is recognized that in-depth counseling cannot be expected in the screening setting; however, a simplified, clear message as well as factual answers to questions should be provided.

- The staff members should be thoroughly familiar with ATP II.

Screening Environment

Overall planning of the screening environment is important. Understanding of the community, its resources, and liaison with its health-care agencies are critical initial steps. These are especially important for enhancing recruitment, participation, and compliance with referral recommendations.

The physical environment of screening is important. Well-planned patterns for smoothly handling the flow of participants leave them with good impressions of the screening experience and lead to improved measurement quality. The numbers of staff and instruments should be appropriate to the expected flow rates. It is best to have a facility that allows privacy for screenees for both blood sampling and confidential counseling about the results. Laboratory technicians also work more effectively and are best able to adhere to quality-control procedures in such privacy.

Although it is not the purpose of this document to define comprehensively the organization and operation of public screening programs, certain elements are important.

Environment Recommendations

Screening programs need to make provisions for the following environmental considerations:

- The selection of settings that are conducive to handling the flow of participants, privacy during blood sampling, confidentiality of results, and discussions between participants and staff.

- Adequate staffing and equipment to anticipate expected respondent flow rates and to minimize the likelihood of the stressed, hurried environment that is associated with poor quality.

- A manual of operations that documents all procedures, including laboratory methods, within the screening center.

- Documentation of participants' results, quality-control procedures, and other relevant information in logbooks that are available for review.

Referral and Followup

A major purpose of cholesterol screening is to assist in the detection of people at high risk for CHD on account of high blood cholesterol and other CHD risk factors. The NCEP recommends that all adults 20 years of age and older should have their total and HDL-cholesterol checked at least once every 5 years. For initial testing to be complete, an accurate measurement of both total cholesterol and HDL-cholesterol is needed. However, if the HDL-cholesterol is not available, the total cholesterol level is still useful.

The effect of screening, education, and referral programs on blood cholesterol levels of populations is being studied in several research programs. In these few studies, individuals with elevated levels of blood cholesterol who complied with referral advice had significantly lower cholesterol levels on followup, and this effect remains after taking into account the statistical phenomenon of regression to the mean. Populations that receive general education on cholesterol in community health promotion programs also show a modest lowering of blood cholesterol levels at followup. This lowering appears to occur throughout the entire population range of cholesterol values and is not limited to individuals with high blood cholesterol levels. These early results suggest that public screening, counseling, and referral can lead to lower cholesterol in those who have elevated levels and to a reduction in cholesterol in populations.

One of the major goals of screening is to identify high-risk individuals for subsequent medical management. These screening guidelines recommend that the ATP II advice be followed for referral recommendations. Other considerations also are recommended below to make that referral advice effective. Before cholesterol testing, the person should fill out the risk factor questionnaire (Table 40.4). If any of the conditions under #1 are checked, indicating the presence of atherosclerotic disease, the person should be referred to a physician. Cholesterol testing should not be used as part of the decision making in referral of such an individual. In fact, a relatively low cholesterol in such a person may give a false sense of security, and in patients with established CHD or other atherosclerotic disease, cholesterol screening should be deferred for physician evaluation. Persons with established atherosclerotic disease as outlined under #1 require lipoprotein analysis and, in all probability, specific cholesterol-lowering therapy. The answers to the questions posed under #2 may be useful in referral if the person has a borderline-high total cholesterol level (200 to 239 mg/dL). The following outlines what is acceptable and appropriate advice to give to adults undergoing cholesterol screening outside the medical setting.

1. **Total cholesterol of 240 mg/dL or higher.** Any person found to have a total cholesterol 240 mg/dL or higher should be referred to a physician within 2 months for further evaluation and lipoprotein analysis. This referral should be made regardless of the presence or absence of other risk factors.

2. **HDL-cholesterol less than 35 mg/dL.** A person found to have an HDL-cholesterol level less than 35 mg/dL should be referred to a physician within 2 months for further lipoprotein analysis. The presence or absence of other risk factors or the level of total cholesterol does not affect the decision to refer.

3. **Total cholesterol between 200 and 239 mg/dL.** Determine the number of risk factors from question #2 of the risk factor questionnaire. Risk factors include current cigarette smoking, hypertension (or on drug treatment for hypertension), diabetes,

family history of premature CHD, and age 45 years or older for a male or 55 years or older for a female. If HDL-cholesterol is available, add an additional risk factor if HDL-cholesterol is less than 35 mg/dL and subtract one risk factor if HDL-cholesterol is 60 mg/dL or greater.

   a. If the person has two or more CHD risk factors, refer to medical care within 2 months.

   b. If the total cholesterol is between 200 and 239 mg/dL and less than two risk factors are present, it is still prudent to advise the patient to have further cholesterol testing in the medical setting. NCEP recommends repeating total cholesterol within 1 to 2 years for individuals in this category. An earlier repeat measurement by a physician within 1 year seems appropriate when the first value is obtained through screening. This is particularly the case if the HDL-cholesterol value is not available. In the meantime, the opportunity should be taken to reinforce nutrition and physical activity education.

4. **Total cholesterol below 200 mg/dL.** If an accurate HDL-cholesterol measurement is available, it should accompany the total cholesterol measurement. If an HDL-cholesterol test is not available, the person should be informed of the importance of an HDL-cholesterol measurement to complete the initial assessment of CHD risk. If the HDL-cholesterol level is available and is 35 mg/dL or higher, and the total cholesterol level is desirable (less than 200 mg/dL), the person can be advised of the potential benefit to be derived from healthy eating patterns, weight reduction (if the person is overweight), and regular physical activity. The importance of a regular cholesterol check (every 5 years) should be stressed, and it should be pointed out that cholesterol screening is not a substitute for regular medical care.

A concern about public screening is that a substantial proportion of screenees who have high blood cholesterol levels may not seek physician followup or may not heed the advice given them by a physician. This is an issue of considerable importance that should continue as a priority of screening programs and the health-care community.

In well-managed screening programs that emphasized compliance and education, as many as one-half to two-thirds of individuals identified as having high blood cholesterol (greater than or equal to 240 mg/dL) sought advice from physicians. Specific strategies such as followup letters and telephone calls increased compliance with referral advice even more and suggested that, on average, such strategies can improve the rate of followup physician visits by 10 to 15 percent. Another approach is to mail a letter containing cholesterol

Table 40.4. Risk Factor Questionnaire

1. Have you ever had any of the following conditions? (Check if yes)

A. Been told by a doctor that you have coronary heart disease?

B. Heart attack (myocardial infarction)

C. Angina pectoris (chest pain due to insufficient blood flow to the heart)

D. Coronary bypass surgery

E. Coronary angioplasty (coronary "balloon" procedure)

F. Abdominal aortic aneurysm

G. Blockage of arteries to the legs

H. Transient ischemic attacks (TIAs; transitory strokes)

I. Blockage of a carotid artery

2. Which of the following pertain to you? (Check if yes)

A. Current cigarette smoker

B. History of high blood pressure (or taking blood pressure medication)

C. History of diabetes (high blood sugar)

D. Heart attack in first-degree relative (mother, father, sisters, brothers, children)—if a male relative before age 55 or female relative before age 65

E. Male 45 years or over

F. Female 55 years or over

results directly to the individual's physician. This approach has the advantage that it provides a direct link between the screening process and the clinical management of patients with cholesterol disorders. If the patient does not have a physician, the screening procedure can be used as an impetus to have the patient be checked periodically by a physician for CHD risk factors.

According to followup self-reports from referred high-risk individuals who visited a doctor, most were receiving appropriate attention. The majority had their cholesterol level rechecked in the physician's office.

Referral Recommendations

• Maintain liaison with sources of health care, including hospitals, clinics, and public health agencies. These provide resources for consultation and development of mechanisms for referral.

• The referral levels mentioned above should be used.

• Screening centers should have available lists of community resources that can give additional health information.

• Methods should be developed so that the majority of screenees with elevated cholesterol seek referral and medical care. Screening programs should utilize methods such as mail followup, telephone calls, or other approaches to ensure that referral advice is taken. A minimum goal is that 50 percent of referred participants are seen by their physicians within a 2-month period.

Other Issues

Cholesterol Testing in Children and Adolescents. The NCEP Expert Panel on Blood Cholesterol Levels in Children and Adolescents, in its 1991 report, noted that blood cholesterol levels of childhood tend to reflect those of adulthood, but the association is imperfect. To identify children whose elevated cholesterol levels are likely to be clinically significant, the panel recommended selective screening, in the context of continuing health care, of children and adolescents likely to become adults with high blood cholesterol levels and increased risk for CHD, i.e., those with a family history of premature cardiovascular disease or with a parent who has been found to have high blood cholesterol (240 mg/dL or greater). The panel did not recommend universal screening of children and adolescents or cholesterol testing outside the health care setting.

Home Testing. Devices are being developed for personal (self-testing) screening and monitoring of cholesterol levels. One of these has been recently approved by the Food and Drug Administration (FDA) for home use without prescription. There is little information regarding the utility of these devices for screening cholesterol levels in the field; their acceptability, precision, and accuracy in the hands of their intended users; and the consequences of their use. Until more information is obtained about their value and potential utility, they cannot be recommended for the purpose of screening

Direct LDL-Cholesterol. After measurement of total and HDL-cholesterol, LDL-cholesterol is the primary decision parameter for treatment and followup. Convenient methods for directly measuring LDL and suitable for the screening environment are expected to become available in the near future. Such methods would offer the possibility of measuring LDL- and HDL-cholesterol as an alternative to measuring total cholesterol.

Currently most routine clinical laboratories estimate LDL-cholesterol by the Friedewald equation, after measurement of total and HDL-cholesterol and triglycerides. Concerns about the reliability of the estimation have led to a recommendation for the development of direct LDL methods, using a pretreatment step to remove other lipoproteins with quantitation of the LDL by cholesterol measurement. Researchers and the diagnostics industry have responded by developing direct LDL methods. For example, the most common commercial method that is FDA-approved and compatible as a pretreatment step with a variety of analytical systems employs immunochemical separation. A mixture of antibodies specific to epitopes on the apolipoproteins of very low density lipoprotein (VLDL) and HDL is immobilized on latex beads. The specimen is added to the beads in a microfiltration device, and it is mixed and subjected to centrifugation. VLDL and HDL are retained by the filter, whereas LDL passes through and is quantitated by assaying cholesterol in the filtrates. This method is becoming common in routine clinical laboratories. In the future, similar techniques will likely be adapted to the compact analyzers used in onsite cholesterol screening programs.

Chapter 41

Peripheral Vascular Disease (Peripheral Atherosclerosis)

Diseases of the arteries may cause narrowing or blockage of blood vessels, which can lessen blood flow. When the blood flow is decreased, less oxygen reaches the tissues, which causes pain.

When the arteries of the heart are narrowed, the condition is called coronary artery disease. When the narrowing occurs in blood vessels other than those supplying the heart, the condition is known as peripheral vascular disease. The most common form of peripheral vascular disease occurs in the legs.

Whether in the peripheral arteries or the coronary arteries, the narrowing process happens in about the same way. As people age, they may develop fibrous plaques, which narrow their arteries and eventually reduce the flow of blood. When this happens in the coronary arteries, it can cause chest pain and may lead to a heart attack. When it happens in peripheral vessels, it can cause leg pain.

Peripheral vascular disease is also called atherosclerosis of the extremities or peripheral atherosclerosis. It occurs in about 12 percent of people age 65 to 70 and in about 20 percent of those over age 75. Only a fraction of these people have symptoms.

Risk Factors

Behaviors and health problems that increase the risk of developing coronary artery disease also increase the chance of getting peripheral vascular disease.

An undated fact sheet produced by the National Heart, Lung, and Blood Institute Information Center.

- *Cigarette smoking* is a key risk factor in the development of peripheral atherosclerosis. Evidence shows that when patients quit smoking, the clogging of their arteries slows or even stops.

- *High blood pressure* doubles the risk of developing peripheral vascular disease.

- *High blood cholesterol* can worsen existing peripheral atherosclerosis.

- *Diabetes*, particularly when blood sugar is not adequately controlled, can increase the risk for circulatory problems.

Symptoms

Leg pain is the main symptom of peripheral vascular disease. The pain may be felt up the leg and even in the buttock, depending on the location and severity of the blockage in the blood vessel.

The leg pain is called "intermittent claudication." It is a cramp-like pain that occurs during walking. It may worsen when walking fast or uphill but stops with rest.

Although most often triggered by physical activity, claudication pain may be brought on by other factors, such as exposure to cold or taking certain medications. For example, some beta-blocker drugs narrow blood vessels and decrease peripheral blood flow.

The pain will be in the calf if the blood vessel blockage is low in the arterial branches that supply the legs. If the blockage is higher in the artery, the pain may be in the thigh. If the blockage is even higher—above the groin—the pain may be felt in the leg and buttock and may cause impotence.

Once arteries become very narrowed or completely blocked, leg pain may be felt even during rest. The legs may look normal, but the toes will be pale, discolored, or bluish. Toenails will be thickened, and feet will feel cold to the touch. Pulses in the legs may be weak or undetectable.

In the most severe cases, blood-starved tissues can begin to die. This can lead to painful sores or ulcers on the lower leg, toes, or ankle and may lead to gangrene. If left untreated, toes or a whole foot may need to be amputated. Fortunately, such serious complications are rare.

Diagnosis

A diagnosis of peripheral vascular disease is usually made by the presence of symptoms—pain in the calf or thigh while walking that ends when stopping—and decreased pulses in the arteries in the feet.

The doctor probably will perform some tests to check blood flow.

- Blood pressure measurements may be taken in the ankles or other parts of the legs to see how much blood is getting to the feet. The tests may be taken both before and after exercise.

- A sonogram may be done to see the blood flow in the arteries. Sonograms produce images of the inside of the body using sound waves. It is a costly procedure and not always needed for a diagnosis.

- A magnetic resonance imaging (MRI) may be done to find out a blockage's severity and location. MRI provides a picture of the inside of the body through magnetism and radio waves. MRI also is costly and not always necessary.

- Angiography is usually done only in cases of severe claudication with signs of poor circulation, such as discoloration, absent pulses, and cold legs and feet. In angiography, a catheter (a hollow flexible tube) is inserted into an artery. A dye opaque to X-rays is then injected through the catheter. The X-ray picture then shows the inside of the artery.

Treatment

Both physical activity and medications are used to treat peripheral vascular disease.

Experts agree that long daily walks are the best treatment for people with intermittent claudication. Regular, brisk walks can lengthen the intervals between bouts of pain. Vascular specialists, doctors who specialize in the treatment of circulation disorders, recommend that patients walk 35 to 45 minutes every day, stopping briefly when discomfort occurs and continuing when it lessens. A person should not attempt to "walk through" the pain because muscles are weak when deprived of oxygen.

Often, a walking program can increase the distance of pain-free walking. This is due to improved physical fitness and the development of alternate circulation through small blood vessels, which is called collateral circulation.

People whose legs hurt during physical activity often find it hard to follow a walking program. For this reason, the cardiac rehabilitation departments of some hospitals have created supervised exercise programs that offer support and encouragement. Patients can ask their doctor for the name of such a program or check with a hospital in their area.

Other important lifestyle changes include losing weight if overweight, controlling diabetes if present, and stopping cigarette smoking.

Foot care also is important. When not enough blood reaches the feet, they can become inflamed or infected. People with peripheral vascular disease should wash their feet every day. After washing, a moisturizing lotion or baby oil should be applied at once. Comfortable, breathable shoes that protect the feet also should be worn. Footwear made of plastic or other synthetic materials should not be worn because they do not let air circulate well.

Foot care also means being sure nothing interferes with blood circulation. Feet should be kept warm, and no garters, support stockings, or socks with elastic tops should be worn.

Various medications have been tried in treating peripheral vascular disease, often with little success. At present, the only drug approved for this condition is pentoxifylline (Trental®), which makes blood less viscous or thick so it flows more easily through smaller blood vessels. In about a third of patients, this drug extends the period of pain-free walking; others are not helped or cannot tolerate the medicine's possible side effects, which are dizziness, headaches, nausea or vomiting, and upset stomach.

It is not known whether aspirin and other anti-clotting drugs help in peripheral vascular disease. Some experts feel that aspirin may slow the disease's progression even though it does not relieve pain, but this result has not yet been proven.

Patients who are disabled by pain, whose disease is progressing, or who have pain at rest may need to undergo a procedure to restore blood flow. Both surgical and nonsurgical procedures are possible. Because the potential benefits of such a procedure must outweigh the risks, those with mild pain are advised not to have one of these procedures, described below.

- *Balloon angioplasty* is usually the preferred procedure because it has the lowest mortality rate, produces the fewest complications, and requires the shortest hospital stay. It is usually performed by a radiologist or cardiologist. It involves inserting a balloon-tipped catheter through the skin. The catheter is threaded through the arteries to the site of the blockage. When the balloon is inflated, it flattens the obstructing plaque against the artery walls, widening the passage for blood. Angioplasty is most successful on blockages that are relatively short and well defined, rather than on those that are long and scattered. In about 30 percent of the cases, the leg arteries become clogged again (called restenosis) within a year or two, and another angioplasty or surgery may be necessary.

- Catheters with either a *laser* or a *cutting device* to remove the blockage burn through or shave out plaques, respectively. They are still being studied in clinical trials and are available primarily at large teaching hospitals.

- A *bypass graft* is sometimes used, typically when angioplasty fails or cannot be done. The graft is attached to pass around the blockage. The graft is made of synthetic tubing or a piece of another vein.

- *Endarterectomy* is another possible treatment. In this procedure, the artery is slit open and the blockage and diseased inner lining of the blood vessel are stripped out.

Extreme pain—that felt even at rest—or tissue damage sometimes can be treated only by amputation. It is usually possible to amputate below the knee, which is an advantage in rehabilitation and prosthesis use. Amputation is considered a last resort.

Prognosis

If treated, an estimated 80 to 90 percent of patients with intermittent claudication stabilize or improve in time. About 10 to 15 percent need to undergo a surgical or nonsurgical procedure. Those who continue to smoke have an 11-percent rate of amputation, compared with a negligible rate for those who stop smoking. Fortunately, most people with peripheral vascular disease do very well without surgery—by modifying their risk factors, sticking with a walking program, and taking good care of their feet.

For More Information

More information on peripheral vascular disease is available from the following organizations.

Society of Non-Invasive Vascular Technology
1101 Connecticut Avenue, N.W., Suite 700
Washington, DC 20036
(202) 857-1149

Society for Vascular Nursing
309 Winter Street
Norwood, MA 02062
(617) 762-3630

Chapter 42

Atherosclerosis: More Ways to Clear "Clogged" Arteries

Balloons, routers, scaffolds and lasers. This strange combination has nothing to do with parties, plumbing, painting or sci-fi movies. But they do have something in common: They're all treatments for narrowed or blocked arteries (atherosclerosis).

Most of the techniques are less than 10 years old. If you have atherosclerosis, they're ever-improving options to surgery.

Silent but Serious

Atherosclerosis is the buildup of cholesterol-containing fatty deposits (plaque) on the interior walls of your arteries. As plaque develops, the interior of your artery narrows and blood flow is reduced. When this happens in your coronary (heart) arteries, it can lead to a type of chest pain (angina pectoris).

Growth of plaque also makes the inside of your artery bumpy and rough. A tear (rupture) in plaque can cause a blood clot to form. A blood clot that blocks blood flow to your heart muscle (myocardium) can lead to a heart attack.

For years, a blocked coronary artery required open heart surgery. To redirect blood flow around the blockage, an artery or a vein from another part of your body is attached to the blocked artery as a bypass.

Reprinted from May 1995 *Mayo Clinic Health Letter* with permission of Mayo Foundation for Medical Education and Research, Rochester, Minnesota 55905. For subscription information, call 1-800-333-9038.

But bypass surgery is a major operation. It's costly and requires a hospitalization of about five to 10 days, plus at least two weeks' recovery at home. In the late 1970s and early 1980s, doctors started using new techniques as alternatives to surgery.

Balloons Flatten Plaque

In balloon angioplasty, your doctor first inserts a long, narrow, hollow tube (catheter) into an artery through a small incision made in your arm or groin. Aided by X-ray images on a TV screen, your doctor guides the catheter through the artery until it arrives at the blockage.

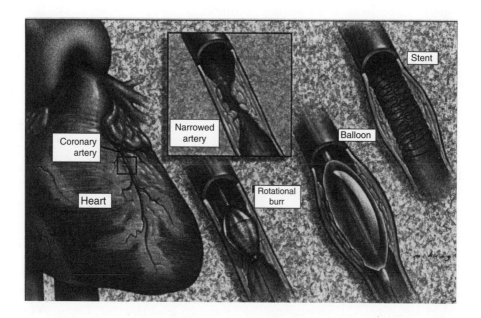

Figure 42.1. To widen narrowed or blocked arteries, a football-shaped burr that rotates up to 200 times per minute is one tool for cutting away cholesterol-containing fatty deposits (plaque). Balloon angioplasty flattens plaque and stretches the artery wall. A stent is typically used to prevent renarrowing after an artery is widened.

Next, a thinner catheter, tipped with a miniature, deflated balloon, is inserted into the first one. A guide wire from inside the catheter is maneuvered past the obstruction, creating a path for the balloon.

Inflating the balloon flattens plaque and stretches the artery wall, widening the path for blood flow. Then the catheters are removed.

Angioplasty is successful more than 90 percent of the time. But it does have limitations:

- **Arteries narrow again.** About one-third of the time, narrowing recurs within six months. When the balloon is inflated, plaque may crack as it's pushed aside. The remaining bumpy edges can allow growth of new plaque.

  Renarrowing may also be the result of elastic recoil, where the stretched artery gradually returns to its original shape. Or it could be growth of tissue from the trauma of balloon angioplasty.

  If renarrowing causes symptoms, the artery must be widened again.

- **It works best for certain blockages.** Although it can be used on total blockages, balloon angioplasty is best for obstructions that aren't too hard, too long or odd-shaped.

Atherectomy Cuts Away Plaque

Instead of flattening and pushing aside plaque, atherectomy (ath-ur-EK-tuh-me) actually removes it.

As in balloon angioplasty, your doctor inserts a catheter in your artery and guides it to the site of the obstruction. A second catheter equipped with a cutting tool is then threaded inside the catheter.

During the six years since atherectomy was introduced, different cutting tools have evolved:

- **Directional.** The second catheter is hollow and has an opening along one side. With the opening over the blockage, a moving blade inside the catheter cuts away plaque. This type of atherectomy works best on new blockages that are confined to a small area.

- **Rotational.** A football-shaped burr at the end of the catheter rotates up to 200,000 times per minute, sanding away layers of plaque. This cutting tool seems to be most effective on hardened (calcified) or irregularly shaped plaque.

- **Extractional.** The catheter has cutting blades attached to the end. The blades cut away plaque and suction removes it.

Atherectomy typically takes one to four hours. During this time, the cutting catheter may be removed and reinserted several times until the obstruction is cleared.

Afterward, the surface of the artery wall is often larger and smoother than with balloon angioplasty. Rarely, the procedure injures artery walls.

Your doctor may recommend you have atherectomy instead of balloon angioplasty because of the type, location and shape of the obstruction in your artery. However, the rate of renarrowing is similar in both procedures.

Stents Support Artery Walls

Despite advanced technology, return of the stretched artery to its original shape and renarrowing are still the Achilles' heel of treating atherosclerosis. One solution may come from the use of stents, a type of scaffold to hold up the interior walls of your arteries.

Stents are small, about the size of a spring inside a ballpoint pen. In 1992, they were approved for emergency use when balloon angioplasty failed. A stent was inserted as a stopgap measure, allowing bypass surgery to be scheduled later.

Last year, the Food and Drug Administration approved the routine use of stents after balloon angioplasty or atherectomy to prevent renarrowing.

After balloon angioplasty or atherectomy, a stent is fed through a catheter to the site that was cleared. The stent holds your artery open. Some stents are self-expanding; others are expanded by a balloon.

A stent attaches to the innermost layer of cells on the artery wall. A thin layer of clotted blood forms over the surface of the stent to promote healing.

However, clotting can become a problem. You may have to take an anticoagulant to reduce clotting. Depending on the medication, you may have to stay in the hospital longer than the one to two days needed after balloon angioplasty or atherectomy alone.

Lasers Destroy Plaque

Lasers use heat or light to destroy layers of plaque. They were introduced for use in coronary arteries in the late 1980s.

Since then, lasers have evolved as a combination treatment with balloon angioplasty to treat total blockages. A laser cuts through an obstruction enough for your doctor to insert a balloon and widen the artery.

No Perfect Choice

Despite their high success rates, balloon angioplasty, atherectomy and stents aren't perfect. There's a slight risk of heart attack during and after any of the procedures.

Renarrowing of your artery may make repeat treatments necessary. And in 1 to 2 percent of cases, emergency bypass surgery is needed if the procedure is unsuccessful.

To improve on each procedure alone, your doctor may combine treatments. Future improvements may give you more choices such as nonmetallic and bioabsorbable stents that may reduce the risk of blood clotting.

Part Six

Blood Transfusions and Blood Supply Safety

Chapter 43

Questions and Answers about Donating Blood

Blood Collection

How much blood is donated each year and how much is used?

Each unit of blood consists of a volume of 450 milliliters or about one pint. Because of the constant demand for blood, about 14 million units of blood are donated every year in the United States by about 8 million volunteer donors. This supply of blood is used by 4 million patients. Blood is given to accident victims, people undergoing surgery and patients with leukemia, cancer and other diseases.

Who gives blood?

Volunteers donate virtually all of this country's supply of blood for transfusion. It is important to encourage all healthy individuals to donate blood.

Where do individuals donate blood?

There are several places where blood donations are given. Bloodmobiles travel to places of employment, high schools, colleges, churches and community organizations. People can also donate blood at community blood centers and hospital-based donor centers.

Is there an age limit for donating?

A donor must be at least 17 years old to give blood. Persons who are older than 65 and in good health may usually donate with the approval of the blood bank physician.

How often can blood be donated?

People in good health who weigh at least 110 pounds can donate a unit of blood as often as every 8 weeks. Some states may further limit the number and/or frequency of donations in a 12-month period.

What is involved in donating blood?

A trained person records the donor's name, address and medical history and verifies his/her identification. The donor must read educational materials describing AIDS (acquired immunodeficiency syndrome) and other diseases that could be spread by transfusion. An interviewer will ask about travel outside the United States and a variety of activities that could indicate increased risk of the donor transmitting one of the infectious agents that can be present in blood. The prospective donor will have his or her temperature, pulse, blood pressure and weight recorded.

Next, a small amount of blood is taken from the prospective donor's finger to measure either the volume of red blood cells (hematocrit) or the amount of hemoglobin in the donor's blood. If a low hematocrit or hemoglobin is found, the donor is temporarily deferred. After the individual is found to be qualified to donate blood, he or she goes to the donation area. Many blood donor areas are equipped with contour chairs; others have flat beds. Much care is taken to make the donor as comfortable as possible. A trained person will swab the donor's arm inside the elbow with an antiseptic solution, which cleans the phlebotomy (needle insertion) area. A sterile, new needle, which is attached to a sterile plastic bag, is inserted into the vein. It usually takes less than 10 minutes to collect the unit of blood. After the donation is completed, the needle is removed from the arm and discarded.

The donor is generally asked to rest for at least several minutes and refreshments such as fruit juices, cookies and crackers are served to supply quick energy. Before leaving, donors are advised to drink plenty of fluids for the next 24 hours and to be cautious about lifting heavy objects.

Are there risks in giving blood?

Almost none. It is not possible to acquire any disease through donating blood because new, disposable, sterilized equipment is used for each donation. A very small number of donors, less than half of one percent, experience slight discomfort during or immediately after donating.

Can you get AIDS or hepatitis from donating blood?

No. Sterile procedures and new disposable equipment are used by all blood donor centers. All items used—the finger lancet, the needle, the cotton balls, swabs and solutions—are discarded after each use.

What is the importance of all the tests performed and questions asked before someone can donate blood?

These tests and questions are meant to protect the person who is donating the blood and to protect the patient who might receive the unit of blood. The required questions and tests lessen the chance of a bad effect from giving or receiving blood. For this reason, it is extremely important that prospective donors answer all questions accurately and thoroughly.

What is plateletpheresis?

Although most blood is donated as whole blood, it is also possible to donate only a portion of blood using a technique called apheresis. Blood is drawn from the vein of a donor into an apheresis instrument, which separates the blood into different portions by centrifugation. By appropriately adjusting the instrument, a selected portion of the blood, such as the platelets, can be recovered, while the rest of the blood is returned to the donor either into the same vein or into a vein in the other arm. This process takes more time than whole blood donation, but the yield of platelets is much greater. Platelets collected by apheresis are particularly useful for patients who require numerous platelet transfusions, for example cancer patients who have received chemotherapy.

Can a patient donate his / her own blood for use in surgery?

Yes. When blood transfusions are anticipated, such as upcoming elective surgery, a person can donate blood for his or her own use.

Autologous blood donation refers to a process whereby the patient provides his or her own blood. There are three types of autologous procedures available for a patient undergoing surgery. Preoperative autologous donation, in which the patient donates his or her own blood prior to the surgery, is the most common form of autologous transfusion. Intraoperative and postoperative cell salvage are two other ways of saving blood lost during or immediately after surgery for return to the donor/patient.

In the preoperative autologous procedure, the surgeon will explain that there may be a possibility that the patient will require blood transfusions during the operation.

Depending on the type of surgery and the health of the patient, the surgeon or medical director of the blood bank will determine whether the patient can donate blood and, if so, how much. When the surgeon is satisfied that the process of donating blood will not harm the patient, an order is written and an appointment is made with the blood bank. The procedure for donating autologous blood is almost identical to that used for volunteer blood donors. The same sterile procedures and precautions are taken. Very careful steps are taken to ensure that autologous blood is carefully identified. A special tag with the patient's name, date of birth, date of surgery and social security number are included on the unit.

A second type of autologous transfusion is called intraoperative salvage. A specialized machine, sometimes called a cell saver, collects blood lost during a surgical procedure, and processes it so it can be returned to the patient's circulation.

The third type of autologous procedure is postoperative cell salvage. This procedure is usually done after the patient leaves the operating room. There are certain surgical procedures, such as hip and knee replacements and chest surgery, where there may be an accumulation of blood in the body. This blood can sometimes be collected with a special device and transfused back into the patient.

What is the difference between the collection of whole blood and the collection of plasma in the United States?

Nearly all the nation's blood supply is provided by volunteers, who receive no payment. These volunteers donate their blood through nonprofit organizations such as hospital and regional community blood banks. Most of the whole blood collected is separated into components including red blood cells, platelets, plasma and other clotting factors. All of these components are transfused to patients. A growing number of volunteers also donate platelets by apheresis. Plasma, the fluid in which red blood cells, platelets and other clotting factors are suspended, can also be collected by apheresis. For this process, whole blood is drawn, plasma is removed and the red blood cells are transfused back into the donor. This plasma collection process takes 1 to 2 hours to complete. Plasma is often collected from donors by a variety of organizations, particularly commercial for-profit organizations, that provide it to companies for manufacture into a variety of blood products. These products usually undergo a purification process to make them safe. Some of these products provide clotting factors for people who suffer from abnormal bleeding disorders. Hemophilia, a hereditary disease generally limited to males, often requires treatment with large amounts of clotting factors to stop bleeding episodes.

Donating Blood for Yourself

What is autologous blood transfusion?

Autologous (au-tol'-o-gous) blood transfusion is a procedure where you are transfused with blood that you have donated for yourself because of a specific need, such as upcoming elective surgery.

How does it work?

The autologous transfusion procedure consists of your blood being collected before surgery, stored and returned to you during or following surgery to replace the blood you have lost.

What are the advantages of autologous transfusion?

Autologous blood is the safest blood available for transfusion. Because you donate your own blood, you eliminate the risk of acquiring infectious diseases that may be transmitted by blood transfusion. Blood from friends, family members, or other volunteer donors may transmit an infectious disease or cause some other undesirable side effect. Though blood from volunteer donors, including friends and family members, is tested to eliminate possible risks, autologous transfusion is the ONLY way to eliminate these risks. In addition, the use of autologous blood leaves more of the community blood supply available for those who cannot participate in autologous blood transfusion programs.

How can I donate for my own blood needs?

If you have a need for blood transfusion, such as upcoming surgery, contact your physician. Your physician will make the necessary arrangements. You will then need to make an appointment with the blood bank. On the day of your donation you will be thoroughly screened. Blood bank personnel will ask for a short medical history and take your pulse, blood pressure and temperature, as well as a small sample of blood to test for anemia.

How can I become an autologous blood donor?

You may become an autologous blood donor if you have a specific need such as elective surgery. There are few age or weight limits for donating autologous blood. The criteria for donating autologous blood are liberal. Therefore, you should not feel you cannot donate because you have not been accepted as a blood donor in the past. Your physician and the blood bank medical director will determine whether your medical condition will allow you to donate blood safely for yourself.

Will the donation affect my health?

You may experience a mild anemia (low blood count) at first, but the donation of blood will stimulate your body to produce more red blood cells. Since red cells contain a large portion of the body's iron stores, your physician may also prescribe iron to help your body make blood.

Can I donate if I am pregnant?

Although blood transfusion is rarely needed during pregnancy and delivery, you may donate for yourself with the approval of your physician and the blood bank medical director.

How often can I give?

You may donate as often as every three to four days up to three days before your surgery date as long as you pass the pre-screening tests. You are usually able to donate the number of units of blood required for your surgery. The physician's orders will depend on how much blood is generally used for your surgery.

Will the blood I donate meet all my transfusion needs?

In many cases, autologous blood will meet all your needs. However, you should ask your physician about the likelihood of needing additional blood components from the community blood supply.

Will I know my blood type after donating?

Yes. You may ask the blood bank when you donate or they may send you a donor card showing your blood type.

What happens to my blood if I do not use it?

If you do not use your blood during your hospitalization and you have met the requirements of a regular blood donor, your blood may be given to another patient who requires blood, depending on hospital policy.

Are there any costs?

Yes. There may be additional costs over and above the usual processing and administration fees.

Are there disadvantages of donating autologous blood?

Each donation requires approximately one to two hours of your time. In rare instances the donation process may cause mild discomfort.
For more information contact your physician.

Chapter 44

Progress in Blood Supply Safety

The blood supply plays a vital role in the American health system. Each year, Americans donate approximately 12 million units of blood, which are processed into 20 million blood products. About 3.6 million Americans receive transfusions of these blood products each year.

Although the blood industry is ultimately responsible for the safety of the blood supply, the Food and Drug Administration is responsible for regulating the blood industry.

"Blood banking has become a manufacturing industry—an industry that must conform to high standards and quality control requirements comparable to those of pharmaceutical companies or other regulated industries," said David A. Kessler, M.D., FDA commissioner.

The technology of blood banking grew slowly in the early years of this century, then was markedly stimulated by the needs of World War II. On May 3, 1946, the Public Health Service issued the first federal license allowing an establishment to manufacture whole blood.

In the United States today, licensed establishments include more than 1,000 donor centers that collect, process and distribute blood and blood products in interstate commerce under federal regulations. Establishments not involved in interstate commerce are not licensed, but they register with and, like licensed establishments, are inspected by FDA and are subject to the same high standards as licensed establishments.

Reprint from *FDA Consumer,* Food and Drug Administration (FDA) Publication No. 95-9013, May 1995.

The United States has the safest blood supply in the world, and FDA is striving to keep it safe by decreasing the risk of infectious disease transmission. The agency is continuously updating its requirements and standards for collecting and processing blood. The Blood Products Advisory Committee, a group of outside experts, provides a broad perspective and state-of-the-art experience to issues confronting FDA, so that the agency's final decision will reflect a balanced evaluation. Although FDA is not bound to follow the advisory committee's recommendations, it usually does.

Ongoing improvements and refinements together with advances in technology and science promise more sophisticated methods of blood collection and more accurate tests to protect the blood supply.

Nonetheless, blood and blood products are not entirely risk-free. There is a remote risk of infection with serious blood-borne viruses such as hepatitis and HIV, the virus that causes AIDS. But for patients who need blood transfusions, the risk of transfusion-associated disease is far less than the risk of dying or becoming more seriously ill without a transfusion. (See "Alternatives to Regular Blood Transfusion" in the July-August 1994 *FDA Consumer*.)

How FDA Regulates Blood Industry

As technology develops and new information about the transmission of infectious diseases becomes available, FDA's Center for Biologics Evaluation and Research issues written guidance to all blood establishments. This guidance sets the standard for the industry and is incorporated into standard operating procedures for all blood facilities.

FDA's guidance generally has also been supported and adopted by blood establishments and all major blood organizations, including the American Red Cross, the American Association of Blood Banks, the Council of Community Blood Centers, the American Blood Resources Association, and others involved in collecting and distributing blood and blood products.

FDA investigators in district offices across the country conduct inspections of all licensed blood establishments each year. Inspections are conducted every other year for those establishments that consistently comply with the agency's standards and regulations. These inspections insure that the blood establishments are adhering to all the proper procedures and regulations. During the inspection, investigators monitor donor screening; blood testing, labeling, storage, and handling; and record keeping and other manufacturing practices. FDA expects the establishment to promptly correct any problems or deficiencies. Furthermore, the investigators may verify resolution of deficiencies through follow-up inspections.

FDA can order a recall of hazardous blood products, issue warning letters, seize products, suspend or revoke the establishment's license, or take other legal actions that can result in civil or criminal penalties against the establishment and its officials.

For example, after repeated failures to comply with federal standards, one blood bank signed a consent decree enjoining it from further collection and manufacturing. The establishment closed in November 1993 until FDA could determine that the infractions—including some that created potential disease transmission hazards—had been corrected. (See "North Carolina Blood Bank Closed" in the Investigators' Reports section of the July-August 1994 *FDA Consumer.*)

FDA has taken action in other cases involving centers in a number of states. These actions include suspending licenses and taking steps to revoke licenses of establishments not complying with regulations and standards to safeguard the blood supply. The agency has also requested recalls of blood, when necessary.

At press time, in all cases, the facilities had taken corrective action to bring firms into compliance with FDA regulations.

Layers of Safeguards

The heart of the blood safety system established by FDA is five layers of overlapping safeguards that start at the blood collection center and extend to the manufacturers and distributors of blood products.

- *Donor screening.* Potential donors must answer questions about their health and risk factors. Those whose blood may pose a health hazard are encouraged to exclude themselves. A trained and competent health professional then interviews potential donors regarding their medical history.

  Donors can be temporarily deferred (excluded from donating blood) for a number of reasons, including having a temperature, cold, cough, or sore throat on the day of donation or taking certain medications, such as Accutane (isotretinoin) or Proscar (finasteride). Reasons potential donors are permanently excluded from donating blood include evidence of HIV infection, male homosexual activity since 1977, a history of intravenous drug abuse, or a history of viral hepatitis.

403

- *Blood testing.* After donation, the blood is tested for such blood-borne agents as HIV, hepatitis and syphilis.

- *Donor lists.* Blood establishments must keep current a list of deferred donors and check donor names against that list.

- *Quarantine of untested blood.* Blood products are not available for general use until the products have been thoroughly tested.

- *Investigation of problems.* Blood establishments must investigate any breaches of safeguards and correct deficiencies. Licensed firms must report to FDA any manufacturing problems, errors, or accidents that may affect the safety, purity, or potency of their products. Registered firms, although not required to report problems, are required to thoroughly investigate problems and maintain accurate records for FDA to review during an annual inspection.

An error or accident can result from improper testing, incorrectly labeled components, improper interpretation of test results, improper use of equipment or failure to follow the manufacturers' directions for its use, or accepting units from donors who should have been deferred.

In addition, products such as immune globulin and clotting factors must be treated to inactivate any virus that may be present with processes such as treatment with heat, solvent, or detergent.

"FDA is committed to holding all blood centers to the highest standards," said Kessler. "When it comes to these vital products, our standards can never be too high."

Because of the potential risks involved, FDA regards blood or blood components unsuitable for use if any safeguard is breached. Unsuitable units are subject to recall because of the potential risk, even if tests do not show definitively that the products are contaminated. Because of the safeguards in the system, recalled blood products generally present only a remote health risk.

Improved Standards

FDA monitors all phases of blood preparation and manufacture. In recent years, the agency has intensified its oversight of blood establishments and taken measures to strengthen standards.

The agency has issued a proposed quality assurance guideline to help blood establishments recognize and prevent recurring problems. The guideline emphasizes that manufacturers of blood and blood components should have written quality assurance programs that will help eliminate the causes of errors, ensure the integrity of test results, implement effective controls for manufacturing processes and record-keeping systems, and ensure adequate employee training. Competency evaluations, equipment validation, and laboratory testing procedures, as well as self-policing audits are designed to prevent accidents and errors that can result in the release of unsuitable blood products.

In addition, under this proposed regulation all licensed and registered blood establishments would have to implement "look back" procedures already followed at most facilities. Under these procedures, blood establishments retrieve and quarantine units previously collected from a donor who at the time of donation tested negative for HIV, but subsequently tested positive. The blood establishment then does more specific tests on a current sample of the donor's blood. If the results are positive, previously donated units cannot be used in transfusions, and people who received such units must be notified.

Another measure to strengthen blood safety is FDA's decision to regulate blood establishment computer software as medical devices. Blood establishments use such software in managing donor registries, testing blood, and storing records and other data. Software also helps identify unsuitable donors and prevents the release of unsuitable blood and blood components.

Recognizing the critical role of software in blood establishment operations, FDA has notified manufacturers of computer software for blood establishments that it considers these products to be devices covered under the Federal Food, Drug, and Cosmetic Act when they are intended for use in the manufacture of blood products. The manufacturers now must register with FDA, list all the products they make, provide FDA premarket notification or submit the product for approval, comply with current good manufacturing practice regulations, and report adverse events.

FDA also notified these manufacturers that it will continue to inspect their establishments. The primary focus of these inspections will be to assess compliance with the good manufacturing practices, including a review of the standards for software development, testing, validation, and quality assurance. FDA will also review and assess manufacturers' procedures for investigating product complaints, including their procedures for correcting problems and for notifying customers and FDA when corrective actions are taken.

As the blood industry has become more complex, FDA's oversight has become more comprehensive and attentive to all aspects of the blood industry. These steps are intended to make the blood supply as safe as possible so that patients can continue with confidence to take advantage of its lifesaving potential.

Testing Blood

One of the cornerstones of maintaining a safe blood supply is testing. FDA requires that all blood establishments test each unit of blood for a variety of blood-borne diseases. Furthermore, FDA reviews and approves all assay test kits used to detect infectious and transmittable diseases in donated blood. Each unit of blood must be tested for:

- hepatitis B, using hBsAg (an indicator of the virus) and hB core antibody (an indicator of the antibody) tests

- hepatitis C, using a hepatitis C antibody test

- HIV-1 (AIDS virus), using an HIV-1 antibody test

- HIV-2 (also causes AIDS, but it is far less prevalent in the United States than HIV-1), using an HIV-2 antibody test

- HTLV-1 for evidence of a rare leukemia virus found mainly outside the United States

- syphilis for evidence of this sexually transmitted disease.

In the early 1970s, the risk of contracting some form of hepatitis from a unit of blood was as high as 6 to 8 percent. Now the risk of contracting hepatitis B per unit of blood is approximately 1 in 250,000, and the risk for contracting hepatitis C is less than 1 in 3,300.

For HIV, the risk of infection has decreased from 1 in 2,500 in 1985 to around 1 in 225,000 today. In 1985, FDA licensed the first test, HIV-1 enzyme immunoassay, capable of detecting HIV antibodies in blood. In 1987, the agency licensed the more precise Western Blot Test, which is used as a confirmatory test.

Screening tests are continually being improved. The test for hepatitis C detects the antibody in about 90 percent of chronic non-A, non-B hepatitis cases. However, more sensitive tests are being developed. The screening test for HIV is among the most sensitive, detecting evidence of infection in more than 99 percent of infectious samples.

—by Monica Revelle

Monica Revelle is an FDA press officer.

Chapter 45

Indications for the Use of Red Blood Cells, Platelets, and Fresh Frozen Plasma

Rationale for Component Use

Blood transfusion can be lifesaving therapy for patients with a variety of medical and surgical conditions. Advances in the use of blood components have made whole blood transfusions rarely necessary. Blood component therapy provides better treatment for the patient by giving only the specific component needed. Such therapy helps to conserve blood resources because components from 1 unit of blood can be used to treat several patients.

Red Blood Cell Transfusion

Red blood cell (RBC) transfusions increase oxygen-carrying capacity in anemic patients. Transfusing 1 unit of RBC will usually increase the hemoglobin by 1 g/dL and the hematocrit by 2-3 percent in the average 70 kg adult.

Adequate oxygen-carrying capacity can be met by a hemoglobin of 7 g/dL (a hematocrit value of approximately 21 percent) or even less when the intravascular volume is adequate for perfusion. In deciding whether to transfuse a specific patient the physician should consider the person's age, etiology and degree of anemia, hemodynamic

Taken from U.S. Department of Health and Human Services, National Blood Resource Education Program's *Transfusion Alert: Indications for the Use of Red Blood Cells, Platelets, and Fresh Frozen Plasma*. NIH Publication No. 91-2974. Revised September 1991.

stability, and presence of coexisting cardiac, pulmonary, or vascular conditions. To meet oxygen needs, some patients may require RBC transfusions at higher hemoglobin levels.

When a treatable cause of anemia can be identified, specific replacement therapy (e.g., vitamin B_{12}, iron, folate) should always be used before transfusion is considered. If volume expanders are indicated, fluids such as crystalloid or nonblood colloid solutions should be administered. RBC transfusions are often used inappropriately as volume expanders.

Table 45.1. Red Blood Cell Transfusion

Transfuse Red Blood Cells:

  To increase oxygen-carrying capacity in anemic patients

Do Not Transfuse Red Blood Cells:

- for volume expansion
- in place of a hematinic
- to enhance wound healing
- to improve general "well-being"

Platelet Transfusion

Platelet transfusions are administered to control or prevent bleeding associated with deficiencies in platelet number or function. One unit of platelet concentrate should increase the platelet count in the average adult recipient by at least 5,000 platelets/μL.

Prophylactic platelet transfusion may be indicated to prevent bleeding in patients with severe thrombocytopenia. For the clinically stable patient with an intact vascular system and normal platelet function, prophylactic platelet transfusions may be indicated for platelet counts of <10,000-20,000/μL. A patient undergoing an operation or other invasive procedure is unlikely to benefit from prophylactic platelet transfusions if the platelet count is at least 50,000/μL and thrombocytopenia is the sole abnormality. Platelet transfusions at higher platelet counts may be required for patients with systemic bleeding and for patients at higher risk of bleeding because of additional coagulation defects, sepsis, or platelet dysfunction related to medication or disease.

Table 45.2. Platelet Transfusion

Transfuse Platelets:

To control or prevent bleeding associated with deficiencies in platelet number or function

Do Not Transfuse Platelets:

- to patients with immune thrombocytopenic purpura (unless there is life-threatening bleeding)
- prophylactically with massive blood transfusion
- prophylactically following cardiopulmonary bypass

Fresh Frozen Plasma Transfusion

Fresh frozen plasma (FFP) transfusions should be administered only to increase the level of clotting factors in patients with a demonstrated deficiency. Laboratory tests should be used to monitor the patient with a suspected clotting disorder. If prothrombin time (PT) and partial thromboplastin time (PTT) are <1.5 times normal, FFP transfusion is rarely indicated.

Patients who have been given the anticoagulant warfarin sodium become deficient in vitamin K-dependent coagulation factors II, VII, IX, and X. If these patients are bleeding or require emergency surgery, they

Table 45.3. Fresh Frozen Plasma Transfusion

Transfuse Fresh Frozen Plasma:

Increase the level of clotting factors in patients with a demonstrated deficiency

Do Not Transfuse Fresh Frozen Plasma:

- for volume expansion
- as a nutritional supplement
- prophylactically with massive blood transfusion
- prophylactically following cardiopulmonary bypass

may be candidates for FFP transfusion to achieve immediate hemostasis when time does not permit warfarin reversal by stopping the drug or administering vitamin K.

Patients with rare conditions such as antithrombin III deficiency and thrombotic thrombocytopenic purpura may benefit from FFP transfusion.

Risks Common to All Blood Components

Infection and alloimmunization are the major complications associated with transfusion of blood components. There is a relationship between these risks and the number of donor exposures. The risk of infection is geographically variable.

- *Hepatitis C virus* can be transmitted by blood transfusion. With the recent introduction of a screening test to detect HCV in donated blood, and the discarding of positive units, the risk of transfusion-related hepatitis C has been greatly lessened, although the exact risk per unit transfused is not yet known.

- *Human immunodeficiency virus(es)* presently pose(s) a relatively small hazard. The wide range of estimated risk (1:30,000 to 1:300,000) reflects geographic variance.

- *Other infectious diseases or agents* may be transmitted via transfusion (e.g., hepatitis B, HTLV-I/II, cytomegalovirus, and those causing malaria).

- *Fatal hemolytic transfusion reactions* can occur. They are usually caused by an ABO incompatibility due to errors in patient identification at the bedside.

- Recipients of any blood product may produce antibodies against donor antigens, i.e., *alloimmunization*. This condition can result in an inadequate response to transfusion.

- *Allergic reactions, febrile reactions, and circulatory overload* may also occur.

References

1. Office of Medical Applications of Research. National Institutes of Health. "Fresh Frozen Plasma: Indications and Risks."

Journal of the American Medical Association 253(4):551-553, Jan 25, 1985.

2. Office of Medical Applications of Research. National Institutes of Health. "Platelet Transfusion Therapy." Journal of the American Medical Association 257(13):1777-1780, Apr 3, 1987.

3. Office of Medical Applications of Research. National Institutes of Health. "Perioperative Red Cell Transfusion." Journal of the American Medical Association 260(18):2700-2703, Nov 11, 1988.

Chapter 46

Infectious Disease Testing for Blood Transfusions

Abstract

Objective. To provide physicians and other transfusion medicine professionals with a current consensus on infectious disease testing for blood transfusions.

Participants. A non-Federal, nonadvocate, 12-member consensus panel representing the fields of hematology, infectious disease, transfusion medicine, epidemiology, and biostatistics and a public representative. In addition, 23 experts in hematology, cardiology, transfusion medicine, infectious disease, and epidemiology presented data to the consensus panel and a conference audience of 450.

Evidence. The literature was searched through Medline and an extensive bibliography of references was provided to the panel and the conference audience. Experts prepared abstracts with relevant citations from the literature. Scientific evidence was given precedence over clinical anecdotal experience.

Consensus. The panel, answering predefined consensus questions, developed their conclusions based on the scientific evidence presented in open forum and the scientific literature.

Infectious Disease Testing for Blood Transfusions. NIH Consensus Statement Online 1995 Jan 9-11;13(1):1-29 at http://text.nlm.nih.gov.

Consensus Statement. The panel composed a draft statement that was read in its entirety and circulated to the experts and the audience for comment. Thereafter, the panel resolved conflicting recommendations and released a revised statement at the end of the conference. The panel finalized the revisions within a few weeks after the conference.

Conclusions. The serum alanine aminotransferase test should be discontinued as a surrogate marker for blood donors likely to transmit posttransfusion non-A, non-B hepatitis infection since specific hepatitis C antibody testing has eliminated more than 85 percent of these cases. Anti-hepatitis B core antigen testing should continue as it may prevent some cases of posttransfusion hepatitis B; it also may act as a surrogate marker for HIV infection in donors and may prevent a small number of cases of transfusion-transmitted HIV infection. Syphilis testing should continue until adequate data can determine its effect on the rarity of transfusion-transmitted syphilis. Vigilant public health surveillance is critical in responding to emerging infectious disease threats to the blood supply.

Introduction

The United States has had an organized national blood collection system for 50 years. During this time, testing has been either mandated, recommended by regulatory authorities, or adopted voluntarily so as to make blood transfusions as safe as possible. Various strategies have been used during the past decade to exclude unsafe units from transfusion. These methods, which incorporate systems to ensure donor confidentiality, include refining and expanding the scope of the medical history, identifying behavior associated with high risk, and increased testing of donated blood. In the last 10 years alone, blood collection agencies have implemented five new tests applied to all donated blood: human immunodeficiency virus (HIV 1 and 2) antibodies, hepatitis B core antibody (anti-HBc), serum alanine aminotransferase (ALT), antibodies to human T-cell lymphotropic virus (HTLV I/II), and, most recently, antibodies to hepatitis C virus (HCV). At the time these tests were introduced, some were indirect tests, or "surrogates," whereas others were specific for a particular infection. These actions have been extremely effective, and today the nation's blood supply is safer than ever.

The continuing contribution of some of these tests to the safety of blood transfusions is uncertain. The epidemiology of a disease may change with time, as may immunization status and other factors, so that the optimum combination of donor screening tests is also likely to change. Now that more specific assays are available, the continuing need for certain surrogate assays has been questioned. Both ALT and anti-HBc were introduced as surrogates for an infection that is now subject to more specific testing. Both of these nonspecific tests have a low positive predictive value with frequent false positive results. This leads to disposal of blood from normal donors and to deferral of the donors from future donation. False positive values not only contribute to the present blood shortage but also result in emotional, psychological, and financial costs to the donor. Another test, the serological test for syphilis (STS), was introduced to protect against transfusion-transmitted syphilis; at the present time it is retained primarily as a sign of risky behavior rather than as evidence for infection. STS, too, has a substantial false positive rate, leading to discarding blood and rejecting the donor with resultant distress. Moreover, the costs of these tests may make blood processing and blood transfusions needlessly more expensive.

To maintain the safety of blood transfusion, it is also important to be alert to the possible introduction of new infectious diseases that may be blood-borne and therefore a hazard of transfusion. Thus, whereas one aim is to eliminate tests that are no longer useful, it is equally important to introduce whatever new screening procedures may be necessary to maximize the safety of blood transfusions. An example of such a challenge is the possibility of Chagas disease in donors. Because of immigration from Mexico, South America, and Central America and reports of several cases of Chagas disease resulting from transfusions, testing of donors for *T. cruzi* infection is now being considered by many blood banks. No general plans are in place, however, to deal with the introduction of agents that might threaten the safety of the blood supply.

The purpose of this consensus conference was twofold: (1) to evaluate the need for continued use of ALT, anti-HBc, and STS tests in volunteer blood donors and (2) to develop a proposal for determining mechanisms to cope with the introduction into the community of an infectious agent that might threaten the blood supply.

To address these issues, the National Heart, Lung, and Blood Institute, together with the Office of Medical Applications of Research of the National Institutes of Health, convened a Consensus Development Conference on Infectious Disease Testing for Blood Transfusions. The conference was cosponsored by the Transfusion Branch of the NIH Clinical Center and the National Institute of Allergy and Infectious Disease.

After 1½ days of presentations and audience discussion, an independent, non-Federal consensus panel composed of specialists and generalists from medical and other related scientific disciplines considered the evidence and formulated this consensus statement in response to the following four previously stated questions:

- To what extent does the alanine aminotransferase test contribute to transfusion safety? Should its use as in current practice continue or should its use be modified?

- To what extent do tests for hepatitis B core antibody and for syphilis contribute to transfusion safety? Should their use as in current practice continue or should their use be modified?

- To manage potential threats to transfusion safety from emerging infectious diseases, what are the appropriate ways to identify of important diseases, to change in blood donor screening practices, and to introduce of new laboratory tests?

- What are the highest priorities for research to improve transfusion safety by reducing the transmission of infectious disease?

Background for the Role of ALT and Anti-HBc Testing

ALT and anti-HBc tests were introduced in 1986-87 in an effort to identify donors at risk of transmitting posttransfusion non-A, non-B (PT-NANB) hepatitis. Two major studies in the late 1970's indicated that the rate of non-A, non-B hepatitis in transfusion recipients was higher in those receiving units from donors with high ALT levels than in those receiving units from donors with low ALT levels. In the Transfusion Transmitted Virus Study (TTVS) 45 percent of recipients of blood from donors with ALT in a high range (60-284 IU/L) developed PT-NANB hepatitis, whereas only 5 percent of recipients of blood from donors with ALT in a low range (1-14 IU/L) developed PT-NANB hepatitis. Intermediate rates of PT-NANB hepatitis were observed in recipients of units from donors with intermediate levels of ALT. In addition, recipients of units of blood from anti-HBc positive donors experienced a two- to threefold greater risk of PT-NANB hepatitis compared with recipients of units from donors without anti-HBc. A similar correlation between posttransfusion hepatitis and elevated ALT and the presence of anti-HBc in donors was observed at the National Institutes of Health. These two studies suggested that anti-HBc testing of donors, in concert with ALT testing, might eliminate 30-50 percent of PT-NANB hepatitis. Based on these studies, testing of volunteer donors for ALT and anti-HBc was begun by blood banks to reduce PT-NANB hepatitis. Several years later, HCV was identified, an anti-HCV test was developed, and HCV was shown to be responsible for most, if not all (> 90 percent) cases of PT-NANB hepatitis. The more sensitive second-generation test for anti-HCV combined with improved donor selection has effectively eliminated 85-90 percent of posttransfusion hepatitis due to HCV. It is likely that newer tests for anti-HCV will improve this level of protection against posttransfusion hepatitis C. The issue at present is whether these two surrogate tests (ALT and anti-HBc) continue to contribute to transfusion safety.

To What Extent Does the Alanine Aminotransferase Test Contribute to Transfusion Safety; Should Its Use as in Current Practice Continue or Should Its Use Be Modified?

The panel reviewed the background data of changes in the risk of hepatitis following blood transfusion resulting from implementation of increasingly sophisticated tests for HCV infection. Also reviewed were data regarding the interpretation of an elevated ALT level in otherwise healthy blood donors.

The potential utility of ALT testing is as follows:

- To reduce the risk of posttransfusion hepatitis C not prevented by screening of donors for antibody to HCV;

- To reduce the risk of posttransfusion hepatitis caused by other known hepatotropic viruses, such as hepatitis A and hepatitis B;

- To reduce the risk of putative infectious agent(s) associated with posttransfusion non-A, non-B, non-C hepatitis.

Now that sensitive tests for HCV infection in donors are available, the value of ALT must be questioned. In addition, the current policy of ALT testing results in the elimination of many acceptable donors and causes additional cost.

Setting criteria for discarding units of donated blood because of ALT elevations has been problematic because modest elevations of serum ALT are common in healthy blood donors. Elevations may reflect acute or chronic liver disease of infectious or noninfectious etiologies. However, frequent alcohol consumption, obesity, or other factors not related to transfusion-transmitted diseases may cause ALT to rise to levels that lead to unnecessary exclusion of donors. Furthermore, studies in the United States and Europe have confirmed that values of ALT in normal males are considerably higher than those in normal females so that a single cutoff value for ALT rejects a higher proportion of men than women.

Because several different methodologies are available to measure ALT activity, some variation in ALT results will occur even if the same sample is tested in different laboratories. Thus, the interpretation of an ALT level is affected by the assay and by the laboratory in which the determination is made. The lack of standardized interpretation of test results and cutoff values for these results contributes to inconsistent rules regarding the inclusion and exclusion of donors. ALT is a continuous variable, but the decision to discard a unit of blood is a binary one. Thus, healthy donors with borderline elevations of ALT may be deferred or permanently excluded from donating blood.

Prior to the introduction of anti-HCV testing, surrogate markers including ALT may have reduced the overall posttransfusion hepatitis rate by 30-40 percent on a per unit basis. Improved donor recruitment and selection also contributed to this reduction. However, the preponderance of the available data indicates that, in the presence of anti-HCV testing, retention of ALT testing of blood donors has little additional value. Several observational studies failed to demonstrate an additional benefit of ALT testing in the prevention of posttransfusion hepatitis C. This conclusion was further supported by a prospective randomized study. With specific anti-HCV testing, the risk of posttransfusion hepatitis was equivalent in groups receiving blood screened with or without surrogate markers, pointing to the redundancy of ALT testing.

ALT elevation has been proposed as a surrogate marker of HCV infection in the "window period" prior to anti-HCV seroconversion, because ALT rises approximately 4 weeks prior to production of anti-HCV. Implementation of newer, unlicensed anti-HCV tests (HCV 3.0) is expected to reduce this 4-week window period. In spite of the theoretical window period, there are no data from clinical studies indicating that ALT screening would improve the margin of safety of blood transfusion.

Even with anti-HCV testing of blood donors, a small but measurable risk of posttransfusion hepatitis remains (< 0.8 percent in both U.S. and Canadian studies). Possible explanations for this residual posttransfusion hepatitis include infection with new agents or known viruses presenting in an atypical fashion. Examples of the latter might include serotypic variants of HCV not currently detected by standard assays, HBV variants with mutations in the envelope protein that are not identified by standard HBsAg testing, and window period infections with HBV not detected by standard assays. In addition, some cases of apparent posttransfusion hepatitis may have a noninfectious etiology. Although the potential benefit of ALT for early detection of unknown hepatotropic viruses is intriguing, current data suggest that such testing will rarely, if ever, be helpful. The potential benefit of ALT for the detection of posttransfusion hepatitis A infection is also likely to be limited since the brief period of viremia largely precedes the rise in ALT.

The direct cost of the ALT test is low. On the other hand, ALT testing incurs very high costs as measured by lost resources, both of discarded units (approximately 200,000 annually) and of donors temporarily deferred or permanently excluded (approximately 150,000 annually). Moreover, evaluation of donors with abnormal ALT represents an additional fiscal burden to the health care system. A substantial, but underappreciated, consequence of ALT testing is the direct psychological and financial impact on the deferred donor. A donor with borderline elevated ALT may be denied health and life insurance and may suffer from unwarranted anxiety and stress.

Recommendation

ALT testing of volunteer blood donors should be discontinued. Persons previously deferred for an isolated elevation in ALT only may now be reevaluated for donor eligibility.

To What Extent Do Tests for Hepatitis B Core Antibody and for Syphilis Contribute to Transfusion Safety? Should Their Use as in Current Practice Continue or Should Their Use Be Modified?

Anti-HBc

Studies indicate that anti-HBc testing does not identify additional donors capable of transmitting HCV infection when such donors are also screened by the current, sensitive anti-HCV tests. However, anti-HBc screening of donors provides two additional benefits that may warrant its retention as a test used to screen blood donors.

First, it is likely that anti-HBc testing contributes to the safety of blood transfusion by helping to reduce the risk of hepatitis B virus (HBV) infectious units entering the donor pool. Such units may come from two sources: (1) individuals chronically infected with HBV in whom HBsAg is not detectable and (2) donors with acute hepatitis B who are in the window period following disappearance of HBsAg and prior to the appearance of anti-HBs. Whereas relatively few HBV infectious units are likely to be excluded solely on the basis of anti-HBc testing, current use of anti-HBc screening probably contributes to the low rates of transfusion-transmitted hepatitis B in the United States. In addition, anti-HCV positivity may act as a surrogate marker for HBV infectious donors who are HBsAg negative.

A second rationale for retention of anti-HBc testing relates to its activity as a surrogate marker for HIV infection. Its ability to serve as a surrogate marker for HIV is due to the overlapping epidemiology of HIV and HBV with common parenteral and sexual transmission risk factors. Given the availability of sensitive serologic markers for HIV infection, the value of anti- HBc as a surrogate marker of HIV infection is restricted to recently infected donors who are in the window period of HIV infection prior to the detectability of HIV antibodies. Although window period donors are extremely rare (presently approximately 1:210,000–1:1,140,000), the severe consequence of transfusion-transmitted HIV infection supports the retention of the anti-HBc test for this purpose. Anti-HBc testing may currently be eliminating as many as one-third of HIV window period units. However, the value of anti-HBc testing as a surrogate for HIV is likely to decline with expanding HBV immunization and changing HIV epidemiology.

Despite these potential benefits of anti-HBc screening, the present test for anti-HBc has many false positive results leading to the unnecessary deferral of tens of thousands of donors. This results in the loss of a large number of units of blood that are otherwise suitable for transfusion. In addition, donors are provided with confusing test results and are subjected to needless anxiety and medical expense, brought about by the mistaken thinking that they may have a contagious disease.

Anti-HBs testing is helpful in confirming the specificity of anti-HBc testing: anti-HBc positivity in donors who also test positive for anti-HBs usually indicates prior HBV infection. Present data suggest that such donors are not likely to be infectious. On the other hand, a small proportion of donors who are anti-HBc positive in the absence of anti-HBs are HBV DNA positive and likely to be infectious. An argument may be made that donors positive for both anti-HBs and anti-HBc have a low probability of transmitting HBV and thus could be returned to the donor pool, but such a strategy would eliminate the potential value of anti-HBc screening in preventing HIV transmission. It would also complicate donor management. Thus the panel concluded that anti-HBs testing should not be a part of donor screening, although it will be useful in the medical evaluation of donors found to be anti-HBc positive.

The value of the anti-HBc test in improving the safety of the blood supply is tempered by the impact of high false positive rates. Its positive predictive value for past or present infection with the hepatitis B virus must be improved.

Anti-HBc Recommendation

Although there is no reason to retain the anti-HBc test to prevent posttransfusion hepatitis C, it is recommended that the anti-HBc test be retained for donor screening for the following purposes:

- Prevention of posttransfusion hepatitis B.

- Prevention of some cases of transfusion-transmitted HIV from donors who test negative for anti-HIV because they are in the window phase of the infection.

Syphilis

Syphilis is one of the oldest recognized infectious risks of blood transfusion, and serologic tests for syphilis have been routinely carried out on blood donors for more than 50 years. In recent years, transfusion-transmitted syphilis has become exceptionally rare, with very few cases reported in the literature. In 1985, an FDA advisory panel proposed eliminating the requirement for serologic testing for syphilis. This proposal was not acted upon because of the possible value of the test as a surrogate marker of HIV. Given this, is it reasonable to continue donor screening for syphilis?

Several factors probably contribute to the absence of reported cases of transfusion-transmitted syphilis. These include improved donor selection processes, the uniform application of serologic tests for syphilis to all donors, and a general shift from transfusion of fresh blood to transfusion of refrigerated blood components. The relative role of these three factors in excluding syphilis as an infectious hazard of blood transfusion is difficult to ascertain because of a paucity of data that specifically address these issues. In addition, uncertainty exists concerning the extent to which current surveillance practices would detect occasional cases of transfusion-transmitted syphilis. Antibiotics received by many hospitalized, transfused patients may partially treat transfusion-transmitted syphilis, obscuring the diagnosis but not necessarily preventing long-term complications of the infection.

The general use of refrigerated blood for transfusion is often cited as an important factor in reducing the risk of transfusion-transmitted syphilis, as *Treponema pallidum* loses its viability within a few days in whole blood stored at 4 degrees C. However, available data indicate that a small proportion of viable organisms may survive up to 96 hours under such storage conditions, and many units of blood are refrigerated for shorter time periods prior to transfusion. In addition, platelet concentrates are stored at room temperature and no data are available concerning the survival of *T. pallidum* under these conditions.

Thus, current blood storage conditions would not appear to provide an adequate margin of safety against transfusion-transmitted syphilis, should the donor screening test be eliminated. Further information concerning *T. pallidum* survival under blood and platelet storage conditions, and the application of molecular techniques to assess the presence of *T. pallidum* DNA in serologically positive units, would allow better assessment of this question.

An alternative rationale often cited as a reason for retaining serologic testing of donors for syphilis is the potential ability of such tests to serve as surrogate markers of other transfusion-transmissible infections, especially HIV. However, cross-sectional studies and examination of prior donations from donors undergoing HIV seroconversion indicate that serologic tests for syphilis have very little value as surrogate markers for HIV infection in recently infected persons who have not yet developed detectable antibodies to HIV. Syphilis testing is likely to identify less than one such donor annually within the United States. This low efficacy of syphilis testing as a surrogate marker of HIV is not sufficient by itself to warrant its application to all blood donors. Low positive predictive values for HBV, HCV, or HTLV infections similarly do not support retention of syphilis testing as a surrogate for these infections.

Syphillis Recommendation

Because the contribution of serologic tests for syphilis in preventing transfusion-transmitted syphilis is not understood, the panel concludes that testing of donors for syphilis should continue.

What Are the Appropriate Ways to Manage Potential Threats to Transfusion Safety from Emerging Infectious Diseases, Considered in Terms of Identification of Important Diseases, Changes in Blood Donor Screening Practices, and Introduction of New Laboratory Tests?

Assurance of transfusion safety relies upon effective public health surveillance for emerging infectious diseases. Appropriate management of newer disease threats requires effective surveillance in combination with the rational use of screening measures to eliminate or minimize the risk of transfusion-associated disease transmission.

Decisions regarding the appropriate response to a new infectious disease involve many considerations. The answers to the following three questions will direct a logical approach to a control strategy.

Is the disease potentially transmissible through blood products?

Not every existing or emerging infectious disease is potentially transmissible through transfusion. On the other hand, diseases with a long and relatively asymptomatic period during which microorganisms are present in the blood are of particular concern to transfusion safety.

Potential threats to transfusion safety from emerging infectious diseases can be identified in a number of ways. Case reports of infection following transfusion or infections appearing in patients who have received blood from multiple donors should prompt epidemiologic investigation. Even in the absence of such reports, if the disease has a significant period during which the causative microorganism is present in the bloodstream, it may be important to institute surveillance systems to detect transfusion-acquired infections. The potential survival of the organism in an infectious form during blood processing and storage should also be investigated.

Is the disease an important public health problem?

The effort expended and resources committed to the disease threat will be determined by the severity, incidence, prevalence, and potential for secondary spread of infection. HIV infection, when it first appeared, affected only a small number of patients, yet the dire consequences of infection triggered a focused effort to exclude HIV from the blood supply. CMV infection is an example at the other end of the spectrum. CMV antibody is present in approximately 50 percent of donors, representing active infection in some, which can in turn be transmitted to recipients. CMV antibody-positive donors are retained since infection in immunocompetent adult recipients is usually mild, and exclusion of CMV positive donors would drastically reduce the nation's blood supply. Only in immunocompromised patients is CMV potentially fatal, and in these patients blood components lacking CMV infection are preferentially transfused.

The incidence and prevalence of the infection in the donor population are also critical determinants. The approach to a widespread infection will require strategies different from those required for a rare or regionally concentrated infection. An example of the latter is *T. cruzi* infection, a proven transfusion threat currently limited to blood from donors who were born in or resided for prolonged periods in Mexico, Central America, or South America. Thus, regionality, habits, travel history, country of birth, medical history, and perhaps other indices of donor behavior are important considerations in the potential of any infectious agent to emerge as a threat to the blood supply. Another consideration in evaluating the public health importance of an emerging infection is the potential of that infection for secondary spread.

What are the appropriate responses to the threat?

Identification of an emerging transfusion-transmitted infectious disease and assessment of its magnitude will determine the balanced response required to ensure the continuing safety of blood components while maintaining an adequate supply. Management of an emerging threat to the blood supply involves refinement of donor recruitment and selection practices, donor testing, and blood processing. Recipient surveillance may also be important. The appropriate strategy is based on careful assessment of the risk:benefit ratio, cost-effectiveness, and availability of procedures to remove that threat from the donor pool. Each intervention must be tailored to the epidemiology and microbiology of the infection.

The intervention strategy that may have the greatest potential efficacy is refinement of the donor history. Data from the early 1980's demonstrate that a substantial reduction in the incidence of posttransfusion hepatitis B, hepatitis C, and HIV transmission occurred following redesign of donor recruitment and selection practices as well as improved transfusion practice. The efficacy of this approach is further corroborated by recent studies on Chagas disease, which show that careful design and validation of historical questions can separate high-risk from low-risk donors. Further studies on the development and validation of this instrument should be encouraged.

The next step in screening for potential transfusion-transmitted infection is implementation of new laboratory tests of donor blood. Ideally such tests should be very sensitive, in order to lead to the rejection of all dangerous donors, and also very specific, in order to achieve a strong positive predictive value and minimize unnecessary deferral of otherwise acceptable donors. In the absence of reliable assays specific for the infection in question, it may be necessary to institute surrogate testing as was done for posttransfusion hepatitis. Implementation of revised donor questionnaires and introduction of laboratory testing must be accompanied by evaluation of outcomes demonstrating that the interventions favorably influence component safety and supply. Ineffective or inefficient interventions should be discontinued if their impact is negative or neutral.

Implementation of a response to an emerging infectious disease threat to the blood supply requires a wide range of activities. Once a strategy is adopted, personnel must be trained, equipment and supplies obtained, procedures and policies prepared and validated, and appropriate documentation prepared. In view of the fact that any change per se may induce a higher error rate for some time, close supervision is critical at this phase. Numerous other effects result from changes in donor screening strategy. For example, the donor will now be required to answer additional or different questions, or may receive notification of the result of unfamiliar tests. Planning must include these considerations.

Recommendations

In the absence of any formal mechanism by which transfusion medicine evaluates the threat of a potential transfusion-transmitted infection, it is recommended that:

• The blood transfusion community arrange for periodic communication with the Centers for Disease Control and Prevention to proactively review emerging infectious disease threats to the United States and its borders.

• The appropriate responses once a potential threat to transfusion safety is identified include:

a. evaluation of transmissibility by transfusion

    b.   assessment of public health significance

    c.   definition of responses appropriate to the potential transfusion safety risk.

What Are the Highest Priorities for Research to Improve Transfusion Safety by Reducing the Transmission of Infectious Disease?

The panel believes that the following issues represent important needs in improving transfusion safety. Recognizing that research is already under way in most of these areas, the panel wishes to provide a comprehensive list of research issues, not in any priority.

- *T. pallidum* in relation to transfusion
- Definition of the incidence and causes of bacterial contamination of blood
- Better methods for eliminating or inactivating infectious agents in blood components
- Improved direct tests for infectious agents
- Definition of the biology and natural history of non-A, non-B, non-C, posttransfusion hepatitis
- Prevalence of residual hepatitis B and hepatitis C posttransfusion hepatitis; large-scale, prospective donor repositories and recipient surveillance
- Implications of transfusion-transmitted diseases in neonates
- Evaluation of the risk of nonenveloped viruses in patients receiving plasma derivatives
- Epidemiology of Chagas disease in the United States
- Design of questionnaires to elicit evidence of risk in donors
- Impact of deferral on donors
- Improved understanding of donor motivation and recruitment practices
- Development of artificial blood components

Conclusions

- Since the determination of ALT has not been shown to be a useful surrogate marker in the present setting, the panel recommends that it be discontinued.

- Anti-HBc testing does have the potential to prevent some cases of posttransfusion hepatitis B. It may also act as a surrogate marker for HIV infection in donors and may prevent a small number of cases of transfusion-transmitted HIV infection. However, it has a high false positive rate, which results in the deferral of many acceptable donors. The panel therefore recommends that the test be continued but that its specificity be improved. Since disease prevalence in populations is in constant flux, the accuracy of direct and indirect tests for disease also changes. The panel therefore also recommends periodic critical reevaluation of the utility of these tests.

- The test for syphilis has been used for many years, and data are inadequate to ascertain whether it accounts for the rarity of transfusion-transmitted syphilis. The panel therefore recommends that use of the test continue, but also recommends that research be done to determine if seropositivity is predictive of spirochetemia and to define the extent to which the organism remains viable and infective in blood components.

- Public health surveillance, and collaboration between public health and transfusion medicine specialists, is critical in responding to emerging infectious disease threats to the blood supply.

An organized multidisciplinary approach to these threats must be formulated (including Federal and State public health agencies, the medical community in general, and the transfusion medicine community).

Statement Availability

Preparation and distribution of this statement is the responsibility of the Office of Medical Applications of Research of the National Institutes of Health. Free copies of this statement and bibliographies prepared by the National Library of Medicine are available from the Office of Medical Applications of Research, National Institutes of Health, or the NIH Consensus Program Information Service by 24-hour voice mail. In addition, free copies of all other available NIH Consensus Statements and NIH Technology Assessment Statements may be obtained from the following resources:

NIH Consensus Program Information Service
P.O. Box 2577
Kensington, MD 20891
Telephone 1-800-NIH-OMAR (644-6627)
Fax (301) 816-2494

NIH Office of Medical Applications of Research
Federal Building, Room 618
7550 Wisconsin Avenue MSC 9120
Bethesda, MD 20892-9120

Full-text versions of all these statements are also available online through an electronic bulletin board system and through the Internet:

NIH Information Center BBS
(301) 480-5144

Internet

Gopher
gopher://gopher.nih.gov/Health and Clinical Information

World Wide Web
http://text.nlm.nih.gov

ftp
ftp://public.nlm.nih.gov/hstat/nihcdcs

About the NIH Consensus Development Program

NIH Consensus Development Conferences are convened to evaluate available scientific information and resolve safety and efficacy issues related to a biomedical technology. The resultant NIH Consensus Statements are intended to advance understanding of the technology or issue in question and to be useful to health professionals and the public.

NIH Consensus Statements are prepared by a nonadvocate, non-Federal panel of experts, based on (1) presentations by investigators working in areas relevant to the consensus questions during a 2-day public session, (2) questions and statements from conference attendees during open discussion periods that are part of the public session, and (3) closed deliberations by the panel during the remainder of the second day and morning of the third. This statement is an independent report of the panel and is not a policy statement of the NIH or the Federal Government.

Chapter 47

Risks Associated with Blood Transfusions

Background

Widespread concern about the safety of the blood supply has led to many changes in the way blood is collected, processed, and transfused. Consequently, the risks of contracting certain diseases, such as AIDS and hepatitis, are lower today than they were in the mid-1980s, when the public became increasingly aware that blood transfusions are not risk free. In this chapter, we address the risks of contracting AIDS and hepatitis from blood as well as other known risks of blood transfusion. [An evaluation of the Food and Drug Administration's (FDA's) layers of safety and its ability to ensure the safety of the blood supply in light of changes in the blood industry is provided in a report entitled *Blood Supply: FDA Oversight and Remaining Issues of Safety.*[1]]

On June 30, 1992, 4,619 persons had been reported with suspected transfusion-associated AIDS, representing about 2 percent of the 222,418 U.S. residents reported with AIDS. The number of suspected transfusion-associated AIDS cases rose every year from 56 for patients transfused in 1978 to 714 for patients transfused in 1984 (Selik, Ward, and Buehler, 1993). Then, in 1985, when HIV antibody screening of donors began, the number declined sharply to 288 cases, and it fell

Excerpted from the United States General Accounting Office Report to the Ranking Minority Member, Committee on Commerce, House of Representatives. *Blood Supply: Transfusion Associated Risks*, GAO/PEMD-97-2 (Washington, D.C.: 1997).

below 20 cases per year from 1986 through 1991.[2] The number of new HIV infections definitively associated with transfusions is even smaller. Only 38 cases of AIDS have been attributed to transfusions of blood screened negative after March 1985.

Measuring Risk

Meanwhile, researchers at the Centers for Disease Control and Prevention (CDC) and within the blood industry were developing and implementing new methods to measure transfusion-associated risks. As a result, the risk estimates that have been presented in the literature vary considerably, depending on when a study was published, the area of the country it considered, and the assumptions underlying its methods. For instance, early studies employed less-sensitive tests than are currently available, were conducted in high-risk areas rather than nationally, and used measurements that were less precise than those used today.

Moreover, the donor pool is safer today than when early studies were conducted because donors who have tested positive for certain viruses or who have acknowledged risk factors for disease have been removed from the donor pool. Indeed, testing may be the mostly widely cited, and is perhaps the most important, step in protecting the public from the risks of blood transfusions. Tests performed on every unit of blood include tests for antibody to hepatitis B core antigen (anti-HBc), hepatitis B surface antigen (HBsAg), antibody to hepatitis C virus (anti-HCV), human immunodeficiency virus (antibody for HIV-1 and HIV-2, and antigen for HIV-1), human T-lymphotropic virus type I (HTLV-I), and syphilis.[3]

Because the scientific community has focused primarily on the risks of contracting specific diseases from blood transfusion, the state of knowledge is quite advanced for some risks such as hepatitis and HIV. Less is known about bacterial contamination and some noninfectious risks such as circulatory overload. No systematic analysis has been published regarding the overall risks of blood transfusion compared to its potential benefits.

Donated Blood and Its Products

About 8 million people donate approximately 14 million units of whole blood each year. This blood—blood in its natural state—is rarely transfused into patients. Instead, the blood industry separates each unit of whole blood into an average of 1.9 specialized products that, in blood-banking terminology, are "components" consisting of various types of blood cells, plasma, and special preparations of plasma.[4] Health care facilities transfuse these components—usually 4 to 5 units at a time—into as many as 4 million patients to treat anemia, bleeding disorders, and low blood volume. Donors give an additional 12 million units of plasma each year, for a total of approximately 26 million annual blood and plasma donations prior to testing for viral infections.

In an increasingly common procedure called apheresis, specifically desired components of a donor's blood are removed and the undesired components are given back to the donor. Whole-blood donors must wait 8 weeks between donations to allow the body to replenish its red blood cells. Apheresis collection of plasma, platelets, or white blood cells (leukocytes) may be performed more frequently, however, if red blood cells are returned to the donor. As we discuss later in this chapter, apheresis often minimizes transfusion risks for the recipient without compromising safety for the donor.

Results in Brief

The blood supply is safer today than any time in recent history. Improved donor screening and education have removed from the donor pool many persons who are at high risk for disease. Tests used to screen blood for viruses are considerably more sensitive than previous versions. Repeat donors constitute most of the donor pool, which means that they have been tested for viruses on earlier donations. Thus, the window of opportunity for infection is considerably smaller than for first-time donors who have never been tested. Viral inactivation techniques for plasma derivatives eliminate most viruses that may escape detection on testing. And changes in transfusion practices have eliminated some of the circumstances that may have led to unnecessary transfusions in the past.

Nevertheless, because blood is a biological product, some risk remains. Eight of every 10,000 donated units of blood carry some kind of potentially serious risk to the recipient, including allergic reactions, bacteria, reactions to incompatible blood transfusions, and viruses. We calculated that 4 of every 1,000 patients who receive the average transfusion of 5 units of blood are at risk of receiving an implicated unit and thus may be exposed to conditions with the potential for the development of serious (chronic, disabling, or fatal) outcomes.[5] While these risks may appear to be substantial when considered outside a medical context, it is commonly understood that transfusion provides substantial benefits. We reasoned that as many as 50 percent, or 500, of the 1,000 recipients would be at serious risk of dying immediately if they did not receive transfusions.[6]

Not all recipients of a contaminated unit acquire the disease it contains. Moreover, many recipients die soon after transfusion from the underlying condition for which the blood was prescribed. Finally, the likelihood that a patient will develop chronic disease or die is small for some diseases. We determined that the overall risk of developing chronic disease or dying as a direct result of a blood transfusion is about 4 in 10,000, which translates into about 1,525 of the 4 million patients who receive transfusions each year.

The risk that a general surgery patient will require blood and develop a chronic disease or die as a result of that blood is 5 in 100,000. For the average person in the United States who has no foreseeable plans for surgery, the annual risk of developing a need for surgery, requiring blood, and developing a chronic disease or dying from the transfusion is 5 in 1 million.

We concluded that in context these risks are very small, particularly considering that many patients would die without blood transfusion. The risks from transfusing blood to recipients in general and surgery patients specifically are considerably smaller than other hospital-related risks. Furthermore, the annual risk to an average person in the United States with no foreseeable plans for surgery is more than 250 times less than the annual risk of hospitalization from accidental poisoning by drugs and other medicines and nearly 600 times less than that of other diseases or events of high public concern, such as heart disease.

We took a worst-case approach in our analysis. That is, we used the most conservative risk estimates among current comprehensive studies published in the scientific literature. Consequently, the actual risks of transfusion may be somewhat lower, but are not likely to be higher, than the risks we present.

Objectives, Scope, and Methodology

Our objective in this report was to quantify the current risks associated with blood transfusion. To respond to your request, we reviewed data on the current risks of blood transfusion in the United States, evaluating the content and quality of the data. We analyzed the theoretical and research foundations underlying current and past risk estimates and held extensive interviews with industry and government epidemiological experts.

Our analysis assumed that all the layers of safety are working properly. That is, our risk estimates are for units of blood from donors who were properly screened, who were checked on the deferral registry, whose blood was tested for viruses, and so on.

We included risks of receiving units contaminated by eight viruses (HAV, HBV, HCV, HIV-1 and HIV-2, HTLV-I and HTLV-II, non-ABC hepatitis), various bacteria, and one parasite-transmitted disease (Chagas'), as well as four complications of transfusion itself (ABO incompatibility, acute lung injury, allergic reaction, and circulatory overload). We did not include the risks of some diseases that are known to be present in blood but that have very low prevalence rates (such as Leishmaniasis), that have already high prevalence rates in the general population with few complications (such as cytomegalovirus, or CMV, and B19 parvovirus), or that have no scientific proof of transfusion transmission (Creutzfeldt-Jakob disease, or CJD).[7]

Unless otherwise noted, our risk estimates are for whole-blood products from unpaid allogeneic donors. Allogeneic donors include volunteer donors for the general supply and directed donors for friends and family.[8] Autologous donors, who donate their blood for their own use, can be infectious but cannot transmit a virus to themselves. A small portion of unused autologous blood is "crossed-over" into the general supply. We included these units.

Limited data are available concerning the risks posed by paid donors of plasma; therefore, we did not include plasma derivatives in our analysis. Although the disease rates of paid donors are thought to be higher than those of volunteer donors, most plasma-derived products undergo viral inactivation processes during manufacturing, which eliminates most but not all viruses. Few cases of disease transmission have been reported since testing and inactivation began. We discuss relevant issues in Chapter 49, Plasma Products.

Our analysis consisted of several estimates for each of the diseases above or complications: (1) risks per donated unit, (2) annual number of infectious or otherwise implicated component units released for transfusion, (3) risks that the transfusion recipient would receive an implicated unit, (4) number of recipients who would contract the disease present in the blood transfusion, (5) number of recipients who would not die from the underlying disease or trauma necessitating the transfusion before problems associated with the blood transfusion manifest, and (6) the number of recipients who would die or develop chronic disease as a result of the disease or other transfusion complication. These numbers are for patients who have a blood transfusion. We also considered the risks for general surgery patients who may or may not require a transfusion and the annual risks for a person in the general population who does not foresee a plan for surgery. [See

Appendix II of the original document for information on the studies used in the analysis and the calculations.]

No risk estimate can be properly interpreted in isolation. Therefore, we compared our risk estimate for death or chronic disease from a blood transfusion with other known hospital-related risks, as well as with those for death by other common diseases.

Finally, we reviewed means currently or soon to be available by which the risks of blood transfusion may be further reduced.

Wherever possible, we included in our analysis the most recent, nationally representative studies that used state-of-the-art viral tests. For example, we did not include some of the older studies on HIV risk that employed donors from geographical areas that at the time were of high risk and are, therefore, less useful as predictors of current risk at a national level. However, we do recognize their value as the first controlled studies of HIV risk and we note that they are the models upon which newer, more relevant studies are conducted. In Chapter 48, Blood Transfusion-Associated Complications, we discuss the details of the major studies we reviewed, including their relative strengths and weaknesses.

We used one overarching principle when choosing between studies that we considered equally sound and that were a matter of continuing debate in the research community: we chose to include the studies with the higher risk estimates. In other words, ours is a worst-case analysis. Thus, the actual risks for some of the agents and activities we discuss may be somewhat lower but are not likely to be higher given the available research. Using some of the more variable estimates, we conducted sensitivity analyses for our final analysis of the number of recipients likely to die or develop chronic disease; we found the results to be highly robust. That is, even when using different estimates for individual diseases or complications, the resulting final estimate changed very little.[9]

We conducted our review in accordance with generally accepted government auditing standards.

Principal Findings

In the context of other health-related risks, the risks of blood transfusion are extremely small, especially considering the often fatal consequences of refusing a medically necessary transfusion. Moreover, these risks are continually decreasing as a result of advances in donor screening, improved viral tests, viral inactivation techniques, and changes in transfusion medicine practices.

Five Factors That Help Reduce Risk

The risk of contracting a disease from blood transfusion continues to decrease. We identified five factors that have helped reduce the risk of contracting viral diseases from blood transfusions.

First, better donor screening and education efforts have refined the volunteer whole-blood donor pool to one comprising primarily persons with lower risk than those who donated blood before such screening was introduced. The frequency of positive HIV test results among blood donors is now much lower than that of other tested groups, such as military recruits, inner-city emergency room patients, and randomly selected newborns. Moreover, the current rate of positive HIV test results is about 8 per 100,000 blood donors, which is 50 times lower than the rate of 400 per 100,000 in the general population.

Second, state-of-the-art viral screening tests can detect infected blood donations. For example, before anti-HCV testing, the rate of transfusion-associated hepatitis was 4.4 percent. After first-generation anti-HCV tests were introduced, the rate fell to about 1 percent—nearly an 80-percent reduction. Second-generation tests identified an additional 10 percent of infected donors for an overall reduction of 90 percent in transfusion-associated hepatitis C.

Third, because FDA regulations and industry practices prevent the use of blood from infected, behaviorally risky, or test-positive donors, the donor pool comprises primarily repeat donors who have been deemed safe. These repeat donors have a narrower window of opportunity of infection (defined by the interval between tested donations) compared to first-time donors whose blood has never been tested and who, therefore, have a substantially longer window of opportunity of infection.

Indeed, a recent collaborative study by the CDC and the American Red Cross (ARC) revealed that 7 million donations, or 80 percent of all donations collected by ARC in 1991 through 1993, were from repeat donors (Lackritz et al., 1995). Of these donations from repeat donors, less than 2 of every 100,000 donations (142) tested positive for HIV. The remaining 20 percent of the donor pool were first-time donors who provided only about a fourth as much blood, or 2 million donations. Donations from first-time donors were 9 times more likely to be HIV-positive than those of repeat donors: 18 of every 100,000 donations (349) from first-time donors tested positive for HIV.

Fourth, viral inactivation techniques are used whenever possible in the manufacture of plasma derivatives. This is particularly important for the plasma derivatives that hemophiliacs routinely use (see

Chapter 49, Plasma Products). Recent research suggests that new inactivation techniques may be available in the future for other blood products, such as red blood cells, that are too fragile to withstand most heat or chemically based inactivation.

And fifth, as physicians have become more aware of changes in the practice of transfusion medicine, they have moved away from routinely prescribing whole blood. Instead, they have moved toward prescribing specific blood components to alleviate specific complications, using plasma volume expanders wherever appropriate, collecting a patient's own blood before an operation, and salvaging and reinfusing a patient's own blood during surgery. See Chapter 50, Reducing Transfusion-Associated Risks, for additional discussion of new technology and medical practice changes that could further reduce risk.

Risks of Blood Transfusion

We evaluated the overall risk of blood transfusion by synthesizing the risks of a number of different adverse outcomes that could result from receiving blood (see Table 47.1).[10] Because estimates of risk are better understood in context, we compared them to other known health-related risks.

[See Appendix II of the original document for a discussion of the method of analysis in detail, including citations for the estimates in Table 47.1.]

Although the risk of receiving HIV-contaminated blood is the public's greatest fear, other diseases transmitted through blood are far more common than HIV. For example, we found that the risk of contracting HCV infection is more than 100 times greater than that of contracting HIV. After screening and testing, the likelihood that a unit of blood infected with hepatitis C virus would remain undetected and be released for transfusion is 1 in every 4,100 units of blood; for HIV, the likelihood is 1 in every 450,000 units.[11] A more sensitive anti-HCV test that detects more infected units is available in Europe and has been licensed in the United States during the past year. Its use is widespread but not universal.

The likelihood that a unit of blood may become contaminated by bacteria ranges from 1 in 500,000 for red blood cells to 1 in 10,200 for random donor platelets, the blood component used to treat certain bleeding disorders. As we discuss in *Blood Supply: FDA Oversight and Remaining Issues of Safety*, cited above, bacteria can enter a unit during collection as a result of either poor aseptic technique or donor bacteremia. Bacteria present in a unit can proliferate during storage.

Table 47.1. Individual and Overall Risks of Adverse Outcomes From Allogeneic Blood Transfusion[a]

Agent or activity	1. Risk estimate per unit (12.057 million units donated)	2. Patient risk per transfusion of 5 units	3. Annual number of implicated component units if 23.19 million components available and 19.23 million transfusions	4. Number of recipients affected (likelihood of seroconversion) Number	Percent	5. Number of recipients who do not die of underlying disease or trauma first (30% die within 2 years)	6. Number of recipients who develop chronic disease or die as a result of transfusion (likelihood) Number	Percent
Virus[b]								
HAV	1:1,000,000	1:200,000	23	21	90%	15	0	0.2%
HBV	1:63,000	1:12,600	368	258	70	181	18	10
HCV	1:4,100	1:820	5,656	5,090	90	3,563	713	20
HIV-1 and -2	1:450,000	1:90,000	52	47	90	33	33	100
HTLV-I and -II	1:50,000	1:10,000	464	125	27	88	4	4.75
Non-ABC hepatitis	1:5,900	1:1,180	3,931	3,538	90	2,477	372	15
Bacterium								
Platelet contamination[c]								
Random donor	1:10,200	1:1,700	460	460[d]		460[e]	120	26
Apheresis	1:19,500	1:19,500	31[d]	31[d]		31[e]	8	26
Yersinia[f]	1:500,000	1:100,000	24	24[d]		24[e]	6	26
Parasite[g]								
T. cruzi	1:42,000	1:8,400	552	55	10	39	12	30
Subtotal risk of infection	5:10,000[g]	2.7:1,000[g]	11,561	9,649		6,911	1,286	
Transfusion[h]								
ABO incompatible[i]	1:12,000	1:2,400	895[j]	322[k]		322[e]	19	6
Acute lung injury	1:10,000	1:2,000	1,923	1,923[d]		1,923[e]	96	5
Anaphylaxis	1:150,000	1:30,000	128	128[d]		128[e]	26	20
Circulatory overload	1:10,000	1:2,000	1,923	1,923[d]		1,923[e]	96	5
Subtotal risk of transfusion reaction	3:10,000	1.5:1,000	4,869	4,296		4,296	237	
Total			16,430	13,945		11,207	1,523	
Risk	8:10,000[l]	4.2:1,000[l]	3.5:1,000[m]	2.8:1,000[m]			4:10,000[m]	

Notes for this table are presented on the following two pages.

Table 47.1 NOTES.

[a]Although donors may carry more than one disease, the likelihood that a unit will escape detection by multiple tests is almost nonexistent. Therefore, the individual risks presented here are independent, and the total risk is calculated by summing individual risks. Numbers may not be exact because of rounding. An example using HIV across columns 1-6 is as follows:

1. The risk of HIV is 1 in every 450,000 donated units. That is, of the 12.057 million units donated, 27 will be HIV positive (12.057 million/450,000 (not shown)).

2. Assuming each patient receives an average of about 5 units of blood (except platelets noted below), then the risk to the patient is 450,000/5, or 1 in 90,000.

3. Each allogeneic unit is made into an average of 1.87 transfused components. Hence, 12.057 million units = 22,583,000 components plus 607,000 apheresis platelets = 23,190,000 total components. The 27 units of HIV-positive blood become 52 different components.

4. Not all recipients will develop the disease present in the blood (seroconvert); 90 percent of the 52 recipients of HIV blood will seroconvert (47 patients). This concept applies only to viruses.

5. Most patients receiving blood are at great risk of dying from their underlying conditions; 30 percent die within 2 years. For HIV, 33 of the 47 patients will survive.

6. Not all agents and activities lead to chronic disease or death. The likelihood that HIV will is nearly 100 percent, so all 33 patients who survive their underlying conditions will die.

[b]The number of virus- and parasite-contaminated units is based on the number of allogeneic units donated (12.057 million) and the number of components made (23.190 million).

[c]A total of 8.330 million individual units of platelets were transfused. Patient risk and available components are based on 4.688 million random donor platelets transfused (56 percent of total platelet transfusions) and 607,000 single donor apheresis platelets transfused (each apheresis unit has 6 individual units collected from 1 donor, totaling 3.642 million platelets, or 44 percent of total platelet transfusions). For

example, patient risk for a random donor unit is the risk for each donor unit divided by the average number of units pooled into a therapeutic dose, 10,200/6, or 1 in 1,700 in Morrow's (1991) research on platelet contamination. The number of implicated random donor units is 4.688 million/10,200, or 460 units. The patient risk for apheresis platelets is the same as the per-unit risk (1:19,500) because the platelets are collected at the same time from a single donor. Number of implicated apheresis units is 607,000/19,500, or 31 units.

dSeroconversion not relevant. Numbers carried over from column 3.

eNot relevant for bacterial contamination or transfusion-related outcomes that are near-term events.

fRisk is based on 12.057 million red blood cell units because Yersinia occurs only in these units.

gRisk is based on sum of viral risks plus Yersinia risk plus a weighted sum of platelet risks based on proportion transfused ((random platelet risk x 0.56) + (apheresis platelet risk x 0.44)).

hThe number of units associated with transfusion problems is based on the number of units actually transfused (4.688 million random donor platelets, 607,000 apheresis platelets, 10.741 million whole blood and red blood cells, and 3.194 million other components). Risk is based on 19,230,000 total transfusions. [See Appendix II of the original document for supply and transfusion calculations.]

iRisk is based on 10.741 million red blood cells and whole blood transfused because compatibility is an issue only for these units.

jAssumes a 64-percent chance that a random transfusion to an unintended recipient would be compatible and 100-percent reporting of incompatible erroneous transfusions.

kSeroconversion not relevant. Assumes 36-percent incompatible.

lRisk is based on sum of viral risks plus Yersinia risk plus a weighted sum of platelet risk based on proportion transfused ((random platelet risk x 0.56) + (apheresis platelet risk x 0.44)) plus transfusion-related risks.

mNumber of affected patients/total number of transfusion recipients (4 million).

Platelets are at high risk because they are stored at room temperature; the risk of their contamination greatly increases over their storage life of 5 days. Bedside tests for bacterial contamination could greatly mitigate this problem and may soon be presented to FDA for approval.

We estimated that about 1 in every 2,000 units may be infected by a virus, bacterium, or parasite.[12] Certain noninfectious risks are also associated with blood transfusion. One such problem is the immune reaction associated with the inadvertent transfusion of blood that contains red blood cells that are incompatible with those in the recipient's blood. Other risks include acute lung injury, circulatory overload, and allergic reactions to certain blood proteins. Some of these risks (for example, acute lung injury) cannot be eliminated without advances in the state of knowledge about how they occur.[13] The overall likelihood of noninfectious complications is difficult to ascertain, because estimates are based on voluntary hospital reports and because they are likely to remain undiagnosed in the hospital setting. We estimated that some type of noninfectious complication may occur in 1 of every 3,448 units of blood.[14]

Using current risk estimates for individual adverse outcomes, we determined that as many as 8 of every 10,000 units of blood carry a potentially serious risk to the patient, including incompatibility, allergic reactions, bacteria, and viruses. About 11,560 of the 23.19 million components available are infected by bacteria, viruses, or parasites, and about 4,870 of the 19.23 million components that are transfused may lead to an adverse, noninfectious outcome, such as circulatory overload. We calculated that an individual patient's risk of receiving an implicated unit is 4.2 in 1,000, or 1 in 238 patients.[15]

In order to fully understand the risks of blood transfusion, one must consider three additional factors. First, even if a unit of blood is contaminated, the likelihood of acquiring the disease it contains is less than 100 percent, ranging from 10 to 90 percent. Second, blood is typically prescribed for patients who have very serious trauma or disease. Indeed, there is a 30-percent chance that a patient will die within 2 years from the underlying condition for which the blood is prescribed and, therefore, never experience some of the possible negative consequences from the blood transfusion itself.[16]

Third, only HIV-contaminated blood leads to nearly certain fatal outcomes; the likelihood that a patient would develop clinically serious chronic disease or die as a result of blood transfusion ranges from 0.2 to 30 percent for all other possible complications. When we included all these facts in our analysis, we determined that only 10 percent of exposed recipients are ultimately harmed seriously by their blood transfusions. Indeed, the overall risk of developing chronic disease or dying as a direct result of a blood transfusion is about 4 in 10,000, which translates into 1,523 of the 4 million patients who receive transfusions each year.[17]

Surgery patients numbered 23 million in 1993. Given that there are 3 million surgical transfusion patients annually, we estimated that 13 percent of the surgery patients received blood. Therefore, discounting the fact that some patients had multiple surgeries, a maximum of 9 percent underwent surgery and 1 percent both underwent surgery and received blood among the 260 million in the general U.S. population.[18]

Given these estimates, we calculated that the risk of a general surgery patient's requiring blood and then developing a chronic disease or dying as a result of that blood is 5 in 100,000 (see Table 47.2). For an average person in the general population who does not foresee a plan for surgery, the annual risk that he or she would develop a need for surgery, require blood, and develop a chronic disease or die as a result of that blood is 5 in 1 million.

Blood Transfusion Risks in Perspective

In order to determine whether these risks are small or large, we compared them to other health-related risks. Data from the Medical Practice Study suggest that more than 1 million patients are injured in hospitals each year, and approximately 180,000 die annually as a result of these injuries (Brennan et al., 1991; Leape et al., 1991). A recent study

Table 47.2. Risks of Surgery and Blood Transfusions[a]

Likelihood of problem if patient	Risk
Receives blood	40:100,000
Is a surgery candidate	5:100,000
Has no plans for surgery	5:1,000,000

[a]Assumes 23 million surgeries in 1993, or 9 percent of the U.S. population, with an estimated 13 percent of the surgeries using blood and 0.012 probability of surgery and blood transfusion occurring together. Assumes further that only 3 million of the 4 million patients who received transfused blood were surgery patients; the remaining 1 million received transfusions for cancer therapy, hemophilia, and other disorders.

at two large Massachusetts hospitals found that 6.5 percent of admitted patients suffered an injury resulting from medical intervention related to a prescribed drug during their hospital stay (Bates et al., 1995).

The risks to blood transfusion recipients and general surgery patients are considerably smaller than the risk of dying as a direct result of surgery, the risk that a hospital stay will result in death or chronic disability, the risk of suffering an injury from hospital drug therapy, and the risk of developing an infection of unknown cause in intensive care (see Table 47.3).

Table 47.3. Likelihood of Various Health Outcomes

Outcome	Per 100,000 patients or hospitalizations[a]
Chronic disease or death from blood if:	
General surgery patient	5
Received blood transfusion	40
Hospital stay ends in death or disability	600[b]
Death as direct result of surgery	1,333[c]
Injury related to drug therapy during hospital stay	6,500[d]
Infection of unknown cause in intensive care	7,500[e]

[a]We were unable to determine whether some of these figures include the risk of dying from transfusion. However, that risk is a very small proportion of the other risks.

[b]T. A. Brennan et al., "Incidence of Adverse Events and Negligence in Hospitalized Patients: Results of the Harvard Medical Practice Study I," *New England Journal of Medicine*, 324:6 (1991), 370-76.

[c]C. B. Inlander et al., *The Consumer's Medical Desk Reference* (New York: Stonesong Press, 1 995).

[d]D. W. Bates et al., "Incidence of Adverse Drug Events and Potential Adverse Drug Events: Implications for Prevention," *Journal of the American Medical Association*, 274:1 (1995), 29-34.

[e]B. N. Doebbeling et al., "Comparative Efficacy of Alternative Hand-Washing Agents in Reducing Nosocomial Infections in Intensive Care Units," *New England Journal of Medicine*, 327 (1992), 88-93.

Furthermore, the annual risk from transfusion to an average person in the United States who foresees no plan for surgery is the same as or lower than the annual risk of dying from tuberculosis or from accidental electrocution or drowning, and it is as much as nearly 600 times less than the annual risk of dying from other diseases or events of great public concern (see Table 47.4). These differences are particularly striking considering that the risk estimate for blood transfusion includes both chronic disease and death, whereas some of the other risk estimates include only death; estimates that included chronic disease would be substantially higher. Perhaps most importantly, the risks associated with blood transfusion must be compared to the risk of dying from having refused a blood transfusion that physicians believed to be medically necessary—a risk that could approach 100 percent in some cases.

Conclusions

We found that the current risks from blood transfusion are small compared to transfusion's overwhelming benefits in saving lives. Blood transfusion is the most common therapy using human tissue in the world. As a tissue, blood retains the medical history of its donor. Because it is a biological product, the risks can approach but may never reach zero.

Medical testing and manufacturing technologies continue to improve blood safety. Medical practice is being transformed to accommodate new knowledge about the risks and benefits of blood transfusion. Ultimately, each patient benefits from these advances. However, because the risks are already so low, incremental increases in safety may be difficult to achieve. Therefore, the potential outcomes of alternatives for reducing blood transfusion risks may require careful consideration in order to identify areas of improvement that would maximize safety with reasonable costs.

The analysis we present here incorporates what is known today about infectious agents in the blood supply. New infectious agents are always emerging, and there is always the possibility that they could be transmitted by blood. Continued safety, therefore, depends on the scientific and medical communities' detecting and identifying new threats to the blood supply.

Table 47.4. Annual Rates of Various Health Outcomes

Outcome	Condition	Per 100,000 population
Chronic disease or death by transfusion without surgery plans		0.5
Hospitalization for:	Septicemia (bacteria infection in bloodstream)	105
	Accidental poisoning by drugs, medicines, and biologicals	128
	Drugs and other phar-maceuticals causing adverse effects in therapeutic use	142
	Infections or parasitic diseases	311
	Cerebrovascular disease	328
	Pneumonia	462
	Malignant tumor	578
	Injury and poisoning	1,060
	Heart disease	1,541
Death from:	Electrocution	0.5
	Tuberculosis	0.8
	Drowning	2.8
	Hardening of arteries	9
	Motor vehicle crash	15
	Pneumonia or influenza	32
	Stroke	59
	Cancer	206
	Heart disease	296

Notes to the Text in This Chapter

[1]U.S. General Accounting Office, *Blood Supply: FDA Oversight and Remaining Issues of Safety*, GAO/PEMD-97-1 (Washington, D.C.: 1997).

[2]Within the human body's disease-fighting capabilities, it can develop antibodies that are specific to each viral infection. The initial HIV-1 tests detected the HIV antibody in blood donated by infected persons.

[3]Antibody tests detect antibodies that the human body produces in its immune response to a virus, whereas antigen tests detect a component of the actual virus. Because it takes time to develop antibodies, antigen tests detect infection earlier than antibody tests. HTLV is a retrovirus that can lead to neurologic disease or adult T-cell leukemia and lymphoma. Tests currently available are specific for antibodies to HTLV-I, although there are varying degrees of cross-reactivity with antibodies to HTLV-II. Nevertheless, it is the closest test for HTLV-II at this time. We discuss transfusion-associated diseases further in Chapter 48, Blood Transfusion-Associated Complications.

[4]In addition to separating whole blood into component products, other facilities manufacture plasma derivatives by fractionating plasma chemically into concentrated proteins. These include albumin, used for blood volume expansion; immune globulin, used to prevent certain infectious diseases and to treat deficiencies of protein; clotting factor concentrates, used to control bleeding in patients with clotting factor deficiencies, such as hemophilia; and specific immune globulins, prepared from plasmas collected from donors with antibodies to specific diseases and then used to prevent those diseases in others. Derivatives are commonly made by commercial manufacturers from plasma collected from paid donors. Depending on the product, they may pool plasma from as many as 60,000 donors for fractionation in order to produce sufficient amounts of the final concentrated material cost-effectively.

[5]We present an overall risk for all types of blood components. Strictly speaking, different blood components carry different risks. This is especially true for a therapeutic dose of apheresis platelets, which, because it contains only 1 donor's platelets, carries a much lower risk to the patient than a typical therapeutic dose of random donor platelets (6 donors) or red blood cells (5 donors). [See Appendix II of the original document for a detailed discussion of these differences.]

[6]The ethical concerns surrounding a study of differences in survival rates between groups of patients who have and have not received blood make collecting such data difficult. However, Jehovah's Witnesses who refuse blood on religious grounds are natural case study controls. Research on this population suggests that the mortality rate is between 38 and 53 percent among severely anemic patients who refuse transfusion (Spence et al., 1990 and 1992). Mortality is higher (7.5 percent) for those with active bleeding who require emergency surgery (Carson et al., 1988).

[7]No cases of transfusion-transmitted Leishmaniasis have been documented in the United States. In 1991, a new form of the disease, Leishmaniasis tropica, was detected in seven Desert Storm veterans, leading to deferral of individuals who had been in the Persian Gulf in or after 1990. With the absence of any data substantiating transmission of this parasite, the ban was lifted in January 1993. CMV is a type of herpes virus. Estimates suggest that between 60 and 90 percent of the general population have been infected by the time they are adults. Primary infection is usually the result of respiratory or sexual contact, and the acute phase of the virus usually passes without symptoms. Once infected, however, blood carries antibodies for a lifetime. Only blood transfusion recipients with weakened immune systems (such as leukemia patients) and newborns are thought to be at risk for severe complications from CMV-positive blood. Therefore, units for these types of patients are routinely screened for CMV antibodies. Parvovirus, like CMV, causes a clinically mild, short disease state in all but severely immunocompromised patients. It can be severely detrimental to fetuses. About 50 percent of adults show evidence of past infection and no licensed screening test is available. The neurological disease CJD is caused by an unidentified infectious agent and has no cure. However, there is no evidence at this time that it can be transmitted by transfusion.

[8]Directed donors are donors who are, for example, relatives or friends of a patient and who donate blood because the patient has asked them to.

[9]For example, we used a risk estimate of 1 in 4,100 units for HCV based on research suggesting that the anti-HCV screening test misses some infected donors. Using this estimate, we predict that 4 in 10,000 patients will develop serious chronic disease or die. Some researchers do not accept this theory, believing that the risk is closer to 1 in 103,000. Using this estimate changes the prediction only slightly to 2 of every 10,000 patients.

[10]Our analysis did not include risks associated with plasma products. See Chapter 49, Plasma Products, for a discussion of plasma.

[11]Precise numbers such as these are known as point estimates. Their precision is necessary for calculating purposes but should not be construed as definitive. Scientists know that statistical measurement is not perfectly precise. Thus, they calculate a range, or confidence interval, of estimates that is wide enough that they are confident in believing that the real number is somewhere between the two endpoints of the range. For example, the confidence interval for HBV risk ranges from 1 in 31,279 to 1 in 146,662, meaning that the real risk almost certainly lies somewhere in the middle. In the case of HBV, the point estimate is 1 in 63,171 units. We used point estimates in our analyses. We include confidence intervals in Chapter 48, Blood Transfusion-Associated Complications, wherever they are available.

[12]See Table 47.1, note g, for calculation method.

[13]Graft-vs-host disease is one example of a problem that has been virtually eliminated as scientists discovered how it acts. Donor lymphocytes engraft and multiply in the recipient, who is usually immunocompromised. The donor cells react against the "foreign" tissues of the recipient. The reaction occurs most often in blood received from first-degree family members. These blood donations are now irradiated, thus making graft-vs-host disease from blood transfusion very rare in the United States.

[14]Estimated by summing transfusion-related, noninfectious risks from the second column of Table 47.1: 1/12,000 + 1/10,000 + 1/150,000 + 1/10,000 = 0.00029, or 2.9 in 10,000 units, or 1 in 3,448 units.

[15]The average patient risk is calculated by dividing the per-unit risk by the average number of units in a transfusion. But it must be noted that patient risk depends on the number of units transfused. For example, if the risk per unit for a disease is 1 in 500,000, then a patient who has received an average transfusion of 5 units would have a risk of 1 in 100,000 (500,000 divided by 5). That is, if 1 of every 500,000 units is contaminated, then 1 of every 100,000 patients who receive 5 units could receive a contaminated unit. Similarly, 1 of every 5,000 patients who receive 100 units could receive a contaminated unit (500,000 divided by 100).

[16]This is to say not that there is a causal relationship between receiving blood and dying but, rather, that those who receive a blood transfusion

are typically quite ill or traumatized and, consequently, may die from the underlying reason for which the transfusion was administered. The mortality rate may be even higher for platelet recipients, who are often extremely ill with cancer or other life-threatening problems.

[17]The risk for HIV we present does not include the expected reduction resulting from the introduction of the new p24 antigen HIV test. Although no confirmatory data have been collected, it is estimated that the risk of HIV in blood screened by the new test will be 1 in 700,000. When we used this risk estimate in our analysis, we concluded that it would detect an additional 19 of the 52 contaminated components in the supply and ultimately prevent 12 (less than 1 percent) of the 1,523 cases of chronic disease and death associated with transfusion.

[18]Among the estimated 260 million U.S. population, 9 percent underwent surgery (23 million divided by 260 million). Furthermore, 13 percent of those surgery patients received blood (3 million estimated surgery transfusions divided by 23 million surgeries). The likelihood that an average U.S. citizen with no plans for surgery would undergo surgery and receive blood is 1 in 100 (probability of surgery and blood = 0.09 x 0.13 = 0.01).

Chapter 48

Blood Transfusion-Associated Complications

In this chapter, we discuss factors important for understanding the nature of blood transfusion risks. Specifically, we highlight epidemiological disease factors, present and evaluate the data from blood-supply-risk and transmission-by-transfusion studies, and discuss what is known about the clinical prognosis for each virus, bacterium, and transfusion complication we include in our risk analysis.

HIV-1 and HIV-2

Disease Factors

HIV-1 is widely distributed throughout the world, 21.8 million cases having been reported by July 1996. Sub-Saharan Africa is home to 63 percent, South Asia and Southeast Asia to 23 percent, and North America to 3.7 percent of all reported cases. HIV-2 is endemic only in West Africa, although cases have appeared in other parts of Africa and in Europe, North America, and South America.

The mode of transmission and the course of immunological destruction are similar in HIV-l and HIV-2. The rate of disease progression, however, may be substantially slower in HIV-2, as may be the likelihood of secondary transmission. HIV-2 is rare in the United States:

From the United States General Accounting Office Report to the Ranking Minority Member, Committee on Commerce, House of Representatives. *Blood Supply: Transfusion Associated Risks*, GAO/PEMD-97-2 (Washington, D.C.: 1997).

by 1991, CDC had confirmed only 17 cases, of which 13 had migrated from West Africa, where it was first identified.

HIV cases in the United States were initially clustered among homosexual males, intravenous drug users, prostitutes, and transfusion recipients. However, distribution patterns have changed in the past 10 years to include more cases of infection acquired from heterosexual sex and from perinatal transmission to newborns. CDC reported in July 1996 that 1 in every 300 Americans carries the HIV virus. According to its most recent data, 650,000 to 900,000 Americans were infected by 1992, and 40,000 more become infected each year. More than 325,000 persons had died of AIDS in the United States through 1994; 50,000 more die each year. Experts point to five factors that contribute to HIV's emergence: urbanization, changes in lifestyles, increased intravenous drug abuse, international travel, and blood and tissue transplantation.

In July 1996, CDC announced the discovery in California of the first person in the United States known to carry a rare strain of HIV (group O) that is not consistently detected by current HIV screening tests. Fewer than 100 cases of this virus have been reported worldwide from West and Central Africa, Belgium, France, and Germany. The source of infection of the patient in Los Angeles is not known, but she is originally from Central Africa, and CDC officials believe that she contracted the disease before coming to the United States. The patient has never donated blood, and FDA is working with industry to improve HIV screening tests to detect HIV group O reliably. A second case of HIV-1 group O infection has been identified in the United States under CDC's surveillance activities for unusual HIV-1 variants.

The incubation period from exposure to antibody seroconversion for HIV ranges from days to months before the virus is detectable in blood. It is thought that the average time between infectiousness (when a recently infected blood donor can transmit disease) and seroconversion is 22 days, with a 95-percent confidence interval of 6 to 38 days. It takes an average of 10 years after infection for clinical signs of HIV disease to emerge.

The period of communicability is not well established but is presumed to begin early after the onset of HIV and to extend throughout life. Recent advances in treatment using a combination therapy, which may include new "protease-inhibitors," appear promising. The drugs work by blocking an enzyme critical to HIV replication and can reduce the amount of HIV in the blood to levels that cannot be detected by even the most sensitive tests available. However, success depends on strict compliance with the treatment program.

Prevention and control measures include blood and tissue screening, avoidance of any form of sexual intercourse with persons known or suspected of infection, use of latex condoms and spermicide to reduce risk of sexual transmission, avoidance of shared needles by intravenous drug users, and universal precautions by health care workers.

Blood-Supply-Risk Studies

In a study carried out between 1985 and 1991 in Baltimore and Houston (both areas of high HIV risk), Nelson and colleagues (1992) directly tested the blood of patients before and after cardiac surgery to determine their risk of acquiring HIV from blood donations screened negative for the antibody to HIV. Two cases of HIV were documented in 11,532 recipients after the transfusion of 120,312 units of blood, for an estimated risk of 1 per 60,000 units (upper limit of confidence interval 1 in 19,000). A direct approach was also taken in San Francisco, another high risk area, using donations made between November 1987 and December 1989. Busch and colleagues (1991) first pooled units of blood that had been screened for HIV antibodies and issued for transfusion and then they tested for evidence of the actual virus. This study estimated the risk of HIV-1 as 1 per 61,171 units, with a 95-percent upper confidence bound of 1 in 10,695. In a subsequent analysis of pools of screened blood donated between October 1990 and June 1993, researchers reported a risk of 1 in 160,000 units (upper bound of 95-percent confidence interval, 1:128,000) (Vyas et al., 1996).

Statistical modeling techniques have replaced most of the direct measurement methods of collecting transfusion risk data. The first such method estimated risk based on data on the incidence of seroconversion among donors (the total number of new infections in a given time period) and assumptions about the sensitivity of tests and the length of the window period. Using this method, Ward and colleagues (1988) estimated the HIV risk at about 1 per 40,000 units.[1] Ward's groundbreaking reasoning was as follows.

From May 1986 to May 1987, 0.012 percent of repeat blood donors and 0.041 percent of first-time donors in the United States had HIV antibody.[2] If we assume that all HIV infections detected in repeat blood donors are new, or incident, infections and that those in first-time donors are preexisting, or prevalent, infections, then we can estimate the number of persons who are infected with HIV after they have received transfusions screened as negative for antibody. We can do this by assuming the following: a test sensitivity of 99 percent, the development of detectable HIV antibody 8 weeks after infection, an equal probability of infection throughout time, a repeat donation rate of 1.5 times per year (about every 32 weeks), and the collection of 14.4 million of the 18 million components transfused annually (or 80 percent) from repeat donors. In other words,

- for repeat donors, $(14,400,000 \times [0.00012 \times (8/32)]) + (14,400,000 \times [0.00012 \times (24/32) \times 0.01]) = 445.$[3]

- For first-time donors: $3,600,000 \times (0.00041 \times 0.01) = 15.$

- Transmission by HIV seronegative blood: $445 + 15 = 460$ units of 18 million = 1 per 39,130, or about 1 per 40,000.

Cumming and colleagues (1989) used similar methods but with more refined rates of donor infectivity that accounted for differences between males and females and between first-time and repeat donors and a lower estimate of test error (0.1 percent). They reported the risk of an HIV positive unit at 1 per 153,000 units if the window period was 8 weeks (as was then thought, using first-generation HIV tests), a 1-in-300,000 risk with a 4-week window period, and 1 in 88,000 with a 14-week window period.

Kleinman and Secord (1988) improved the mathematical model by employing "look-back techniques" to estimate the number of HIV-infected units that would be donated by repeat donors in the window period. That is, they looked back at recipients who had received test-negative donations from repeat donors who later gave test-positive donations. With this technique, Kleinman and Secord calculated the rate of recipient infection from these preseroconversion donations, estimated the duration of the window period, and found the HIV risk in Los Angeles in 1987 to be 1 per 68,000.

Petersen and colleagues (1994) used the lookback method to refine the estimate of the window period. They evaluated the HIV status of recipients who had received screened negative donations from 182 repeat donors who later tested positive for HIV. The study reflected donations from a large portion of the United States and conditions from 1985 to 1990. These researchers found 20 percent of recipients of preseroconversion units infected. Moreover, the rate of disease transmission in recipients was found to be higher as the interval between the negative and positive donations decreased. Mathematical modeling showed that the infectious window period averaged 45 days (95-percent confidence interval, 34 to 55 days).[4] Subsequently,

Petersen combined the 45-day window period with measures of the rate of seroconversion among repeat donors in a large donor population with estimates of seroconversion rates for first-time donors to arrive at the first national HIV risk estimate of 1 in 225,000.

Today, newer HIV antibody tests have reduced the window period to between 22 and 25 days. Using the 25-day window estimate and nationally representative data from a total of 9 million ARC donations in 1992 and 1993, Lackritz and colleagues (1995) used a laboratory error rate of 0.5 percent, which predicted the erroneous release of 1 in every 2.6 million positive donations. An additional factor in this model was the elimination of the window-period units that would have been discarded because they were positive on other test results, such as hepatitis, syphilis, and liver enzymes. Indeed, 15 percent of HIV preseroconversion (HIV test-negative) donations from repeat donors and 42 percent of HIV test-positive donations were positive on other tests. This study concluded that there was a residual risk of HIV transmission in 1 of every 450,000 to 660,000 transfusions of a unit of screened blood.[5]

In discussing the implications of their findings, the researchers noted several limitations. First, scientists are unable to measure directly the number of window-period donations that are discarded for positive results on other screening tests, and it is not known what pattern of positivity on other tests window-period donors might display. Second, because current data on the incidence of HIV among first-time donors is unavailable, researchers must rely on 1985 data collected when HIV testing began that showed that the prevalence among first-time donors was 1.8 times higher than the prevalence among repeat donors. It was assumed that the incidence rates would show a similar relationship. Whether this has changed in the past 11 years is a question still outstanding. Third, although the study is based on a large sample of donations from 42 different ARC regions that together collect nearly half of the nation's blood, it is not certain that they represent non-ARC centers.

Schreiber and colleagues (1996) studied the donations of 586,507 repeat donors who donated 2,318,356 units at five metropolitan blood centers between 1991 and 1993. Using a window estimate of 22 days, the researchers estimated the likelihood that a repeat blood donor would donate a unit in the window period at 1 in 493,000 (95-percent confidence interval, 202,000 to 2,778,000).[6] Schreiber did not adjust for the first-time donors who constituted 20 percent of the donor pool or for laboratory error. When we did so, using the method that Lackritz and colleagues published, we calculated the risk at 1 in

412,000. Our revised estimate is higher than Lackritz's. However, the study population for Schreiber's research is in Baltimore, Detroit, Los Angeles, Oklahoma City, and San Francisco—metropolitan areas that collect only 9 percent of the nation's blood and that would be expected to pose higher risks than the national average.[7]

To date, no cases of transfusion recipients infected with HIV-2 have been reported in the United States and only 2 HIV-2 positive units have been detected among nearly 60 million screened units. In Europe, however, a sizable number of infected blood donors have been detected on screening, and some cases of transfusion transmission have been documented. Thus, the United States may see cases of transfusion-transmitted HIV-2 in the future.

Transmission-by-Transfusion Studies

Donegan and colleagues (1990) retrospectively tested 200,000 blood component specimens stored in late 1984 and 1985 for HIV antibody and contacted recipients of positive donations to determine their status. Of the 124 recipients with no known risk factors for HIV, 111 (89.5 percent) were positive for HIV. The recipients' gender, age, underlying condition, and type of component did not influence infection rates. The rate of progression to AIDS within the first 38 months after infection was similar to that reported for homosexual men and hemophiliacs. A later study by Donegan and Lenes (1990) suggested that washed red blood cells and red blood cell units stored more than 26 days had lower transmission rates than other components. Rawal and Busch (1989) have demonstrated that filtering leukocytes from blood components reduces HIV infectivity.

Clinical Prognosis

Despite the encouraging findings of recent research on AIDS treatment, it is currently believed that 50 percent of persons testing positive for HIV will develop AIDS within 10 years after contracting the virus and, because AIDS is currently incurable, it is expected that all will succumb to it eventually.

Hepatitis A

HAV is almost always transmitted by the fecal-oral route. Commonly reported risk factors among patients with HAV include household exposure (about 24 percent of all patients), contact with young children in day care (18 percent), homosexual activity (11 percent), foreign travel in endemic areas (4 percent), and illicit drug use (2 percent), but in about 40 percent of cases no risk factors can be identified. The infection does not lead to chronic disease and mortality is 0.2 percent or less. A vaccine was introduced in 1995.

HAV is very rarely found in donated blood because the virus circulates in blood for only 7 to 10 days before an infected person becomes symptomatic. The risk of hepatitis A by blood transfusion is estimated at 1 per 1 million, and only 25 cases of transfusion transmission had been reported in the literature by 1989.[8]

Hepatitis B

Disease Factors

HBV, a DNA virus, has a worldwide distribution. In the United States, an estimated 1 to 1.25 million persons have chronic HBV infection, with 200,000 to 300,000 new infections each year. HBV is diagnosed by elevated levels of certain liver enzymes and by serological antigen and antibody tests, such as those used in blood donor screening. Antigen tests are 99.9-percent sensitive; antibody tests are 99-percent sensitive. Antibody tests remain positive even after infectious viremia has subsided, and positivity is considered a surrogate for persons with lifestyle behaviors that place them at risk for HIV or hepatitis C.

Symptoms include the gradual onset of anorexia, abdominal pain, or jaundice (yellowing of the skin as a result of decreased liver function). Sometimes, patients experience joint pains, a rash, or itching. HBV is acquired when the virus enters the body through breaks in the skin or mucous membranes. The virus has been isolated in many different body fluids but has been shown to be at infectious levels only in blood, semen, and saliva. The virus is spread by sharing contaminated needles, sexual contact, occupational exposure to blood or body fluids, transmission from an infected mother to her newborn during the perinatal period, and blood transfusions. Although 30 percent of all infected persons have no identifiable risk factor, most have other high risk characteristics (that is, history of other sexually transmitted diseases, noninjection drug use, incarceration) or belong to minority populations of low socioeconomic levels.

Blood-Supply-Risk Studies

Transfusion-associated HBV infection has not been studied to the same extent as transfusion-associated HIV. Few direct measures exist. Most estimates are based on statistical modeling of the window period or on mathematical modeling of the incidence rates and test sensitivities.

The current estimate of the window period for detecting HBV is 59 days, with a range of 37 to 87 days. Blood containing the virus is infective many weeks before the clinical onset of symptoms and remains infective during the acute phase of the disease. Chronic carriers who may exhibit no symptoms are also infectious. Often, the amount of virus is too low to be detected on the antigen test; therefore, positivity on antibody tests (anti-HBC) also helps detect chronic carriers.[9]

Transmission-by-Transfusion Studies

No direct measures of HBV transfusion risk exist. In the ARC system, 100 cases per year are reported among 2 million recipients. Surveillance studies indicate prior transfusion as a factor for 1.1 percent of the 23,000 cases of hepatitis B reported each year, or 250 cases.

M. J. Alter of CDC (1995) estimates the transfusion risk of HBV at about 1 per 200,000 units. Her analysis is based on the theory that a certain proportion of infectious cases of HBV (and other hepatitis viruses as we discuss below) among blood donors are not detected by current tests. In the case of HBV, the relevant figures are as follows: HBV is found in 0.03 percent of blood donors (3 in 10,000). The antigen test is 99.9-percent sensitive and the antibody test is 99-percent sensitive, meaning that as many as 1 percent of infected individuals test false negative. After testing, 1 in 233,000 units (0.00043 percent) are still infectious.[10] The risk from transmission of missed units is 100 percent.[11] Among patients who receive 4 units of blood, 1 in 58,000 are at risk.

More recently, Schreiber and colleagues (1996) used data on 2,318,356 allogeneic blood donations from 586,507 donors who had donated more than once between 1991 and 1993 at five blood centers. Among donors whose units passed all screening tests, the risks of giving HBV-contaminated blood during the infectious window period was estimated to be 1 in 63,000 units (confidence interval from 1 in 31,000 to 1 in 147,000).

Clinical Prognosis

M. J. Alter (1995) assumed that half of the 4 million annual transfusion recipients die of their underlying disease.[12] Using these assumptions, Alter predicts 34 HBV infections among the 2 million transfusion recipients who survive long enough to develop HBV.

The development of chronic infection occurs in 5 percent to 10 percent of HBV-infected adults (M. J. Alter, 1995). An estimated 15 percent of persons with chronic HBV acquired after early childhood die of either cirrhosis or liver cancer. There is no treatment for HBV. Factors that facilitate the emergence of the virus are increased sexual activity and intravenous drug abuse.

Interferon treatment of adults with HBV-related chronic hepatitis has been shown to achieve long-term clearance of infection in upward of 40 percent. Routine hepatitis B vaccination of infants and adolescents and vaccination of adolescents and adults in high-risk groups has begun to prevent transmission of HBV.

Hepatitis C

Disease Factors

HCV, a flavi-like virus, has a worldwide distribution and is relatively common among dialysis patients, hemophiliacs, health care workers, and intravenous drug users. In 1995, CDC estimated that there are 35,000 to 180,000 (average 120,000) new HCV infections each year in the United States. Diagnosis is by an antibody test that is 90- to 95-percent sensitive. Symptoms include gradual onset of anorexia, nausea, vomiting, and jaundice. Its course is similar to that of HBV but more prolonged.

Most HCV is acquired in the community and much needs to be learned about modes of transmission. CDC reports among documented cases in 1992 that 2 percent were associated with health care occupational exposure to blood, 4 percent with blood transfusion, 12 percent with exposure to a sexual partner or household member who had hepatitis or multiple sexual partners, 29 percent with injection drug abuse, 46 percent with low socioeconomic level, and 6 percent with other high-risk behavior (that is, noninjection illegal drug use, history of sexually transmitted diseases, imprisonment, sexual partners or household contacts who inject drugs, or no identifiable risk factors).

Blood-Supply-Risk Studies

Before an antibody-specific test for HCV was implemented, blood donors were tested for surrogate markers of the disease using tests to detect antibody to HBV (anti-HBc) and elevated alanine aminotransferase, a liver enzyme that, when levels are high, may indicate liver problems such as those associated with HCV. Donahue,

Nelson, and other colleagues in Baltimore and Houston evaluated the risk of HCV at four different phases of blood donor screening in 12,146 cardiac surgery patients who had been transfused (Donahue et al., 1992; Nelson et al., 1992, 1995). Prior to surrogate testing, these researchers estimated the risk of transfusion-associated HCV at 1 in every 222 units of blood. When surrogate testing was implemented, the risk decreased to about 1 in every 525 units. The first-generation anti-HCV test further reduced the risk to 1 in 3,333 units. When the second generation HCV test was introduced in 1992, these researchers found 15 cardiac surgery patients infected with HCV among a study population who together had received 22,008 units of blood for a per-unit risk of about 1 in 1,470.

In another study, Kleinman and colleagues (1992) concluded that second generation HCV tests reduced HCV risks to between 1 in 2,000 and 1 in 6,000 component units.

The current estimate of the window period is 82 days with a range of 54 to 192 days. Blood containing the virus is infective from 1 week after exposure into the chronic stage. Screening is inhibited by several factors: current second-generation tests may not detect 10 percent of persons infected with HCV; acute, chronic, and resolved infections cannot be distinguished on the basis of test results; the window period can be quite prolonged; and in populations with low prevalence (such as blood donors), the rate of false positives is high.

Two factors currently contribute to the risk of HCV in the blood supply. First, donors in the window period do not yet have any antibodies to be detected on screening tests. Schreiber and colleagues estimate that the risk posed by these donors is 1 in every 103,000 units (95-percent confidence interval, 28,000 to 288,000).

A much bigger risk stems from the possibility that the relatively low sensitivity of current antibody tests results in false negative tests in 10 percent of donors actually infected by HCV. Assuming that the prevalence of HCV among donors is 0.244 percent and test sensitivity is 90 percent, M. J. Alter (1995) at CDC estimates that 0.0244 percent of all units (1 in 4,100) are HCV infectious after screening.[13] Using the 50-percent mortality rate for transfusion, M. J. Alter predicts 1,955 infections in the 2 million surviving recipients.

M. J. Alter's estimate is based on observations in community-acquired hepatitis, identified as a result of active surveillance. It has not been independently confirmed, it is based on second-generation tests, and it is unclear whether it applies to asymptomatic blood donors. Nevertheless, because it represents the most conservative risk estimate in the current literature, we chose to use it in our overall risk analysis.

Transmission-by-Transfusion Studies

Studies from around the world suggest that between 80 and 90 percent of transfusion recipients who receive antibody positive blood seroconvert to HCV.

Clinical Prognosis

Approximately 25 percent of persons infected with HCV become acutely ill with jaundice and other symptoms of hepatitis, and each year more than 4,000 patients require hospitalization. About 600 die of fulminant disease.[14]

Much still needs to be learned about the long-term effects of HCV infection. Eighty-five percent or more develop persistent HCV infection, and while about 70 percent of infected individuals develop chronic hepatitis, long-term follow-up studies suggest that only 10 to 20 percent develop clinical symptoms of their liver disease over a 20-year period following transfusion. (Farci et al., 1991; Seeff et al., 1992; Koretz et al., 1993; Iwarson et al., 1995). Many persons who are affected suffer no symptoms.

Until recently, no treatment was available for hepatitis C. Recent evidence now suggests that interferon may be helpful in treating chronic hepatitis C. Studies by DiBisceglie and colleagues (1989) and Davis and colleagues (1989) demonstrated marked improvement of liver enzyme activity in about half of all treated patients. In many, the liver itself improved. However, liver enzyme activity was sustained in only 10 to 51 percent of patients, and the effect of long-term therapy had not been determined.

Other Hepatitis Viruses

Disease Factors

Hepatitis E has been identified in developing nations around the world. Like HAV, it is transmitted by the fecal-oral route (and also by contaminated water) and its course of symptoms parallels that of HAV. HEV, however, is associated with a high rate of fulminant hepatic failure among pregnant women, in whom the death rate may be as high as 20 percent.

In 1995, researchers announced the discovery of a new hepatitis virus not previously identified as hepatitis A, B, C, D, or E. Labeled hepatitis G virus (HGV), it is not yet known if this strain is associated with acute and chronic hepatitis. Between 0 and 16 percent of cryptogenic (non-A,B,C,E type) hepatitis patients and between 28 and 50 percent of patients with fulminant hepatitis were HGV-positive. HGV may also lead to aplastic anemia (decreased bone marrow mass); 3 of 10 such patients were HGV positive (Alter, 1996). Persistent infection has been observed for up to 9 years. In 1995, the National Institutes of Health (NIH) reported that 3 of 13 hepatitis patients (23 percent) enrolled in an ongoing study had acquired HGV from their blood transfusion. In the NIH study, HGV was also detected in 12 percent of transfusion recipients who had minor symptoms that were not clinically identified as hepatitis, in 10 percent of those with HCV-related hepatitis, in 8 percent of those with no symptoms, but in only 0.6 percent of the 157 nontransfused patients enrolled as study controls.

Blood-Supply-Risk Studies

The prevalence of HGV in blood donors as measured by HGV RNA detected by PCR is higher than that of HCV. The HGV virus was identified in the blood of 24 of 1,478 (1.6 percent) of the NIH donors, and a small study of 200 Midwestern blood donors found that 4 (2 percent) were reactive for HGV ("New Hepatitis G Virus," 1995; "Abbott Announces Discovery," 1995). Although no antibody tests have been developed to detect HGV, HGV frequently coexists with HBV or HCV; therefore, tests that detect either of the latter viruses help eliminate HGV from the blood supply.

Both HBV and HCV tests help detect non-ABC hepatitis in blood donors. Using the same methods and assumptions as for HCV, M. J. Alter (1995) estimates the risk of transfusion-transmitted non-ABC hepatitis at 1 per 5,925 units.

Transmission-by-Transfusion Studies

Despite the relatively high risk estimates of hepatitis in the blood supply, hepatitis researchers assert that the residual risk of hepatitis from transfusion is very small and no different from the risk of background hepatitis found in nontransfused hospitalized patients. For example, analyses from two large transfusion-related hepatitis studies conducted in the United States in the late 1970s and in Canada in the 1980s suggest that the risk of non-ABC hepatitis from transfusion (3.6 percent of patients) is similar to that of control groups of nontransfused hospital patients (3 percent) (Aach et al., 1991). The Canadian Red Cross found the same rate of non-ABC hepatitis (0.6 percent) between patients receiving volunteer supply blood and patients receiving their own blood.

HTLV-I and HTLV-II

Disease Factors

HTLV-I is endemic in southern Japan, the Caribbean basin, and Africa. Populations in Japan have rates of HTLV-I infection ranging from a low of 1.1 percent in Tokyo to a high of 37.5 percent in males and 44 percent in females from Okinawa. Populations native to the Caribbean basin have HTLV-I seroprevalence rates of 2 percent to 12 percent. HTLV-II, which is detected by the HTLV-I-based laboratory tests currently used to screen the blood supply, is endemic among Indian populations in the Americas, including populations in Florida and New Mexico (Levine et al., 1993; Hjelle et al., 1990) and among intravenous drug users in the United States and Europe. The rate of infection in the United States blood donor population has been estimated to be between 0.009 and 0.043 per cent (Williams et al., 1988; Lee et al., 1991; Sandler et al., 1990). Dodd reports that the ARC observes a donor seropositivity rate of 0.006 percent to 0.008 percent.

The most common modes of transmission are from mother to child by breast feeding, by transfusion of contaminated cellular blood products, by needle sharing among intravenous drug users, and through sexual activity.

Blood-Supply-Risk Studies

The current estimate of the window period for HTLV-I and HTLV-II is 51 days with a range of 36 to 72 days (Manes et al., 1992). When blood screening for HTLV was introduced in 1988, nearly 2,000 U.S. donors were found to be positive. The HTLV infections among blood donors in the United States are nearly evenly divided between types I and II.[15] Most HTLV-I positive donors were born in or report sexual contact with a person from the Caribbean or Japan, while nearly all HTLV-II positive blood donors report a past history of intravenous drug use or sex with an intravenous drug-using partner. Because the current blood screening tests use HTLV-I antigens to detect both types, the sensitivity of detection of HTLV-II is lower than that for HTLV-I antibodies. Hjelle and colleagues (1993) reported that the screening ELISA test misses 20 percent of HTLV-I infections and 43 percent of HTLV-II infections. Thus, low test sensitivity, especially for HTLV-II, is the primary reason that infected blood remains in the blood supply.

Schreiber and colleagues (1996) estimate that the risk of receiving an HTLV-contaminated unit from a repeat donor in the infectious

461

window period is 1 in 641,000 (confidence interval from 1 in 256,000 to 1 in 2,000,000).

Dodd (1992) has calculated the residual risk of transfusion transmission at 1 in 50,000 units based on current seroprevalence rates among donors and screening test sensitivity.[16]

Transmission-by-Transfusion Studies

Data from the Transfusion Safety Study (Donegan et al., 1994) show that, overall, 27 percent of recipients who received anti-HTLV-positive blood became infected. The rates of infectivity varied by blood product and storage time. Only cellular blood products (red blood cells and platelets) appear to transmit HTLV; no plasma products have been implicated in disease transmission. Moreover, the longer the blood was stored, the less likely it was to transmit HTLV: the transmission rate for products stored 0 to 5 days was 74 percent; 6 to 10 days, 44 percent; 11 to 14 days, 0 percent. The transmission rate in the United States appears to be much lower than in other countries, where rates of 45 to 63 percent have been reported. The most likely explanation for the lower infectivity of U.S. blood is its typically longer storage time.

Clinical Prognosis

Two diseases have been associated with HTLV-I: adult T-cell leukemia and lymphoma (ATL) and a chronic degenerative neurologic disease called HTLV-I-associated myelopathy and tropical spastic paraparesis (HAM/TSP).

ATL is a malignant condition of T lymphocytes, a form of white blood cell produced by the lymph nodes and important for immunity. The clinical features of ATL include leukemia, swelling lymph nodes, enlarged and impaired functioning of the liver, enlarged spleen, skin and bone lesions, and increased calcium in the blood. Conventional chemotherapy is not curative, and the median survival after diagnosis is 11 months.

ATL occurs in 2 to 4 percent of individuals infected with HTLV-I in regions where the disease is endemic and early childhood infection is common. The typical patient is 40 to 60 years old, which suggests that several decades may be required for the disease to develop. Only one case of ATL has been documented as having been acquired by transfusion (CDC, 1993).

HAM/TSP is characterized by slowly progressive chronic spastic paraparesis (slight paralysis of the lower limbs), lower limb weakness, urinary incontinence, impotence, sensory disturbances (tingling, pins and needles, and burning), low back pain, exaggerated reflexes of the lower limbs, and impaired vibration sense. Fewer than 1 percent of persons infected with HTLV-I develop HAM/TSP. The interval between infection and disease is much shorter than that for ATL, and cases of HAM/TSP as a result of blood transfusion have been documented with a median interval of 3.3 years between transfusion and development of the disease.

Despite sporadic case reports, HTLV-II had not been definitively associated with any disease until recently. In November 1996, Lehky and colleagues (1996) reported on the clinical and immunological findings of 4 HTLV-II positive patients with spastic paraparesis, whose disease progression resembles that of HTLV-I-infected patients with HAM/TSP. HTLV-II was first isolated in 2 patients with hairy cell leukemia, although no virus has been isolated from additional cases of this disease.

Parasites

Disease Factors

Several bloodborne parasites can be present in donated blood. Few direct measures of risk exist; therefore, estimates are based on reported cases. With the exception of one parasite, the risk of transfusion-associated parasite transmission is less than 1 in 1 million.[17]

Chagas' disease is caused by the parasite *T. cruzi*. Typically, humans become infected following the bite of a reduviid bug, otherwise known as the kissing bug. The bug favors poverty conditions, particularly in rural areas where wood and adobe housing is cracking or decaying. Infected bug feces either contaminate the bite wound or enter by other mucous membranes. Chagas' disease is endemic in large parts of South America, Central America, and Mexico. Estimates are that as many as 100,000 *T. cruzi*-infected persons are in the United States (Shulman, 1994).

Blood-Supply-Risk Studies

Four cases of transfusion-transmitted Chagas' disease have been reported in the United States and Canada. Risk of blood donors infected with *T. cruzi* varies in the United States, depending on the number of Hispanic immigrants in a given area. Brashear et al. (1995) reported that 14 of 13,309 (10.5 percent) donors in Texas, New Mexico, and California had evidence of infection. Kirchhoff et al. (1987) reported that as many as 5 percent of the Salvadoran and Nicaraguan immigrants in the Washington, D.C., area may be infected. In some U.S. areas, about 1 in 600 eligible blood donors who have Hispanic surnames and 1 in 300 eligible blood donors who are Hispanic immigrants or refugees might be infected (Kerndt et al., 1991; Pan et al., 1992).

Most blood banks now ask donors whether they have a history of Chagas' disease and questions about risk factors that are linked to possible infection with *T. cruzi*. ARC has conducted seroepidemiological studies of blood donors in Los Angeles and Miami, where 8 percent and 12 percent of prospective donors reported having been born in or having traveled for more than 4 weeks to areas in which Chagas' disease is endemic.[18] Additional screening questions ARC asked these donors included a history of sleeping in rural areas where the bugs are prevalent, a history of transfusion in an endemic area, and a history of a positive test for Chagas' disease. Of those at risk, 0.1 percent tested positive for the antibody to *T. cruzi*. Dodd estimates that 1 in about 8,500 units in Miami and Los Angeles may contain *T. cruzi*.

Furthermore, about 2.4 percent of donors nationally report risk factors, or about one fourth the risk in Miami and Los Angeles, where large numbers of Hispanic immigrants reside. If the same rate of seroprevalence (0.1 percent) exists among all U.S. donors who report behavioral risk, then Dodd estimates that the national risk for *T. cruzi*-contaminated blood is 1 in about 42,000.

Transmission-by-Transfusion Studies

Schmunis (1991) reports that the risk of transmitting *T. cruzi* through infected blood ranges from 14 to 49 percent in South America. ARC has found no evidence of transmission among 15 recipients of infected blood, suggesting that transmission rates in the United States are no higher than 10 percent.[19]

Clinical Prognosis

Following the bug bite, a characteristic lesion may form but usually passes unnoticed. If the bug feces fall onto mucous membranes directly, the classic Romana sign (conjunctivitis and swelling of the eye area) develops. During the acute phase, the parasite can be seen in the blood for a few weeks. Acute infection with *T. cruzi* can be asymptomatic, or it can be fatal. More typically, after a 10-to-14-day incubation period, fever, swollen lymph nodes, and enlarged spleen and liver develop.

Between 20 and 30 percent of infected individuals develop chronic Chagas' disease, often years to decades following infection. Rapid and erratic heartbeats signify cardiac involvement. The parasite has an affinity for cardiac cells and for the smooth muscle of the esophagus and colon. As the disease progresses, the heart, esophagus, and colon (and occasionally, the stomach, gallbladder, and bladder) enlarge (Shulman, 1994).

Treatment of acute infections with the drugs nifurtimox and benznidazole is successful in at least 70 percent of cases. In July 1996, Venezuelan scientists announced success in eradicating Chagas' disease in 70 percent to 90 percent of infected laboratory mice using the antifungal drug DO870 (Urbina et al., 1996).

Bacteria

Disease Factors

Bacteria can enter donated blood at one of several points (Yomtovian, 1995). Bacteria can be introduced during the manufacture of the bag used to collect blood. During collection, bacteria from the skin can contaminate blood, especially if the donor's arm is not disinfected properly. Donors who are suffering from a bacterial disease—even common food-induced digestive infections—can unknowingly donate a contaminated blood unit. In a review of the research on transfusion-associated bacterial sepsis, Wagner and colleagues (1994) point to several reports of bacteria already present in the collection bag proliferating during processing or storage of the blood. Finally, bacteria can be introduced while preparing for transfusion, particularly if the entry port of a thawing container for a frozen blood component comes in contact with contaminated water in the warming bath. Although fresh plasma and cryoprecipitate can harbor bacteria, contamination of red blood cells and platelets is the most significant problem. Bacterial contamination is one complication that cannot be eliminated by donating blood for self use.

Red blood cells are refrigerated, which reduces the viability of most bacteria, such as the one that causes syphilis. However, certain cold-loving bacteria, such as *Yersinia enterocolitica* and *Pseudomonas florescens*, thrive under refrigerated conditions. *Yersinia* is present in the digestive tract or lymph nodes of humans and can cause diarrhea and other gastric symptoms that may be mild enough to be overlooked by blood donors. *Pseudomonas florescens* is one of several common skin bacteria that can enter blood during collection.

Platelets run a greater risk of bacterial contamination because they are stored for up to 5 days at room temperature. Skin contaminants, such as *Staphylococcus epidermidis*, are the most frequently isolated bacteria from platelets. In the United States, platelets can be administered as either apheresis single-donor units or pooled random donor units collected from 6 to 10 donors. Bacterial sepsis can occur if any of the pooled units are contaminated. Indeed, Morrow and colleagues (1991) found that the rate of sepsis was 12 times higher for pooled units than for single-donor units. Today, single-donor units are increasingly replacing pooled units.

Blood-Supply-Risk Studies

Wagner and colleagues (1994) report that the frequency of bacterial contamination is measured three ways—through laboratory culture, hospital surveillance programs, and fatalities. Laboratory culture techniques measure bacteria directly but are subject to lapses in sterile techniques that can introduce bacteria into samples. In addition, many quality control studies reporting bacterial contamination have found that the number of bacteria in the sample was far below the level that would be expected to cause problems to the recipient. Nevertheless, culture methods of bacterial detection suggest that blood component units—particularly platelets—run a significant risk of contamination.

Most episodes of bacterial sepsis are associated with platelets late in the storage period. Yomtovian (1995) conducted a 4-year hospital-based surveillance program in which platelets were cultured for bacteria. The reported contamination rate of platelets 4 days old or less was 1.8 per 10,000 units, whereas the contamination rate for 5-day-old platelets was significantly higher, at 11.9 per 10,000 (p < .05). Morrow et al. (1991), also found that the contamination rate was five times higher in 5-day-old platelets than in 1-4–day-old platelets (Morrow et al., 1991). Earlier findings such as this led FDA in 1985 to reverse its 1983 decision to extend the shelf life of platelets from 5 to 7 days.

In 11 percent of all reported patient fatalities (10 of 89 deaths) between 1986 and 1988, bacteria in the patient's blood matched that of the donated units. During this period, about 60 million units of blood components were transfused. Thus, about 1 death per 6 million transfused units was definitively caused by bacterial sepsis. However, researchers acknowledge that bacteria-induced transfusion fatalities are only rarely diagnosed and reported, because physicians fail to attribute patients' deaths to the possibility of bacteria in blood transfusions.

Similarly, nonfatal outcomes of sepsis are believed to be greatly underdiagnosed and, therefore, underreported. Common, nonthreatening reactions of a patient's immune system to transfusion include fever and chills that may mask underlying bacteremia. Morrow and colleagues of Johns Hopkins Medical Institutes (1991) reported platelet transfusion-associated sepsis in 1 out of every 4,200 platelet transfusions. Bacterial contamination associated with fever following transfusion occurred once in about 1,700 pooled platelet units or once in 19,519 single-donor platelets. This is undoubtedly an underestimate because only patients exhibiting clinical symptoms were evaluated.

More recently in Hong Kong, Chiu and colleagues (1994) conducted a 3-year prospective study of bone marrow transplant recipients for clinical evidence of platelet transfusion reactions. These researchers found 10 episodes of symptomatic bacteremia with 4 leading to septic shock. A total of 21,503 random-donor platelet units were pooled into 3,584 doses administered to 161 patients. Each patient received an average of 20 pools. The frequency of bacteremia was calculated three ways: 1 in every 2,100 platelet units, 1 in every 350 transfusions, and 1 in every 16 patients.[20] Again, this is probably an underestimate, because Chiu and colleagues looked only for symptomatic bacteremia.

In sum, there is no reliable estimate of the frequency of bacterial sepsis among transfusion recipients across the United States. Culture methods probably yield overestimates while reporting mechanisms probably yield underestimates of clinically relevant bacterial contamination. CDC is initiating a prospective incidence study in collaboration with AABB, ARC, and the Navy in an attempt to quantify this risk. For the purpose of our analysis, we include the Morrow estimate of documented bacterial sepsis (not all febrile reactions) because the researchers prospectively monitored patients and obtained bacterial cultures from implicated units in the United States.

Although it is now well documented that refrigerated red blood cells can harbor bacteria, we could find no studies that directly estimated the likelihood that red blood cells are contaminated by bacteria. Dodd (1994) estimates that 1 in every 500,000 red blood cell units may be contaminated by *Yersinia* or other bacteria.[21]

Transmission-by-Transfusion Studies

Many surgical patients who are otherwise healthy can sustain a small amount of bacteria introduced by transfusion. However, immunocompromised patients, such as those with leukemia, are very susceptible to foreign organisms. Unfortunately, these patients are the primary users of platelets.

Clinical Prognosis

In transfusion-associated bacterial sepsis, the onset of symptoms usually occurs within the first few hours following transfusion but may occur during the transfusion or following an extended delay (Greene, 1995). The initial signs are typically fever and chills and may include nausea, vomiting, diarrhea, chest or back pain, low blood pressure, rapid heartbeat and breathing, and cyanosis from lack of blood oxygen. Patients with advancing bacterial sepsis rapidly progress to acute renal failure, respiratory distress, disseminated intravascular coagulation (uncontrolled internal bleeding), and death. Death may occur from 50 minutes to 17 days following transfusion (Morduchowicz et al., 1991; Tipple et al., 1990). Goldman and Blajchman (1991) reported that 26 percent of identified transfusion-associated sepsis cases ended in death.

Noninfectious Complications of Transfusion

Transfusions can result in serious or fatal complications as a result of serological or clerical errors in blood typing, mismanagement of the transfusion, or unanticipated reactions in the recipient to elements of the donor's blood. Many of the unanticipated reactions are unavoidable within current understanding and practice of transfusion medicine. Few comprehensive assessments of the incidence of such outcomes can be found in the literature. Thus, estimates of the frequency of noninfectious transfusion risks are based on studies by a small number of transfusion services, summation of the number of such occurrences reported in the literature, or from regulatory reports of errors, accidents, and deaths (Dodd, 1994).

Transfusion-Related Acute Lung Injury

Transfusion-related acute lung injury (TRALI) has only recently been recognized as a potential complication of blood transfusion. No known risk factors have been identified among recipients who develop TRALI.

Cases have been evenly distributed between males and females and among recipients of all ages. No underlying conditions necessitating transfusion have been identified, and most patients have no prior history of transfusion reactions.

Implicated blood components include whole blood, red blood cells, fresh frozen plasma, and cryoprecipitate. It is the plasma portion of the blood that causes TRALI, and even red blood cells contain small residual amounts of plasma.

In TRALI, specific white blood cell antibodies present in the donor's blood react with the entire circulation of the recipient's white blood cells. The result is the release of various components that cause severe damage to lung tissue, which in turn leads to acute respiratory crisis. Most cases of TRALI have been traced back to blood donated by women who have been pregnant more than once, because pregnancy causes the mother's blood to develop specific antibodies to elements of the fetus's blood that her body considers foreign (Popovsky and Moore, 1985).

Walker (1987) estimated the risk of TRALI to be 1 in 10,000 units.[22] However, Popovsky argues that TRALI is rarely diagnosed and reported. Therefore, Walker's figure is probably an underestimate. Popovsky et al. (1992) report that, prior to 1985, only 31 cases of TRALI had been reported. By 1992, additional reports involving over 40 recipient reactions had been published. At the time of their publication, Popovsky and colleagues were aware of an additional 35 unreported cases.

TRALI presents with acute respiratory distress within about 2-4 hours following transfusion (Boyle and Moore, 1995). Fever, low blood pressure, chills, cyanosis from lack of blood oxygen, nonproductive cough, and shortness of breath or difficulty breathing are common symptoms. In most instances, TRALI improves within 48 to 96 hours, provided that prompt diagnosis and respiratory support is initiated. For those who recover, there appear to be no long-term consequences. Death may be the outcome in approximately 5 percent of cases.

ABO Incompatibility

ABO incompatibility is the result of improper serological typing or clerical recording of the major blood groups in donor or recipient blood, mislabeling of donor units, or improper verification of donor or recipient blood type.

A study of errors reported to New York State in 1990-91 found 104 cases of erroneous transfusions out of 1,784,641 (0.006 percent) red cell transfusions, over half of these (54, or 0.003 percent) related to ABO incompatibility (Linden, Paul, and Dressler, 1992). This is important because transfusion of ABO-incompatible blood is one of the major causes of serious noninfectious risks for transfusion recipients.

Most of the 50 other errors were related to the transfusion of a wrong unit of blood that was fortuitously ABO-compatible with the recipient's blood type and transfusion of ABO-incompatible fresh-frozen plasma.

It was also found that 61 incidents (59 percent of the 104 cases) were the result solely of errors outside the blood establishment. The majority of these stemmed from the failure of the person administering the transfusion to verify the identity of the recipient or the blood unit. However, there were 25 incidents (25 percent) in which the errors were attributable to the blood establishment and 18 cases (17 percent) in which both the blood bank and hospital service made errors in administering incorrect blood or in giving blood to someone other than the intended recipient.

From this information, the study's authors calculated an incidence rate of ABO-incompatible errors of 1 in every 33,000 transfusions (0.003 percent). The study concluded that three persons died from acute transfusion reactions, for a death rate of 1 per 600,000 red cell transfusions. The overall true rate of ABO errors, accounting for instances in which errors were made but the blood was fortuitously compatible, was calculated at 1 in 12,000 units.

Transfusing ABO-incompatible blood usually—but not always—leads to a hemolytic transfusion reaction (HTR), the result of the immune system's destruction of red blood cells. It presents with fevers, chills, low blood pressure, destruction of red blood cells, kidney failure, blood in the urine, uncontrolled internal bleeding, shock, and death. Occasionally, initial symptoms are deceptively mild with the patient experiencing a vague sense of unease or an aching back. There are no known long-term effects. In the Linden study, death occurred in 6 percent of cases.

Anaphylaxis

Anaphylaxis is a serious allergic reaction that can occur in recipients who are deficient in IgA, a type of antibody normally present in humans. Approximately 1 in 700 individuals are IgA-deficient, but anaphylaxis occurs only in those who have developed antibodies to IgA as a result of pregnancy or prior blood transfusion and then receive a blood transfusion that contains IgA. Therefore, cases of transfusion-induced anaphylaxis are generally unanticipated and unavoidable. Walker (1987) estimates that 1 in 150,000 blood units transfused results in anaphylaxis in the recipient.[23]

Anaphylaxis occurs immediately after transfusion begins, sometimes after the infusion of only a few milliliters of blood or plasma.

The onset is characterized by coughing, bronchospasm, respiratory distress, vascular instability, nausea, abdominal pain, vomiting, diarrhea, shock, and loss of consciousness. We found no estimates of the likelihood of death as a result of anaphylaxis. Because of its seriousness and the possibility that it can be overlooked or not diagnosed rapidly, we used a fatality rate of 20 percent in our analysis. Patients with a history of anaphylaxis should receive plasma from an IgA-deficient donor.

Circulatory Overload

Rapid increases in blood volume are not tolerated well by patients with poor cardiac or pulmonary functioning. Even the transfusion of small amounts of blood can cause circulatory overload in infants. Patients with chronic anemia or active hemorrhaging are also susceptible. Walker estimates that 1 in 10,000 transfused units leads to circulatory overload.[24]

Circulatory overload presents with rapid breathing, severe headache, swelling of hands and feet, and other signs of congestive heart failure. Other symptoms include coughing, cyanosis from lack of blood oxygen, discomfort in breathing, and a rapid increase in systolic blood pressure. No long-term effects have been noted when transfusion is stopped promptly at the first signs of circulatory overload. We found no estimates of the likelihood of death. Because the symptoms typically develop over the course of the transfusion, we assume that most instances are diagnosed before permanent damage ensues. We used a fatality estimate of 5 percent in our analysis.

Notes to the Text in This Chapter

[1]Ward did not report confidence intervals.

[2]Personal communication from Roger Dodd of the American Red Cross.

[3]That is, [number of donors x (the HIV positivity rate x the proportion of the time between donations when the donor could be in the window period)] + [number of donors x (the HIV positivity rate x the proportion of the time between donations when the donor would be outside the window period x the probability that the test result is false negative)], the latter probability being 100 percent minus 99 percent.

[4]By 95-percent confidence interval, we mean that the researchers have established a range of values for which they are confident that in 95 out of every 100 measurements (in this case of the window period),

the true value would fall somewhere between the two endpoints of the stated interval. These researchers found preliminary evidence suggesting that antibody tests used after March 1987 had a smaller window period of 42 days, a finding that was later confirmed.

[5]No point estimate is reported.

[6]Schreiber's calculation of the window period is 3 days less than that of Lackritz's. They are considered equally valid estimates. The choice of one over the other does not significantly change the outcome of the calculations.

[7]For similar reasons, we did not use Schreiber's estimates for HTLV-I risk (1 in 641,000, confidence interval from 1 in 256,000 to 1 in 2,000,000) or for HCV (1 in 103,000, confidence interval from 1 in 28,000 to 1 in 288,000). But we did use his estimate for HBV despite the lack of adjustment for testing sensitivity and errors, because it was more conservative than the estimate that did.

[8]HAV is a very stable virus capable of withstanding considerable heat in dry conditions. In 1992, hemophiliac patients receiving factor VIII concentrates of plasma were exposed to HAV because the method used for inactivating viruses (solvent-detergent washing) did not affect HAV in the plasma. The outbreak led to swift recall of this product. A heat-inactivation process should eliminate this risk.

[9]Delta hepatitis (HDV) is an incomplete virus that requires the help of HBV to replicate in the human body. Persons coinfected with HBV and HDV may have a more severe acute illness and a higher risk of fulminant hepatitis than others infected only with HBV. No direct measure of the incidence of HDV is available, but CDC's models suggest that HDV accounts for 7,500 infections annually. Its prevalence among HBV-infected donors is estimated at between 1.4 and 8 percent Hepatitis B immunizations prevent HDV infections, too.

[10]After antigen screening, 0.00003 percent of units are infectious; after antibody screening, 0.0004 percent. In sum, 0.00043 percent of all units are infectious. Note that Alter rounds this last figure to 0.00040 percent in table 2 of her article. We use 0.00043 percent, which changes the estimate slightly.

[11]The risk of transmission among donors who test positive on the antibody test alone is 4 percent, because in most cases a positive antibody test indicates an old, resolved infection.

[12]The 50-percent fatality rate for transfusion is based on a study by Ward et al. (1989) that traced back selected recipients of transfusions and found that 50 percent of a transfusion control group that had not received HIV-infected blood had died within a year and that 63 percent of recipients of HIV-infected blood had died by the time investigators could locate them. However, other researchers have noted that these study participants were not representative of a general surgery population as they were often referred from a subspecialty surgical area and had a poorer prognosis for survival. In a more recent study, Vamvakas and Taswell (1994) enrolled all residents of a U.S. county who underwent transfusion in 1981. While this group cannot be directly generalized to all U.S. surgeries, the enrollment of all transfusion patients without any selection bias better characterizes actual transfusion practices. These researchers found a 30-percent fatality rate within 2 years following surgery.

[13]No confidence interval reported.

[14]These figures include all cases of HCV, not transfusion-associated cases alone.

[15]More than 80 percent of HTLV-I and HTLV-II seropositivity among intravenous drug users stems from HTLV-II infection. HTLV-II also appears endemic among North American Indians in Florida and New Mexico.

[16]No confidence interval reported.

[17]Malaria is caused by the bite of an infected mosquito in endemic areas. An average of 3 cases a year that were acquired by transfusion are reported in the United States. Donor history questions are designed to defer donors who are at risk of malaria as a result of travel. Viscerotropic Leishmaniasis is caused by the bite of an infected sandfly in endemic areas, such as the Persian Gulf. Viscerotropic Leishmaniasis affects the internal organs of the body. Veterans of Desert Storm were deferred from donating blood when 7 cases were discovered among military personnel serving in Desert Storm and Desert Shield. While cases of cutaneous Leishmaniasis have been reported in Texas, this variant of the disease is not thought to be a risk for blood transfusion. No cases of transfusion-transmitted viscerotropic Leishmaniasis have been reported in the United States. Babesiosis is caused by the bite of an infected tick, a problem found mostly in endemic areas of the northeastern United States. To date, CDC

reports 15 cases of transfusion-transmitted babesiosis in the United States. Toxoplasmosis is caused by infection with a parasite whose usual host is the domestic cat. The parasite is transmitted through handling of infected cats or cat litter. Other means of transmission include eating raw or undercooked pork, goat, lamb, beef, or wild game. Recent preliminary data from CDC indicate that about 20 to 25 percent of the U.S. population has been infected. Most cases pass unnoticed. Cases have been reported as transmitted by transfusion only to immunocompromised patients.

[18]Interview with Roger Y. Dodd, American Red Cross, Jerome H. Holland Laboratory.

[19]Interview with Roger Y. Dodd, American Red Cross, Jerome H. Holland Laboratory.

[20]No confidence intervals were reported.

[21]No confidence interval was reported.

[22]No confidence interval was reported.

[23]No confidence interval was reported.

[24]No confidence interval was reported.

Chapter 49

Plasma Products

In this chapter, we describe some of the ways in which the manufacturing of plasma differs from that of blood. We give particular attention to differences that stem from volunteer versus paid, or commercial, donors. We note viral inactivation processes. Finally, we discuss what little information we could find on the differences in viral seropositivity rates of paid and volunteer donors.

Plasma Product Uses

More than 40 million hospital patients use plasma products each year. Plasma is the liquid portion of blood, containing nutrients, electrolytes (dissolved salts), gases, albumin, clotting factors, hormones, and wastes. Many different components of plasma are used, from treating the trauma of burns and surgery to replacing blood elements that are lacking as a result of disease such as hemophilia. Table 49.1 describes plasma components and their uses.

Plasma Donors

Plasma is typically collected from paid donors in a commercial setting. Donors receive between $15 and $20 for the 2 hours required to

From the United States General Accounting Office Report to the Ranking Minority Member, Committee on Commerce, House of Representatives. *Blood Supply: Transfusion Associated Risks*, GAO/PEMD-97-2 (Washington, D.C.: 1997).

Table 49.1a. Uses for Plasma Components

Component	Use
Albumin	To restore plasma volume in treatment of shock, trauma, surgery, and burns
Alpha 1 proteinase inhibitor	To treat emphysema caused by genetic deficiency
Antihemophilic factor concentrate	For prophylaxis and treatment of hemophilia A bleeding episodes
Anti-inhibitor coagulant complex	To treat bleeding episodes in presence of factor VIII inhibitor
Anti-thrombin III	To prevent clotting and thromboembolism associated with liver disease, anti-thrombin III deficiency, and thromboembolism
Cytomegalovirus immune globulin	For passive immunization subsequent to exposure to cytomegalovirus
Factor IX complex	For prophylaxis and treatment of hemophilia B bleeding episodes and other bleeding disorders
Factor XIII	To prevent and treat bleeding in factor XIII-deficient persons
Fibrinolysin	To dissolve intravascular clots
Hepatitis B immune globulin	For passive immunization subsequent to exposure to hepatitis B
IgM-enriched immune globulin	To treat and prevent septicemia and septic shock stemming from toxin liberation in the course of antibiotic treatment

Table 49.1b. Uses for Plasma Components

Component	Use
Immune globulin: intravenous and intramuscular	To treat agamma- and hypogamma-globulinemia; for passive immunization for hepatitis A and measles
Plasma protein fraction	To restore plasma volume subsequent to shock, trauma, surgery, and burns
Rabies immune globulin	For passive immunization subsequent to exposure to rabies
Rho(D) immune globulin	To treat and prevent hemolytic disease of fetus and newborn infant stemming from Rh incompatibility and incompatible blood transfusions
Rubella immune globulin	For passive immunization subsequent to exposure to German measles
Serum cholinesterase	To treat prolonged apnea subsequent to the administration of succinylcholine chloride
Tetanus immune globulin	For passive immunization subsequent to exposure to tetanus
Vaccinia immune globulin	For passive immunization subsequent to exposure to smallpox
Varicella-zoster immune globulin	For passive immunization subsequent to exposure to chicken pox

Source: Adapted from American Blood Resources Association, "Basic Facts About the Commercial Plasma Industry."

remove whole blood, separate the plasma from the cells and serum, and reinfuse the latter back into the donor. People may donate once in 48 hours but no more than twice a week. Prospective paid donors, like volunteer donors, are screened for medical history and risk behaviors, and each one must pass an annual physical examination and tests for total protein and syphilis in the blood every 4 months.

The American Blood Resources Association (ABRA)—a trade association for plasmapheresis collection centers and plasma derivative manufacturers—maintains a national donor deferral registry. Only first-time donors are checked against the registry of known donors deferred for positive test results, disease history, or risky behavior. Repeat donors' records are checked at the plasmapheresis center where the plasma is removed. Most centers ensure that donors are not migrating from one center to another over the 48-hour minimum donation interval.[1]

As with whole blood donated by the volunteer population, first-time donors are known to carry higher viral test positivity rates than repeat donors. One manufacturer reported success with its program to detect and remove first-time donor blood that was found to have positive viral markers (Philip, 1995).

Plasma Fractionation and Product Manufacture

Plasma collected at plasmapheresis centers is shipped in separate collection containers to pharmaceutical manufacturing plants. There the plasma is pooled into processing lots of as many as 60,000 units. A chemical fractionation process separates the various active components of plasma, which are further manufactured into clotting factor products for hemophiliacs, albumin for burn victims, and immunoglobulin preparations for immune-deficient persons.

Most plasma derivatives undergo viral inactivation or removal. The two main methods are heat treatment and solvent-detergent washing. Heat treatment is accomplished either by exposing the lyophilized (freeze-dried) product to dry heat or suspending it in a solution. Alternatively, the completely soluble liquid product is heated with the addition of various stabilizers such as sucrose and glycine. Extensive research has carefully calculated specified temperatures and times for different heat treatment processes.

Another method in use today exposes the product to an organic solvent such as N-Butyl phosphate and a detergent such as Triton X-100 or polysorbate 80 to dissolve the lipid coat of viruses, rendering them inactive. Solvent detergent inactivation cannot eliminate nonlipid-coated viruses such as HAV or parvovirus B-19.

A delicate balance maintains between disabling viruses and retaining adequate concentrations of the unstable components in the plasma. Heat and chemicals are particularly damaging to the plasma. Gentle but potentially safe methods still under investigation include nanofiltration to remove virus particles on the basis of molecular size; monoclonal antibody affinity chromatography to capture the protein of interest while the viruses and unwanted components are washed away; irradiation to inactivate viruses; virucidal agents that, having killed viruses, can then be removed during further manufacturing; and exposure to ultraviolet light.

Genetic engineering techniques are now used to produce recombinant factors VIII and IX, meaning that the genes to produce the proteins have been cloned and can be harvested from genetically engineered Chinese hamster ovary cells in the laboratory. These products have, so far, been found free of human viruses.

History of Disease Transmission from Plasma Products

In the 1980s before the etiology of HIV transmission was understood, many hemophilia patients used plasma products infected with HIV, with 63 percent of all hemophilia patients in the United States becoming infected as a result. Many more contracted HBV and HCV.

Disease has been transmitted in many fewer cases since the introduction of antibody tests and viral inactivation and removal processes for plasma derivatives.

In January 1996, CDC reported the transmission of HAV by plasma derivatives factor VIII and factor IX, which are used to treat hemophilia patients. Both products had been virally inactivated by solvent detergent, but this technique is not completely effective in inactivating HAV or other nonlipid viruses such as parvovirus.

Clinical trials have demonstrated that current heat treatment and solvent detergent viral inactivation techniques are effective against HBV, HCV, and HIV. (Colombo et al., 1985; Horowitz et al., 1988; Kernoff et al., 1987; Manucci et al., 1988; Schimpf et al., 1987.)

In February 1994, Baxter Healthcare announced a voluntary withdrawal of its Immune Globulin Intravenous (IGIV) following reports that the product may have transmitted HCV to 14 patients in Spain, Sweden, and the United States. In July 1994, CDC confirmed 112 reports of possible cases of acute HCV infection from Baxter's IGIV (111 cases) and that of the American Red Cross (1 case). Because these products had maintained a longstanding safety record, they had not been virally inactivated with FDA-approved methods. In the 74 cases

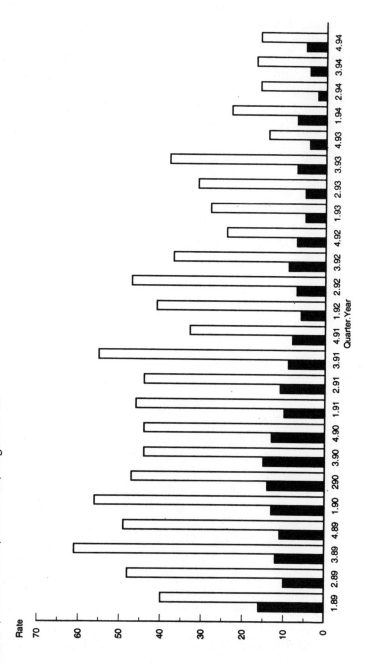

Figure 49.2. *Reported Confirmed HIV Prevalence Rates among Donations in California, 1989-1994. Reported Western Blot Confirmed HIV prevalence rates per 100,000 commercial plasma donations and volunteer whole blood donations in California (1989-1994). Source: California Department of Health Services, Office of AIDS, HIV/AIDS Epidemiology Branch, Sacramento, California, August 1995.*

in which risk-factor data were available, 68 (92 percent) had receipt of IGIV as the only risk factor for infection.

In December 1994, FDA notified manufacturers of immunoglobulin products that it would begin testing for HCV in all products that had not undergone a validated virus inactivation or removal step. FDA further required manufacturers to submit their plans to incorporate the steps into their manufacturing plan. The immune globulins affected by this policy include Rho(D) immune globulin for Rh-negative pregnant women and specific immune globulins for HBV, tetanus, and varicella-zoster. No new cases of HCV transmission by IGIV have been reported to date.

A similar product, immune globulin for intramuscular administration (IGIM), is not virally inactivated. Although no cases of HCV transmission by this means have ever been reported, concerns have been raised about this product, and FDA allows only the manufacturing lots that have been tested for HCV to be distributed.

HIV is a delicate virus in that it is readily inactivated. In 1988, CDC reported on a worldwide survey of 75 suspected cases of HIV transmission by heat-treated factor concentrates. Among the 75 recipients, 18 met the strict criteria for a probable association, including 8 who had received U.S.-manufactured concentrates. Subsequently, the manufacturer withdrew the product and modified its viral inactivation technique (Centers for Disease Control and Prevention, 1988). No cases of HIV transmission by plasma products inactivated according to current standards have been reported.

Rates of Viral Test Positivity among Commercial and Volunteer Donors

Despite the evidence that viral inactivation and removal processes make today's plasma products safer than ever, the fact remains that the paid commercial plasma donor pool has higher rates of viral infectivity than the volunteer whole blood donor pool.

In 1978, FDA required that each blood unit be labeled as either volunteer or paid. In the regulations, FDA concluded that paid blood donors were more likely to transmit hepatitis to recipients than were volunteer donors. Its conclusions were based on the following research evidence: higher rates of HBsAG positivity in commercial donors; higher rates of HBV and non-A, non-B, hepatitis in recipients of paid donor blood; and a highly researched cohort of transfusion recipients in which the elimination of commercial blood resulted in substantially fewer cases of posttransfusion hepatitis.

While the commercial donor pool for whole blood is all but nonexistent in the United States today, the plasma industry continues to rely on paid donors to supply the raw plasma for further manufacturing into plasma derivatives.

We were unable to obtain national data on the viral test positivity rates among paid plasma donors compared to volunteer blood donors. We did, however, find several sources of information pertaining to this issue. First, we found that California requires the reporting of initial and confirmed HIV prevalence rates for both blood banks and plasma collection centers. Figure 49.2 shows that the confirmed HIV prevalence rates per 100,000 commercial plasma donations has decreased in recent years but remains substantially higher than those same rates in volunteer whole blood donations.

Plasma donors can donate much more frequently than blood donors, so fewer plasma donors are needed to collect 100,000 units. Moreover, several plasma units could be donated during the window period, whereas it is unlikely that more than one whole blood unit could be donated in the window period. Comparing donors to donors would probably show an even greater discrepancy.

Second, we analyzed the clinical data that manufacturers submitted to FDA during the approval process for a sample of viral tests. As Table 49.3 shows, the test-positive rates for commercial plasma donors are substantially higher than those of volunteer whole blood donors.

Summary

Clearly, most commercial plasma donors are healthy and free of disease. However, monetary incentives such as those offered by commercial plasma-collection centers may be tantalizing to those who are known to be at risk for infectious diseases, such as intravenous drug users and prostitutes. Screening questions address these risk behaviors, but there is no definitive way to screen out all risky donors, and current tests may not be sufficient to catch all infected units. For example, more than 80 percent of HTLV-I and HTLV-II infections among intravenous drug users stem from HTLV-II, but the HTLV-I antibody test is somewhat less sensitive for HTLV-II infections.

Newly emerging and yet unknown viruses often enter the population through high-risk individuals. Viral antibody tests may not yet exist, and current viral inactivation and removal techniques may be ineffective for new viruses. It is not known for sure whether HTLV-II is present in plasma. Moreover, one infectious donation can contaminate an entire pool of as many as 60,000 units.

Table 49.3. Viral Test Antibody Positivity Rates: Clinical Trial Data[a]

	Blood Volunteer	Plasma Paid
HIV-1 and HIV-2		
Sample size	13,059	3,995
% positive		
	0.09	0.15
HCV		
1st generation (1990)		
Sample size	9,998	10,523
% positive	0.6	6.7
2nd generation (1994)		
Sample size	14,068	6,005
% positive	0.5	10.6
HTLV-I[b]		
1st generation (1990)		
Sample size	13,690	3,850
% positive	0.12	0.55
2nd generation (1994)		
Sample size	6,510	c
% positive	0.29	c
HBcore		
Sample size	2,969	10[d]
% positive	1.1	20.0

[a]Rates are for repeatedly reactive results. That is, initial test positives are retested.

[b]HTLV-I is not present in plasma.

[c]Not evaluated.

[d]Note the small sample size. Also, subjects were designated "paid donors" but some may have donated whole blood rather than plasma.

Without national data on the differences in prevalence and incidence rates between paid and volunteer donors, it is not possible to draw firm conclusions about potential risks posed by plasma derivatives. Such data would be valuable because they could be used to monitor the blood industry in its entirety.

Notes to Text in This Chapter

[1]For example, centers may mark the donors' finger with florescent dye. Nearby centers use different colors.

Chapter 50

Reducing Transfusion-Associated Risks

This chapter covers a number of different approaches used to further reduce the risk of blood transfusion. These include drug therapies to reduce the need for transfusion, alternative products, reducing the use of transfusions, and reducing the risks directly by controlling the sources of donation, extending viral inactivation techniques, genetic engineering, or improving viral testing.

Drug Therapies to Reduce the Need for Blood Transfusion

Physicians are increasingly considering alternatives to blood transfusion. Recombinant human erythropoietin—a growth factor that stimulates the body's manufacture of red blood cells—has been shown to decrease the need for blood as well as increase the yield from patients donating preoperatively for themselves. Clinical studies of anemic patients undergoing long-term hemodialysis who use erythropoietin show hematocrits and hemoglobin levels that are high enough to preclude further transfusions (Stack and Snyder, 1991). U.S. patients with anemia now use 200,000 to 400,000 units of red blood cells a year (Menitove, 1991). Similarly, the antidiuretic hormone, DDVAP, when given preoperatively has been shown to be effective in decreasing blood loss in

From the United States General Accounting Office Report to the Ranking Minority Member, Committee on Commerce, House of Representatives. *Blood Supply: Transfusion Associated Risks*, GAO/PEMD-97-2 (Washington, D.C.: 1997).

cardiac and orthopedic surgery as well as reducing the need for postoperative platelet transfusions. For white blood cells, physicians are prescribing granulocyte, granulocyte-macrophage colony-stimulating factors, and multilineage colony-stimulating factor (interleukin-3) to prevent chemotherapy-induced neutropenia (abnormally low numbers of circulating neutrophils) and to accelerate recovery from this condition. The recently discovered thrombopoietin is rapidly advancing through clinical trials and will undoubtedly reduce the need for platelet transfusions.

Alternatives to Blood

Researchers are also working to develop substitutes for blood. One synthetic red blood cell substitute is made from outdated blood. The product, known as stroma-free hemoglobin solution, has been successful at supporting life for baboons with dangerously low hematocrits with no significant changes in heart rate, cardiac output, oxygen consumption, or mean arterial blood pressure (Gould et al., 1986, 1990).[1] However, recent experiments in Scotland using mice suggest that it may increase susceptibility to bacterial infections (Griffiths, 1995). It appears that bacterial sepsis results when hemoglobin provides bacteria with a source of iron that enhances the bacteria's ability to replicate.

If clinical trials can establish that stroma-free hemoglobin can be a safe and effective treatment for anemia, it will have the advantage over red blood cells of being universally compatible, having a long shelf life, and being free of infectious agents.

Perhaps more promising are recombinant red blood cell substitutes that are artificial in the sense that they are not derived from blood. These products are limited by their short shelf life and as yet undetermined toxicity. A double-blind, controlled Phase III clinical trial of a recombinant red blood cell substitute, HemAssist, is under way for patients suffering from blood loss and shock caused by trauma. The clinical trial will compare the outcomes of accident and trauma victims resuscitated under the current standard of care with those treated with HemAssist plus the current standard of care. It is not clear that HemAssist will substitute for blood at all. The anticipated outcome is survival. At this time, this product is not planned to be used as a substitute for blood in patients with anemia caused by other than acute blood loss. Another blood substitute, PolyHeme(R), is expanding its Phase II clinical trials from infusing the equivalent of 6 units of blood to 10 units, or the equivalent of replacing the total adult blood volume. At the same time, the manufacturer is pursuing FDA approval for Phase III trials of the blood substitute.

Reducing the Use of Transfusions

Avoiding unnecessary transfusions is a primary goal of transfusion medicine specialists. "Transfusion trigger" refers to the clinical events and laboratory data that lead physicians to transfuse blood to patients. In a 1985 study, Ali concluded that 11 percent of red blood cell transfusions were probably of doubtful benefit to the patients (Ali, 1988). The most overprescribed blood component, however, is probably fresh-frozen plasma. In 1986, Blumberg and colleagues indicated that as many as 73 percent of fresh-frozen plasma transfusions were unjustified (Blumberg et al., 1986). Yet, transfusions of plasma numbered 2.056 million in 1987 and increased by nearly 10 percent in 1992 to 2.255 million units (Wallace et al., 1993, 1995).

It is the responsibility of the prescribing physician to evaluate the patient's specific needs and to transfuse only appropriate blood components. This requires a scientific approach based on clinical laboratory results and careful consultation with the resident transfusion medicine specialist. Because many physicians lack knowledge about the specific indications for the use of blood products, many blood banks are tightening their control over the prescription of blood products. Hospital transfusion committees (now required for accreditation by the Joint Commission on Accreditation of Healthcare Organizations) routinely review and control transfusion practices.

Intraoperative blood salvage—a procedure in which patients' own blood is collected during surgery and later reinfused—is becoming a more frequent practice. In 1992, an estimated 427,000 patients had their blood collected and reinfused during surgery. However, little is known about the potential risks associated with this procedure.

Other ways to reduce transfusions include preoperative and intraoperative hemodilution; improving the scrutiny of laboratory tests among premature and newborn infants; improving supportive care (for example, close monitoring of the use of fluids); and expanding the use of crystalloids and colloids for the treatment of acute blood loss in surgery, obstetrics, and trauma.

Controlling the Sources of Donation

Nonemergency patients can theoretically reduce the risks of receiving virally contaminated or incompatible blood by donating their own blood prior to surgery. However, a recent industry survey of 1,829 institutions indicated that autologous transfusion errors occur in nearly 20 percent of all blood banks. In most of these cases, the hospital transfused a regular or directed donor unit before using the patient's own blood. The most serious error—giving an autologous unit to an unintended recipient—occurred in 1.2 percent of responding hospitals.

Only about 60 percent of the surveyed facilities test autologous donations for viruses, and about 40 percent permit the transfusion of autologous units that test positive for viruses. The risk of patients' receiving bacterially contaminated blood that they have donated for their own use is equivalent to that risk within the general blood supply. Moreover, breakage or damage during handling of autologous units was reportedly high. Among 599 question respondents, 201 (34 percent) reported breakage of 308 units during laboratory processing or shipping and 195 of 605 (32 percent) respondents reported the unavailability of 368 autologous units from breakage or damage outside the laboratory. Of the 368 units, 182 were damaged by faulty refrigeration.

Consequently, the overall risk of receiving potentially virally infected, bacterially contaminated blood or blood not tested at all may actually be increased by a procedure designed to decrease risk.

Similarly, some patients request that the blood they receive come from directed donations, believing that this will reduce their risk. However, studies indicate that blood donated by the volunteer population can be safer than blood donated by relatives and friends, who may feel social pressure to donate and therefore do not divulge risk behaviors or disease status.

Also of major importance for reducing risk is the increased use of single-donor apheresis platelets, which is slowly replacing the practice of pooling units from 6 to 8 donors. Exposing patients to fewer donors is clearly a way to minimize risk.

Extending Viral Inactivation to Cellular Components

Promising advances in the inactivation of viruses for plasma have been discussed in Chapter 49, Plasma Products. Research on the viral inactivation of cellular components of blood has been more difficult. Extending storage time, washing, platelet removal, or leukocyte reduction—the elimination of white blood cells—for red blood cells reduces but does not eliminate some circulating viruses. Mild temperature elevation irreversibly destroys red blood cells. Chemical approaches, such as using ozone, have shown variable results.

Photochemical approaches to reduce viruses in red blood cells and platelets have shown more promise. Hypericin, a naturally occurring antiviral agent found in the St. John's wort plant, has shown preliminary success at destroying HIV and other viruses in donated blood ("VIMRx Pharmaceuticals Expects," 1995). More importantly, both viral inactivation and improved cell recovery and survival have been demonstrated using psoralen derivatives and ultraviolet light, particularly when used with the "quencher" rutin, a naturally occurring flavonoid obtained from buckwheat.

Closing the Window Period

The majority of virally contaminated units are donated by persons who have recently contracted a virus and whose immune systems have yet to produce the blood antibodies that allow screening tests to detect infection. New screening tests are constantly narrowing this period of undetectability; however, the costs of implementing them throughout the blood supply are considerable while their predicted effect appears to be quite small. For example, current estimates suggest that the full implementation of a new HIV screening test would eliminate 24 cases of transfusion-transmitted HIV among the 21.6 million transfusions conducted each year. This translates into a cost of $2.3 million dollars per life-year saved compared to the median cost of $19,000 per life-year saved for other medical life-saving interventions (Tengs et al., 1995). In comparison, traditional antibody tests prevent 16,000 cases of transfusion-transmitted HIV per year at a cost of about $3,600 per life year saved ("HIV-1 Antigen Test," 1995).

FDA recommended the use of this test when it became commercially available in early 1996. We were unable to find any studies that systematically compared the likely outcomes of targeting similar funding levels toward other avenues of reducing risk, such as improving donor education and screening or viral inactivation techniques.

In September 1996, Stramer reported the one and, to date, only documented case of HIV that has been detected by the p24 antigen test that was not also positive on the traditional antibody test among nearly 8 million donors tested since March 1996 ("Red Cross Reports," 1996). Researchers have speculated that the models predicting the detection of more donors may have overlooked the possibility that acute illness during the early window period may keep donors from giving blood temporarily.

Remaining unanswered is the possibility that the new antigen test has attracted recently infected "test-seekers" for a more sensitive HIV test that is not available at HIV testing and counseling sites and who actually increase the risks of HIV in the blood supply.

Summary

The risks of transfusion will continue to decrease as a direct result of pharmaceutical advances, changes in medical practice, improved selection of donors, viral inactivation techniques, and improved viral tests. Because the risks of transfusion are already so low, any incremental reductions in that risk will come at some cost either to the blood supply or to the health care system. A rapidly progressing medical field such as that of blood transfusion warrants careful consideration of the costs and benefits of different approaches to reducing risk.

Notes to the Text in This Chapter

[1]Stroma is the structural portion of erythrocytes. The hematocrit is the percentage of the volume of a blood sample occupied by cells.

Chapter 51

Alternatives to Regular Blood Transfusions

The second genetically engineered blood clotting factor and a new drug to stem bleeding in heart surgery last year joined other alternatives to regular "homologous" blood transfusion—blood transfused into someone other than the donor.

New steps by the Food and Drug Administration are helping to make the public blood supply as safe as possible. (See *The Real Scoop on AIDS and Shortages*, below). Alternatives, too, may increase safety for some patients, including those with the clotting disorder hemophilia, who all their lives depend on outside sources for clotting factors they lack.

Genetically engineered Kogenate was licensed February 28, 1993, by the Food and Drug Administration as the second non-blood-derived alternative for people without clotting factor VIII. FDA licensed the first non-blood factor VIII, Recombinate, in December 1992. These products are for patients with hemophilia A. They prevent or control bleeding and prevent bleeding associated with surgery.

Previously, factor VIII could only be obtained from products derived from human plasma, the liquid part of blood. Kogenate and Recombinate are produced by hamster ovary cells into which the gene for human factor VIII has been inserted. The resulting factor is highly purified, eliminating the risk of transmission of viruses such as hepatitis or HIV, the virus that causes AIDS.

FDA Consumer, U.S. Food and Drug Administration, July/August 1994.

The new drug Trasylol Injection (aprotinin), approved last December 29 [1993], decreases the need for transfusion in patients undergoing coronary artery bypass surgery. (For more biological and drug alternatives, see *Approved Alternatives*, below.)

In addition to drugs and biologics, several medical practices are available to lessen the already low risk of disease transmission. These alternatives include using the patient's own previously donated blood, recycling the patient's blood shed during surgery, and diluting the patient's blood before surgery.

Your Own Blood

Patients who are likely to require a transfusion during an upcoming surgery may decide to donate their own blood for possible reinfusion. FDA recommends this practice, called "autologous" transfusion, whenever possible for elective surgery.

Use of the patient's own blood may reduce the chance of infection or other adverse reaction. The practice also decreases demand on the public blood supply. In addition, autologous transfusion allows blood lost during surgery to be replaced more quickly because the process of donating blood, in itself, stimulates the bone marrow to produce new blood cells.

The disadvantages include: increased cost (about $24 more per unit), unnecessary donation if surgery doesn't require transfusion, and sometimes waste of unneeded units. Autologous blood not used by the donor-patient often cannot be used by another patient.

Some hospitals have a program for using autologous units in the public blood supply if the intended patient doesn't use them. These units must meet all FDA's safety standards for regular transfusion. In fact, the agency strongly recommends that all tests routinely performed on regular donations be performed on all autologous donations. Uniform testing is less confusing and safer, because it decreases the chance of releasing for general use an incompletely tested unit of blood. Labeling of an autologous donation must clearly indicate the intended recipient. Liquid blood can be stored refrigerated only 42 days; frozen blood, 10 years.

Autologous blood is most widely used for surgery on the bones, blood vessels, urinary tract, and heart. Nevertheless, any medically stable patient, even a child or pregnant woman, can be a candidate for autologous donation, according to Joseph Fratantoni, M.D., director of hematology at FDA's Center for Biologics Evaluation and Research.

Conditions that might prevent someone from donating blood for others don't necessarily prevent autologous blood donation. For example, people who have had hepatitis may give blood to themselves.

Autologous donation may be inadvisable for some patients, such as those with severe heart and blood vessel disease whose condition may be worsened by donating a unit or two of blood, says Fratantoni. "The decision to use autologous donation," he says, "should be made by the physician and the patient, according to the patient's condition."

For an autologous donation, the patient's doctor will make arrangements with the local blood bank, where the person can give one unit of blood a week for up to six weeks, as needed. A unit is just under a pint, about 10 percent of a person's total blood.

Although the fluid lost from donation replenishes within 24 hours, replacement of red blood cells, with their life-giving oxygen, can take as long as two months. For patients giving multiple autologous donations over several weeks, iron supplements may be prescribed to help increase the red blood cell count.

Recycling Blood During Surgery

When an operation is expected to involve a large loss of blood, the surgical team may recover the patient's blood and reinfuse it during the surgery. This practice, called intraoperative blood collection, or salvage, has been widely used in open-chest surgery, says Fratantoni, and may be done using one of two methods.

One method uses a high-speed centrifuge "specifically designed to handle blood gently," says Catherine Wentz, a biomedical engineer who reviews such instruments for FDA's Center for Devices and Radiological Health. Blood that collects in the surgical cavity is suctioned into the centrifuge, which separates it into components, Wentz says. The centrifuge concentrates the red blood cells, washes them with a saline solution, and pumps the red cell suspension into an infusion bag for return to the patient.

Despite the fact that red cell survival in salvaged blood may be as great as that of regularly transfused blood, the immune system's white cells and clotting substances such as platelets do not remain in salvaged blood in useful amounts. To protect against clotting problems, Wentz says, care must be taken to limit the amount of blood reinfused to a patient within a certain time period.

Another salvage method bypasses the centrifuge and collects the suctioned blood into a reservoir that filters the blood. After filtration, the unwashed blood is transferred into a bag for reinfusion.

"The choice of blood salvage method, washed or unwashed," Wentz says, "is usually based on the type of surgery. For example, knee and hip surgeries tend to 'taint' the suctioned blood with debris such as bone chips, so the choice may be a washed, or centrifuge, system."

Factors that make intraoperative salvage inadvisable include cancer or infection.

Scientists are investigating other blood collection practices.

Conserving Red Cells

Blood dilution (hemodilution) is a practice to prevent loss of red blood cells. The patient has blood drawn before surgery and is immediately given intravenous fluids to make up for the drawn blood, which is saved to be reinfused after the operation.

"The idea," Fratantoni says, "is that during the operation any blood the patient loses will have been diluted, and therefore fewer red cells are lost. Following surgery, reinfusion of the removed blood provides a supply of normally concentrated red cells."

Directed Donations Safer?

In directed donations, friends or family donate blood for a specific patient. Such donors must go through all the standard donor screening and testing procedures. Several states have passed laws establishing directed donation as a procedure that must be followed when requested, except in an emergency.

Some people may feel it's always safer to receive blood from a relative or friend than from the general blood supply, but experts say this is not necessarily the case.

"In fact, the track record on directed donations is mixed," Fratantoni says. "Studies have shown that relatives or friends, feeling pressured to donate, sometimes hide information during screening that they wouldn't under other circumstances, so that they give blood when they shouldn't." (Since the blood is tested the same as all other donations, blood that tests positive for infection or other problems will not be used.)

While matching a patient's blood type may be easier when the donor is a relative rather than someone else, such patients have a high risk of developing graft-versus-host disease, a complication due to the donor and recipient's sharing certain tissue-type substances. In this disease, lymphocyte white blood cells from the transfused blood multiply and react against the recipient's tissues.

When the donor and recipient are both from the general U.S. population, the probability of their sharing a tissue-type substance is very low. Not zero, Fratantoni says, but "somewhere between rare and extremely uncommon."

In the United States, the risk of graft-versus-host disease with blood from a blood relative is about 1 in 7,000 (or higher, depending on the data used). The closer the relatedness, the greater the risk. In a parent-child relationship, the risk is double that in a relationship between grandparent, uncle or aunt.

To reduce the risk, the American Association of Blood Banks recommends irradiating blood derived from all donors who are blood relatives of the recipient. Irradiation suppresses proliferation of lymphocytes contained in the transfused blood. Blood treated this way must meet special FDA licensing requirements, such as permanent labeling that it has been irradiated.

For the Future

A look to the future may envision the ultimate alternative to homologous transfusion to be artificial blood. As blood is extremely complex, however, the dream of a true substitute may never be realized.

Even so, one important blood function has been reproduced artificially: bloodstream transport of life-giving oxygen, the substance all tissues need to survive.

The ideal artificial blood oxygen carrier would pick up oxygen in the lungs and deliver it to all tissues, have a long shelf life with stability at room temperature, be compatible with all blood types, and present no risk of infection, immune reaction, or other health problem.

In 1989, FDA licensed the first artificial oxygen carrier, Fluosol, which used substances called "perfluorochemicals" to temporarily transport oxygen to the heart during coronary artery balloon angioplasty. But the product carried limited amounts of oxygen and had other drawbacks. The manufacturer recently stopped production.

Fratantoni says that two new investigational perfluorochemicals have advantages over Fluosol, including greater oxygen solubility and the capability to be stored at room temperature without being reconstituted before infusion.

Researchers are also experimenting with modifying normal red blood cells so that the cells can be freeze-dried, stored at room temperature, and then reconstituted and infused without concern for blood type.

One modification, by a process called "polymerization," permits high concentration and increases circulation time. Using another technique that encapsulates red cells with a fatty membrane, researchers have supported oxygen requirements in animals with too few red cells to sustain life.

But a major problem with perfluorochemical and red cell oxygen carriers is that the bloodstream retains them only six to 36 hours. Normal red cells survive 100 to 120 days.

There also is an ethical consideration to testing artificial oxygen carriers in human studies in which some participants would get the real biologic while others receive a placebo (dummy) infusion.

According to Thomas Zuck, M.D., director and professor of Hoxworth Blood Center of the University of Cincinnati Medical Center, in *Transfusion Medicine in the 1990's*: "If whole blood or red cells that are known to be effective are available, it would be difficult to contend that participating in blood substitute clinical trials for acute hemorrhage would benefit recipients."

At a meeting in March 1990, members of FDA's Blood Products Advisory Committee expressed concerns about reports of severe, unexplained toxicity of artificial red cell oxygen carriers in patients in clinical trials.

Fratantoni and other CBER experts evaluated the committee's recommendations, as well as animal and human studies of the preparations. In the May 1991 issue of *Transfusion*, FDA published "points to consider" for researchers investigating red cell oxygen carriers. In evaluating risks and benefits of the carriers, the agency recommended "consideration of, and comparison with, the safety profile of approved oxygen carriers, such as red cells [derived from the public blood supply]."

No one knows for sure whether researchers will ever develop an "ideal" artificial oxygen carrier as an alternative to homologous transfusion. But promising possibilities are on the drawing board, and FDA is monitoring those possibilities.

Meanwhile, working alternatives continue in the operating room and the pharmacy.

The Real Scoop on AIDS and Shortages

Two concerns about blood transfusion get a lot of news coverage: AIDS and shortages.

The American blood supply is reasonably safe, and patients who need blood can accept it with confidence, according to Food and Drug Administration experts. But this doesn't mean that blood is entirely risk-free. Blood is human tissue, a biological product, so it carries a degree of risk.

Estimates of the risk of infection with HIV, the virus responsible for AIDS, range from 1 in 61,000 to 1 in 225,000 transfused units—or potentially 90 to 300 infections among some 18 million blood products used each year. The risk from transfusion, however, is far less than the risk of not getting blood when it's needed.

FDA's job is to enforce safeguards, such as questioning potential donors about risk behaviors, testing their blood for infection, quarantining donated blood until tests show it to be safe, and monitoring the blood banking system. Recent steps by FDA to help make the blood supply safer include:

- informing firms making computer software intended for blood product manufacture that the software programs are medical devices

- obtaining a consent degree placing the American Red Cross under court supervision to strengthen its quality control procedures

- proposing guidelines to help prevent recurrent blood center problems by eliminating causes of errors, ensuring integrity of test results, establishing effective controls for manufacture and recordkeeping, and ensuring adequate employee training

- proposing a rule, in conjunction with a Health Care Financing Administration rule, calling for blood centers to provide donor test results to hospitals so that patients who receive units can be notified if the donors later test positive for HIV antibodies.

In other words, FDA regulates blood banking much as it does manufacturers. Blood banks must meet quality control requirements comparable to those of the pharmaceutical industry and must ensure the safety of their commodities.

As for shortages, the blood supply has its ups and downs, like any commodity, but this fluctuation does not mean there's not enough blood for transfusions, says Joseph Fratantoni, M.D., director of hematology at FDA's Center for Biologics Evaluation and Research, which regulates blood banks and blood products. "It's a relative shortage," he says. Last winter, for instance, some 40 U.S. cities reported blood shortages. Contributing circumstances included the Los Angeles earthquake, a severe influenza season, and extremely cold weather over an extended period.

At any one time, Fratantoni says, only 4 to 5 percent of the U.S. population is donating all the blood, with 8 million volunteers donating 12 million units each year. About 20 to 25 percent of Americans, when interviewed, say they want no part of giving blood, he says. Of the rest, a significant percentage are unable to donate because they're anemic—mostly reproductive-age women—leaving about 40 to 50 percent of the total population eligible to donate.

Approved Alternatives

A number of approved drugs and biologicals can lessen the need for or serve as alternatives to blood transfusion:

- Kogenate and Recombinate (recombinant factor VIII)—prevent or control bleeding in patients with hemophilia A and prevent bleeding associated with surgery.

- Amicar (aminocaproic acid)—stabilizes clotting to control urinary tract bleeding and bleeding related to heart surgery, lung or cervical cancer, and other conditions.

- Cyklokapron (tranexamic acid)—controls bleeding in hemophilia and reduces the need for factor VIII replacement after tooth extraction; it is for short-term use (two to eight days).

- DDAVP Injection (desmopressin)—increases clotting factor VIII to control bleeding in patients with mild to moderate von Willebrand disease (a bleeding disorder) or hemophilia A, and prevents bleeding associated with surgery.

- Trasylol Injection (aprotinin)—decreases the need for transfusion in patients undergoing coronary artery bypass surgery.

- Epogen and Procrit (epoetin alfa)—stimulate red blood cell production in patients with anemia related to chronic kidney failure, taking Retrovir (zidovudine) for HIV infection, or receiving cancer chemotherapy.

- Leukine and Prokine (sargramostim)—stimulate the bone marrow, where blood cells form, to produce white blood cells; they are used in patients with non-Hodgkin's lymphoma, Hodgkin's disease, and acute lymphoblastic leukemia.

- Neupogen (filgrastim)—stimulates white blood cell production in cancer patients undergoing chemotherapy.

—by Dixie Farley

Dixie Farley is a staff writer for FDA Consumer.

Part Seven

Additional Help and Information

Chapter 52

Blood-Related Terminology

acute chest syndrome. A serious condition caused by infection or trapped red blood cells in the lungs. Fast or difficult breathing, chest pain, and coughing are signs of acute chest syndrome in the child with sickle cell disease. A child with acute chest syndrome usually will have to go to the hospital for treatment.

acute lymphoblastic leukemia (ALL). A usually rapidly progressive malignant disorder involving the production of immature white blood cells which results in the replacement of normal bone marrow with blast cells. Also called acute lymphocytic leukemia. Appears most commonly in children, but can occur in adults.

acute myelogenous leukemia (AML). A malignant disorder involving the white cells which results in the excessive accumulation of myeloid blast cells in both the bone marrow and the bloodstream. AML occurs in all ages and is the more common acute leukemia in adults. AML affects a different type of white cells than those affected by acute lymphoblastic leukemia (ALL).

The terms in this glossary were compiled from Fact Sheet AR-125, National Institute of Arthritis and Musculoskeletal and Skin Diseases (NIAMS), AMT 6/96, June 1996; Sickle Cell Disease in Newborns and Infants, Department of Health and Human Services (DHHS): AHCPR Publication No. 93-0564, April 1993; "Glossary of Terms," Health Resources and Services Administration (HRSA) at http://www.hrsa.dhhs.gov; and Aplastic Anemia Answer Book, ©1995 Aplastic Anemia Foundation of America, Inc., P.O. Box 613, Annapolis, MD 21404,(800) 747-2820; terms marked with * are reprinted with permission.

acute non-lymphocytic leukemia (ANLL). *See* acute myelogenous leukemia (AML). Terminology for acute leukemias which are not lymphocytic.

allele. Alternate forms of a gene. Some genes, like the ones that control expression of human leukocyte antigens (HLA), have many alternate forms. In HLA, each allele specifies a specific tissue type.

allogeneic bone marrow transplant. Transplant of bone marrow cells from a family member (other than an identical twin) or from an unrelated individual.

anemia. A deficiency in the oxygen-carrying material of the blood, measured in unit volume concentrations of hemoglobin, red blood cell volume and red blood cell number. Decreased red cell production.

antibodies. Special proteins (produced by the body's immune system) that help fight and destroy viruses, bacteria, and other foreign substances that invade the body.

antigen. A protein that is capable of inducing an immune response. In bone marrow transplantation, this immune response is graft-verses-host disease (GVHD) or rejection.

antinuclear antibody test (ANA). A blood test done to find out if the body is producing antinuclear antibodies.

antinuclear antibody. Abnormal antibodies that are often present in people who have connective tissue diseases or other autoimmune disorders. These antibodies target material in the nucleus (the "command center") of healthy cells instead of fighting specific disease-causing agents.

apheresis. Process by which particular blood components, such as platelets, plasma or white blood cells, are obtained for transfusion. The procedure is somewhat more time consuming than routine blood donation and involves separation of whole blood into its component parts. Platelet transfusions are used to prevent and control bleeding in transplant patients.

aplastic anemia. Bone marrow failure with markedly decreased production of white blood cells, red blood cells and platelets leading to increased risk of infection and bleeding.

aplastic crisis. Occurs when a child's bone marrow temporarily stops producing red blood cells. A child with aplastic crisis may appear pale and be tired and less active than usual.

arteries. Large blood vessels that carry blood and oxygen from the heart to all parts of the body.

arterioles. Small blood vessels that branch off from arteries and connect to capillaries.

autologous bone marrow transplant. A portion of the patient's marrow is removed, stored and then returned to the body after the patient receives high doses of chemotherapy and/or radiation therapy.

autonomic neuropathies. Diseases that affect the peripheral nervous system, which consists of nerves outside the brain and spinal cord.

baroreceptor dysfunction. The pressure-sensitive nerve endings that control blood pressure do not work properly.

bacteria. organism that can cause infection.*

biofeedback. A technique designed to help a person gain control over involuntary (independent of the will) body functions, such as heart rate, blood pressure, or skin temperature.

blank. Individuals have the ability to express two human leukocyte antigens (HLA) within each category of antigens (one set being inherited from each biological parent). When an individual has apparently inherited the same antigen type from both parents, the HLA typing of that individual is designated by the shared HLA antigen followed by a blank: (-).

blast cells. Blood cells still in an immature stage of cellular development before appearance of the definitive characteristics of the cell.

blast crisis. The stage of chronic myelogenous leukemia in which large quantities of immature cells are produced by the bone marrow. This stage of Chronic Myelogenous Leukemia (CML) is far less responsive to treatment than the chronic or stable phase.

bone marrow. A substance (with the consistency of thick blood) found in the body's hollow bones, such as legs, arms and hips. It produces platelets, red blood cells and white blood cells, the main agents of the body's immune system. Bone marrow for transplant is invariably harvested from the pelvis.

bone marrow aspiration. test in which a sample of bone marrow cells is removed with a needle and examined under a microscope.*

bone marrow biopsy. procedure in which a small piece of bone marrow tissue is removed with a needle; sample is processed by softening the bone and examining thin slices of the softened bone under a microscope.*

bone marrow transplant. procedure in which bone marrow filled with disease is destroyed by radiation or chemotherapy and then replaced with healthy cells from a donor.*

capillaries. Tiny blood vessels that carry blood between arterioles (the smallest arteries) and venules (the smallest veins). Capillaries form networks throughout the body's organs and tissues. They open and close in response to the organs' needs for oxygen and nutrients.

chemotherapy. Treatment of a disease using chemicals designed to kill cancer cells; used in large doses to help destroy a patient's diseased marrow in preparation for a marrow transplant.

chromosome. a rod-like structure that appears in the nucleus of a cell during division; contains the genes responsible for heredity.*

chronic lymphocytic leukemia (CLL). A malignant disorder involving the over-production of mature lymphocytes which results in the abnormal accumulation of these cells in the bone marrow, the bloodstream and the lymph system. CLL usually involves the lymph nodes. It usually effects older persons, with an average age of 60. It is more common in men.

chronic myelogenous leukemia (CML). A malignant disorder involving the predominance of granulocytes (a particular type of white cell) of all stages of development which results in the abnormal accumulation of these cells in both the bone marrow and the bloodstream.

CML may occur at any age in either sex. It is uncommon before 10 years of age, and occurs most often at an average age of 45.

complete blood count (CBC). The amount or level of blood cells present: white cells, red cells, and platelets.*

conditioning. The process of preparing the patient to receive donated bone marrow. Often done through the use of chemotherapy and radiation therapy.

confirmatory typing (CT). A repeat tissue typing test done to confirm the compatibility of the donor and patient. This is one of the final tests done before transplant.

congenital. Existing before or at birth, though not necessarily detected at that time, but not necessarily hereditary.

congenital disorders. Any disorder present at birth.

connective tissue. The tissue that supports body structures and holds parts together. Some parts of the body, such as tendons and cartilage, are made up of connective tissue. Connective tissue is also the basic substance of bone and blood vessels.

connective tissue disease. A group of diseases that affect the body's connective tissues, including tissue in the joints, blood vessels, heart, skin, and other supporting structures. Some of these diseases are caused by a malfunctioning of the immune system. Connective tissue diseases are fairly common and include systemic lupus erythematosus, rheumatoid arthritis, scleroderma, polymyositis, and dermatomyositis.

Cooley's anemia. Another name for thalassemia major. *See also* thalassemia.

cross match. type and cross; test in which the blood cells of a donor and a recipient are mixed together to determine if they are compatible.*

culture. procedure used to identify the source of infection; specimen of blood, urine, sputum or stool is taken and tested to determine the type of infection and the appropriate antibiotic.*

cyanosis. Bluish, grayish, or dark purple discoloration of the skin that occurs when blood cannot circulate freely and gives up all its oxygen.

cytomegalovirus (CMV). A virus which can cause pneumonia in post bone marrow transplant patients.

deoxyribonucleic acid (DNA). The material in a cell nucleus that carries genetic information.

differential. percentage of different types of blood cells in the blood.*

endocrinologic disorders. Problems with glands (and/or the hormones these glands secrete) of the endocrine system such as the thyroid and pancreas.

erythroblast. an immature red blood cell.*

erythrocyte sedimentation rate (ESR). A blood test that determines how fast erythrocytes (red blood cells) settle out of unclotted blood and is used to detect inflammation in the body. Connective tissue diseases can change blood proteins, which changes how quickly red blood cells settle out of unclotted blood to the bottom of a test tube. Higher ESRs (indicating more rapid settling of red blood cells and the presence of inflammation) are found in all of the connective tissue diseases.

erythrocyte. a mature red blood cell that carries oxygen.*

Fanconi's anemia. A rare form of aplastic anemia. Bone marrow transplantation for Fanconi's anemia would require a less intense conditioning regime than other diagnoses.

gangrene. A condition that occurs when tissue dies. Tissue death is usually caused by a loss of blood supply. Gangrene may affect a small area, such as a finger or toe, or a large portion of a limb.

gene. Basic units of inheritance that control for specific characteristics such as eye color or tissue type. Genes are located on the chromosome and consist of segments of DNA.

genotype. The actual genetic makeup of an individual. For example, a person with brown eyes may have inherited a brown eye color gene

(Br) from one parent and a blue eye color gene (Bl) from the other. This person's genotype would be Br/Bl.

graft-versus-host (GVH) disease. A frequent complication of allo-geneic bone marrow transplants in which donor marrow cells can cause damage to the recipient's skin, intestine and/or liver. In essence, this process represents the counterpart to rejection.

granulocyte. a white blood cell produced in the bone marrow that engulfs and destroys invading organisms.*

Haemophilus influenzae. A type of bacteria that causes infection and can lead to serious problems in the child with sickle cell disease. Babies must receive a special vaccine beginning at 2 months of age to protect them from this condition.

hairy cell leukemia (HCL). A rare type or variant of chronic leu-kemia. Primarily a disease of middle-aged men. HCL infrequently re-quires bone marrow transplantation as a treatment.

hand-and-foot syndrome. Pain and swelling of the hands and feet caused by sickle-shaped red blood cells that plug blood vessels in the hands and feet. Often this will be the baby's first problem caused by sickle cell disease.

haplotype. All the human leukocyte antigens (HLA) inherited from one parent. One half of a genotype.

hematocrit. the percentage of blood that is made up of cells. Nor-mal values for men range from 42-52%, and for females 38-48%.*

hematopoietic. Blood forming. Of, or pertaining to, the formation and maturation of blood cells and their derivatives.

hemoglobin. Hg; iron-containing coloring in the red cells that com-bines with oxygen from the lungs and carries it to the body's cells. Normal values for men are 13-16 gms/100 ml and 12-14 gms/100 ml for women.*

hereditary. A genetic transmission of characteristics from parents to children.

heterozygous antigens. Presence of different alleles on both chromosomes, one inherited from each parent.

histiocytosis. A rare and frequently fatal blood disease that affects the body's immune system, allowing a type of white blood cell called a histiocyte to multiply wildly and attack vital body organs. Its cause is unknown, and its progression is unpredictable.

histocompatibility. Referring to the similarity of tissue between different individuals. The level of histocompatibility describes how well matched the patient and donor are. The major histocompatibility determinants are the human leukocyte antigens (HLA). HLA typing is performed between the potential marrow donor and the potential transplant recipient to determine how close a HLA match the two are. The closer the match the less the donated marrow and the patient's body will react against each other. (*See* Graft-Versus-Host Disease).

Hodgkin's disease. A lymphoma most frequently occurring in young adults. Hodgkin's disease not responding to chemotherapy may be treated by autologous bone marrow transplantation (BMT) and less frequently by allogeneic BMT.

homozygous antigens. Presence of identical alleles on both chromosomes, one inherited from each parent.

human leukocyte antigens (HLA). Proteins found on the surface of white blood cells and other tissues that are used to match donor and patient. Patient and potential donor have their white blood cells tested for three antigens, HLA-A, B and DR. Each individual has two sets of these antigens, one set inherited from each parent. For this reason, it is much more likely for a brother or sister to match the patient than an unrelated individual, and much more likely for persons of the same racial and ethnic backgrounds to match each other.

hypovolemic disorders. Indicate low blood volume.

immunoglobulins. kill microbes directly or make it easier for white cells to kill them.*

immunosuppression. decrease in the ability of the body's normal immune response to the invasion of foreign material.*

ischemic lesion. A sore or other skin abnormality caused by an insufficient supply of blood to the tissue.

leukemia. Any of a group of potentially fatal diseases involving uncontrolled growth of white blood cells. Leukemias are classified based upon rapidity of course of disease and cell type affected.

leukocyte. a white blood cell.*

leukopenia. a low number of white blood cells.*

linkage disequilibrium. An increased frequency of allele associations observed, more than would be expected based on random distribution.

locus. Specific place a gene is located on the chromosome.

lymphocyte. A type of white blood cell subdivided into T-cells and B-cells. T-cells provide cellular immunity and B-cells form antibodies. T-cells are responsible for Graft Versus Host Disease.

lymphoma. Malignant proliferation of lymphocytes, generally within lymph nodes, but sometimes involving other tissues such as the liver and spleen. Lymphoma includes Hodgkin's and non-Hodgkin's diseases.

malignant. The progressive growth of cancerous cells. These cells can spread to sites distant from the initial site.

match. In marrow transplantation, the word "match" relates to how similar the human Leukocyte antigen (HLA) typing is between the donor and the recipient. The best kind of match is an "identical match". This means that all six of the HLA antigens (2 A antigens, 2 B antigens and 2 DR antigens) are the same between the donor and the recipient. This type of match is described as a "6 of 6" match. Donors and recipients who are "mismatched" at one antigen are considered a "5 of 6" match, and may be considered suitable for bone marrow transplantation.

megakaryocyte. a cell in the bone marrow that produces platelets.*

melofibrosis. Also called agnogenic myeloid metaplasia. A chronic disease characterized by fibrous material in the bone marrow, an enlarged spleen and anemia.

mixed lymphocyte culture (MLC). A test which measures the level of reactivity between donor and recipient lymphocytes.

multiple myeloma. A malignant disorder of the plasma cells. Multiple myeloma is frequently associated with bone pain and susceptibility to infection.

myelodysplastic syndrome. Also called pre-leukemia or "smoldering" leukemia, is a disease of the marrow in which inadequate platelets, red blood cells and white blood cells are made. Sometime a precursor to acute myelogenous leukemia (AML).

myeloproliferative disorders. A group of disorders characterized by abnormal proliferation by one or more types of marrow cells. Four disorders are generally included as myeloproliferative disorders. These are polycythemia vera (PV), myelofibrosis, chronic myelomonocytic leukemia (CMML) and primary thrombocythemia. Most commonly seen in people over 50 years of age.

nailfold capillaroscopy. A test used to identify the primary or secondary form of Raynaud's phenomenon. The examiner places a drop of oil on the nailfold (the skin at the cuticle or base of the nail) and uses a hand-held magnifying glass or microscope to look at the capillaries in the nailfold. Certain changes in theses capillaries can be characteristic of connective tissue diseases.

neuroblastoma. A solid tumor of children, which in an advanced wide spread stage may be treated by bone marrow transplantation.

neutropenia. low neutrophil (poly) count.*

non-Hodgkin's. A lymphoma which occurs in a wide variety of growth patterns and with diverse signs and symptoms. Treatment depends upon type of non-Hodgkin's lymphoma.

oligonucleotide. Sequence of nucleic acids used as a probe in DNA based Human Leukocyte Antigen (HLA) tissue typing.

osteopetrosis. A disorder of the bones in which hardening of tissue obliterates the marrow, leading to bone failure which may cause early death.

Pain event or painful episode. Pain caused by plugging of blood vessels by sickled blood cells. Pain is most often felt in the arms, legs, back, and abdomen. The pain may last only a few hours or as long as a week or two. The pain may be mild or so severe that pain medicine is needed. The number of pain events a person has may vary greatly.

pancytopenia. low number of blood cells.*

peripheral blood stem cells (PBSC). A cell with the potential to produce all the components of blood that is obtained from peripheral blood rather than from bone marrow.

peripheral blood. blood in the bloodstream.*

petechiae. tiny red dots on the skin due to bleeding under the skin caused by low platelet counts.*

phagocytosis. "cell eating"; the engulfment and destruction of dangerous microorganisms or cells by certain white blood cells.*

phenotype. The physical expression of genes inherited for a particular characteristic. For example, a person who inherited a brown eye color gene (Br) and a blue eye color gene (Bl) has a phenotype of brown eyes.

platelet. A component of the blood important in clotting. Inadequate amounts of platelets will lead to bleeding and bruising easily.

pre-transplant conditioning. Prior to transplant a patient is given high dose levels of chemotherapy and/or radiation treatments to destroy the tumor and suppress graft rejection.

protocol. A specific plan for treatment of a disease or disorder.

radiation therapy. May be used to help destroy a patient's diseased bone marrow and immuno-suppress the rejection mechanism in preparation for a marrow transplant.

red blood cell. oxygen carrying cell in the blood, which contains the pigment hemoglobin, produced in the bone marrow; erythrocyte.*

refractory (to platelets). the immune system's response to platelet transfusions; platelets are recognized as foreign and destroyed.*

relapse. Recurrence of illness after recovery.

remission. The disappearance of cancer cells following treatment. Also the period during which this reduction or disappearance of symptoms occur.

reticulocyte. an immature red blood cell.*

sarcoma. A malignant solid tumor most frequently found in muscle or bone.

sepsis. The presence of infection in the blood stream.

severe combined immunodeficiency disease (SCID). Congenital defect of the immune system leading to frequent life threatening infection. Marrow transplantation is the current treatment of choice. Most patients have an early onset of SCID detected due to infection, usually by 3 months of age.

sickle cell anemia. The most common form of sickle cell disease. Other types of sickle cell disease include hemoglobin SC disease and sickle beta-thalassemia; there are also other, less common types of sickle cell disease.

sickle cell disease. A group of inherited disorders in which anemia is present and sickle hemoglobin is produced.

sickle cell trait. The condition in which a person has both normal and sickle hemoglobin in the red cells as a result of inheriting a normal hemoglobin gene and a gene for sickle hemoglobin. Sickle cell trait is not a disease and does not change to sickle cell disease. Persons with sickle cell trait may pass the sickle gene to their children.

sickled cells. In children with sickle cell disease, hemoglobin molecules in red blood cells stick to one another and cause the red cells to become crescent or sickle shaped. Sickled cells cannot pass easily through tiny blood vessels.

smooth muscle. The muscles of the body that are not under a person's conscious control. Smooth muscle is found mainly in the internal organs, including the digestive tract, respiratory passages, urinary bladder, and walls of blood vessels.

spasm. An involuntary, sudden muscle contraction. In Raynaud's phenomenon, involuntary contraction of the smooth muscle in the blood vessels decreases the flow of blood to the fingers or toes (which leads to color changes in the skin).

splenic sequestration crisis. Occurs when a large portion of the child's blood becomes trapped in the spleen. Early signs include paleness, an enlarged spleen, and pain in the abdomen.

stem cells. Those cells capable of producing all the components of blood and bone marrow following bone marrow transplantation.

Streptococcus pneumoniae. A bacteria that causes a very serious type of pneumonia in children with sickle cell disease. Twice daily doses of penicillin by mouth, starting at about 2 months of age, can help to prevent this life-threatening infection in children with sickle cell anemia and sickle beta-thalassemia.

syngeneic bone marrow transplant. Transplant of bone marrow cells from an identical twin in which immunosuppression drugs are not required.

thalassemia. A group of chronic, inherited anemias. Particularly common in persons of Mediterranean, African and Southeast Asian ancestry.

thrombocytopenia. a low number of platelets in the blood. When the platelet level falls below 5 (or 5,000/cu.mm) it is considered a life-threatening emergency and may be corrected by a platelet transfusion.*

thymocytes (T cells). white blood cells that have traveled through the thymus.*

tumor. Any abnormal mass resulting from the excessive multiplication of cells. Tumors can be cancerous or non-cancerous.

vascular insufficiency. A term used to describe inadequate blood flow in the blood vessels.

vasodilator. An agent, usually a drug, that widens blood vessels and allows more blood to reach the tissues.

vasospasm or vasoconstriction. A sudden muscle contraction that narrows the blood vessels, reducing blood flow to a part of the body.

white blood cells. blood cells that fight infection.*

Chapter 53

Resources for Patients with Blood and Circulatory Disorders

Organizational Resources

American Association of Blood Banks
8101 Glenbrook Road
Bethesda, MD 20814-2749
(301) 907-6977
(301) 907-6895 fax
e-mail: aabb@aabb.org
http://www.aabb.org

American Autoimmune-Related Diseases Association
15475 Gratiot Avenue
Detroit, MI 48205
(313) 371-8600
(313) 371-6002 fax
e-mail: aarda@aol.com
http://www.aarda.org

American Cancer Society (ACS)
1599 Clifton Road, N.E.
Atlanta, GA 30329
(800) ACS-2345 or (404) 320-3333
http://www.cancer.org

American Liver Foundation
1425 Pompton Avenue
Cedar Grove, NJ 07009
(800) 223-0179 or (973) 256-2550
(973) 256-3214 fax
e-mail: webmail@liverfoundation.org
http://www.liverfoundation.org

Lupus Foundation of America
1300 Piccard Dr, Ste. 200
Rockville, MD 20850
(301) 670-9292
(301) 670-9486 fax
http://www.lupus.org/lupus

American Porphyria Foundation
P.O. Box 22712
Houston, TX 77227
(713) 266-9617
(713) 871-1788 fax

Aplastic Anemia Foundation of America
P.O. Box 613
Annapolis, MD 21404
 (800) 747-2820 or (410) 867-0242
(410) 867-0240 fax
e-mail: aafacenter@aol.com
http://www.aplastic.org

Arthritis Foundation
1330 West Peachtree St.
Atlanta, GA 30309
(404) 872-7100
(404) 872-0457 fax
http://www.arthritis.org

Cincinnati Comprehensive Sickle Cell Center
Children's Hospital Medical Center
3333 Burnet Ave
Cincinnati, OH 45229
(513) 636-4541
(513) 636-5562 fax

Cooley's Anemia Foundation
129-09 26th Avenue
Flushing, NY 11354
 (800) 522-7222
(718) 321-3340 fax
e-mail: ncas@aol.com
http://www.thalassemia.org

The Hemochromatosis Foundation, Inc.
P.O. Box 8569
Albany, NY 12208-0569
(518) 489-0972
(518) 489-0227 fax

Iron Overload Diseases Association, Inc.
433 Westwind Drive, Dept. WWW
N. Palm Beach, FL 33408
http://www.ironoverload.org

Leukemia Society of American (LSA)
600 3rd Avenue
New York, NY 10016
1-800-955-4LSA (1-800-955-4572)
(212) 573-8484
(212) 856-9686 fax
e-mail: infocenter@leukemia.org
http://www.leukemia.org

Howard University
Comprehensive Sickle Cell Center
2121 Georgia Avenue
Washington DC 20059
(202) 806-7930
(202) 806-4517 fax

March of Dimes
Birth Defects Foundation
1275 Mamaroneck Avenue
White Plains, NY 10605
(914) 428-7100
(914) 428-8203 fax
e-mail: resourcecenter@modimes.org
http://www.modimes.org

Sickle Cell Disease Association of America
200 Corporate Point, Suite 495
Culver City, CA 90230
(800) 421-8453
(310) 215-3722 fax

The National Hemophilia Foundation
116 West 32nd St
11th Floor
New York, NY 10001
(212) 328-3700
(212) 328-3777 fax
http://www.hemophilia.org

National Organization for Rare Disorders (NORD)
P.O. Box 8923
New Fairfield, CT 06812
(800) 999-6673 or (203) 746-6518
(203) 746-6481 fax
e-mail: orphan@nord.rdb.com
http://www.nord-rdb.com/~orphan

National Rare Blood Club
99 Madison Avenue
New York, NY 10016
(212) 889-8245

Thrombocytopenia-Absent Radius Syndrome Association (TARSA)
212 Sherwood Drive
Egg Harbor Township, NJ 08234
(609) 927-0418
(609) 653-8639 fax
e-mail: purinton@earthlink.net

United Scleroderma Foundation, Inc.
89 Newbury St
Danvers, MA 01923
(978) 750-4499
(978) 750-9902 fax
e-mail: sclerofed@aol.com
http://www.scleroderma.com

Governmental Resources

Agency for Health Care Policy and Research
AHCPR Clearinghouse
P.O. Box 8547
Silver Spring, MD 20907-8547
1-800-358-9295
http:// www.ahcpr.gov

California State Department of Health
Children's Medical Services Branch
714 P Street, Room 350
Sacramento, CA 95814
(916) 654-0499
(916) 653-4892 fax
e-mail: iwhite@hw1.cahwnet.gov
http://www.dhs.cahwnet.gov

Cancer Information Service
National Cancer Institute
Building 31, Room 1 OA24
9000 Rockville Pike
Bethesda, MD 20892
 (800) 4-CANCER
http://www.nci.nih.gov

Clinical Center Communications
6100 Executive Blvd
Suite 3C01, MSC 7511
Bethesda, MD 20892-7511
(301) 496-2563
(301) 402-2984 fax
http://www.nih.gov

Mississippi State Department of Health
Genetics Division, Room UA-107
P. O. Box 1700
Jackson, MS 39215
(601) 960-7619
(601) 354-6032 fax
e-mail: dbender@msdh.state.ms.us
http://www.msdh.state.ms.us

National Digestive Diseases Information Clearinghouse
2 Information Way
Bethesda, MD 20892-3570
(301) 654-3810
(301) 907-8906 fax
email: nddic@info.niddk.nih.gov
http://www.niddk.nih.gov

National Heart, Lung, and Blood Institute
P.O. Box 30105
Bethesda, MD 20824-0105
(301) 251-1222
(301) 251-1223 fax
e-mail: nhlbiic@dgsys.com
http://www.nhlbi.nih.gov/nhlbi/nhlbi.htm

National Institute of Allergy and Infectious Diseases
Building 31, Room 7A5O
31 Center Dr., MSC 2520
Bethesda, MD 20892-2520
(301) 496-5717
(301) 402-0120 fax
e-mail: niaid@nih.gov
http://www.niaid.nih.gov

National Institute of Diabetes and Digestive and Kidney Diseases
Building 31, Room 9A04
9000 Rockville Pike
Bethesda, MD 20892
(301) 496-3583
(301) 496-7422 fax
http://www.niddk.nih.gov

National Institute of Neurological Disorders and Stroke (NINDS)
Building 31, Room 8A06
31 Center Drive, MSC 2540
Bethesda, MD 20892-2540
(800) 352-9424 or (301) 496-5751
(301) 402-2186 fax
http://www.ninds.nih.gov

National Maternal and Child Health Clearinghouse
2070 Chain Bridge Road, Suite 450
Vienna, VA 22182-2536
(703) 356-1964
(703) 821-2098 fax
e-mail: nmchc@circsol.com
http://www.circsol.com/mch

New York State Department of Health
Newborn Screening Program
Wadsworth Center for Laboratories and Research
P. O. Box 509
Albany, NY 12201-0509
(518) 473-7552
(518) 473-1423 fax

Northern California Comprehensive Sickle Cell Center
Childrens Hospital, Oakland
747 52nd St.
Oakland, CA 94609
(800) 675-6599
(510) 601-3916 fax

The Sickle Cell Disease Program
Division of Blood Diseases and Resources
National Heart, Lung, and Blood Institute
6701 Rockledge Drive
MSC 7950
Bethesda, MD 20892-7950
301-435-0055
(301) 480-0868 fax

Texas Department of Health
Newborn Screening Program
1100 West 49th Street
Austin, TX 78756-3199
(512) 458-7111 or (800) 422-2956
(512) 458-7421 fax
http://www.tdh.state.tx.us

Selected Further Reading

Documents Available

The following additional documents are available from the sources listed. They are presented alphabetically by key terms (bolded).

Anemia: It's More Than Just Too Little Iron. Available from Mayo Health Oasis at http://www.mayo.ivi.com

Newsletter (**aplastic anemia**), a quarterly newsletter available from the Aplastic Anemia Foundation of America.

Your Operation Your Blood (**Autologous Blood Donation**), NIH Publication No. 92-2967, 1992. Available from the National Heart, Lung, and Blood Institute.

Check Your Blood I.Q., NIH Publication No. 92-2991, 1992. Available from the National Heart, Lung, and Blood Institute.

Blood and Its Components, Available from the Johnson Space Center (NASA) on-line at http://jsc.nasa.gov/sa/sd/intro/blood.html

Fifth Disease, December, 1992. Available from the New York State Health Department.

The Human Heart: A Living Pump. NIH Publication 95-1058. Available from the National Heart, Lung, and Blood Institute.

Hemochromatosis, an undated fact sheet available from the National Digestive Diseases Information Clearinghouse.

Hemochromatosis Awareness, a periodic newsletter. Available from the Hemochromatosis Foundation.

What Is Hemophilia, an undated fact sheet. Available along with other literature from the National Hemophilia Foundation or on-line at http://www.infonhf.org/bleeding_info/hemophilia/hemo.html.

Facts about Heart Disease and Women: Reducing High Blood Cholesterol, NIH Publication 94-3658. Available from the National Heart, Lung, and Blood Institute or on-line at www.nhlbi.nih.gov.nhlbi.pubs/hdwmncho/hdwncho.htm

Preventing and Controlling **High Blood Pressure**, NIH Publication 97-3655, 1997. Available from the National Heart, Lung, and Blood Institute.

Ironic Blood (**Iron Overload**), a periodic newsletter. Available from the Iron Overload Diseases Association.

Myelodysplastic Syndromes *Answer Book*, 1996, written by Dr. Lyle Sensenbrenner of the University of Maryland Cancer Center. Available from the Aplastic Anemia Foundation of America or on-line at http://www.teleport.com/nonprofit/aafa/myelodysplasticl.html.

Check Your **Platelet** *I.Q.*, NIH Publication No. 92-3300, 1992. Available from the National Heart, Lung, and Blood Institute.

Raynaud's Phenomenon, NIH Publication 93-2263. Available from the National Heart, Lung, and Blood Institute.

Sickle Cell Anemia, NIH Publication 90-3058. Available from Clinical Center Communications.

Preventing **Stroke**. NIH Publication 94-3440-b. Available from the National Institute of Neurological Disorders and Stroke.

Lifeline, (**thalassemia**) a monthly newsletter available from Cooley's Anemia Foundation.

Varicose Veins *and Spider Veins*. Available from MedicineNet at http://www.medicinenet.com/mainmenu/encyclop/ARTICLE/Art_V/VARVN.HTM

Articles Available

The following articles are available in periodical publications. Check your local library for availability.

"Blood Types," *Science Activities*, Winter 1997 v33, n4, p24(4).

"Blood: How It Works," *American Health*, May 1995, v14, n4, p94(2).

Colucciello, Stephen. "Recognizing and Treating Thromboembolic Disease," *Emergency Medicine*, August 1993, p. 59(9).

Davenport, John. "Macrocytic Anemia," *American Family Physician*, January 1996, v.53, n. 1, p. 155(8)

Ernst, E. "Peripheral Vascular Disease: Benefits of Exercise," *Sports Medicine*, September 1991, v.12, n3, p. 149(3).

Flieger, Ken. "Outlook Brighter for Youngsters with Hemophilia," *FDA Consumer*, July-August 1993, p. 19(5).

"Iron Overload," *Mayo Clinic Health Letter*, January 1998, p7(1).

Kienzle, Michael G. "Syncope: Pursuing the Common and Prognostically Important Causes," *Heart Disease and Stroke*, May/June 1992, p. 123(6)

Malloy, Mary J. and John P. Kane. "Aggressive Medical Therapy for the Prevention and Treatment of Coronary Artery Disease," *Disease-a-Month*, January 1998, v44, n1, p5(35).

Poskus, Deborah B. "Revascularization in Peripheral Vascular Disease: Stents, Atherectomies, Lasers, and Thrombolitics," *AACN Clinical Issues*, November 1995, v6, n4, p. 536(11)

Shionoya S. "Buerger's Disease: Diagnosis and Management," *Cardiovascular Surgery*, June 1993, v. 1, no. 3, p. 207(8).

Vosburgh, Evan. "Rational Intervention in von Willebrand's Disease," *Hospital Practice*, March 30, 1993, p. 31(15).

Williams, Alan E. *et al.* "Estimates of Infectious Disease Risk Factors in U.S. Blood Donors," *JAMA*, March 26, 1997, v277, n12, p. 967(6).

Wolfe, Yun Lee. "Case of the Ceaseless Fatigue" (Hemochromatosis), *Prevention*, July 1997, p. 89(4).

Zamorski, Mark A. *et al.* "Advances in the Prevention, Diagnosis and Treatment of Deep Venous Thrombosis," *American Family Physician*, February 1, 1993, p. 457(13).

Clinical Trials for Blood Diseases

The Hematology Branch at the National Institutes of Health in Bethesda, Maryland conducts clinical research studies on a number of hematologic diseases. For patients to be admitted to the Clinical Center, they must be referred by a physician and meet protocol requirements. There is no charge for medical care at the Clinical Center because patients are participating in research studies. In most instances, patients will be expected to pay the costs of their travel and local lodging.

Current Studies

- Aplastic Anemia
- Myelodysplasia
- Chronic Autoimmune Thrombocytopenic Purpura
- Multiple Myeloma
- T Large Granular Lymphocytic Leukemia
- Bone Marrow Transplantation

In addition, we have a strong interest in evaluating for possible novel therapies patients with the following diagnoses:

- Fanconi Anemia
- Paroxysmal Nocturnal Hemoglobinuria (PNH)
- Post-Hepatitis Aplastic Anemia

Aplastic Anemia

Patients with severe aplastic anemia who are 18 years or older are randomized between two immunosuppressive regimens: antithymocyte globulin combined with cyclosporine verses high dose cyclophosphamide combined with cyclosporine. Patients should not be suitable for bone marrow transplantation or have declined this option.

Children and with aplastic anemia with severe aplastic anemia (less than 18 years of age) are treated with immunosuppression consisting of antithymocyte globulin and cyclosporine.

For refractory aplastic anemia, a number of protocols are offered, including high dose cyclophosphamide; or stem cell factor combined with granulocyte colony stimulating factor.

Myelodysplasia

Patients with subtypes refractory anemia, refractory anemia with ringed sideroblasts and refractory anemia with excess blast are considered for treatment with antithymocyte globulin.

Chronic Autoimmune Thrombocytopenic Purpura

Adult patients with severe refractory idiopathic thrombocytopenic purpura (ITP) are offered intensive immunosuppression using high dose cyclophosphamide followed by autologous peripheral blood stem cell rescue.

Multiple Myeloma

Adult patients to the age of 65 are eligible for autologous stem cell transplantation combined with gene marking.

T Large Granular Lymphocytic Leukemia

Patients with this diagnosis may be eligible for treatment with cyclosporine.

Bone Marrow Transplantation

The Hematology Branch has an active experimental bone marrow transplantation unit. Patients with acute myelogenous leukemia, chronic myelogenous leukemia in stable phase or in transformation, and a variety of other hematologic malignancies may satisfy protocol requirements.

For More Information

Patients can contact Wanda Zamani by email (zamaniw@gwgate. nhlbi.nih.gov) or by phone at 301-402-0764or telefax at 301-402-3088 for more information.

Physicians are welcome to call Dr. Neal Young, Chief of the Hematology Branch or Dr. John Barrett, Chief of the Bone Marrow Transplant Unit at 301-496-5093 or telefax at 301-496-8396.

Index

Index

Page numbers followed by 'n' indicate a footnote.

Page numbers in **bold** indicate a table or illustration

A

Index

family issues
  sickle cell disease 130–31
family members
  bone marrow donors 26, 36, 44, 81–82, 83
  bone marrow transplants 186, 192, 200, 219, 225
  platelet donors 43
  von Willebrand disease diagnosis 254
Fanconi's anemia 508, 527
Fantus, Bernard 12
Farley, Dixie 499
fats
  polyunsaturated 346–47
  saturated 346–47
  trans 347
  see also cholesterol
FDA *see* Food and Drug Administration (FDA)
febrile transfusion reaction 76, 77, 410
Federal Trade Commission (FTC) xi
  varicose veins treatment 297n, 302
ferritin 85, **86**
ferritin tests 157
fetal hemoglobin (HbF) 57–58
  sickle cell disease treatment 129, 130, 151, 153–54
  see also under hemoglobin
fibrin
  clotting 262
  formation 20–21
fibrinogen 8, 19–23
Fifth Disease (NY State) 524
filgrastim 499
finasteride 403
Fluosol 495
folic acid
  bone marrow 92
  deficiency, anemia 35
  pregnancy 89
Food and Drug Administration (FDA) xi
  blood safety 401–6, 429, 491, 496
  Center for Biologics Evaluation and Research 402, 497
  Center for Drug Evaluation and Research 149

Food and Drug Administration (FDA), continued
  gene therapy approvals 249
  hydroxyurea (Hydrea) approval 149
  stents approval 388
  varicose vein treatment 299
fractionation 7, 9
  cold ethanol 12
  hemophilia treatment 14
Fratantoni, Joseph 492–98
fraud, varicose veins treatment 297, 301
Friedewald equation 377
frozen blood cells 8–9
  glycerol cryoprotectant 13
FTC *see* Federal Trade Commission (FTC)

G

gallstones, thalassemia intermedia 94
gamma globulin 264
gangrene, defined 295, 508
GAO *see* General Accounting Office (GAO)
gender factor
  hypertension 331
  leukemia 171
  Raynaud's phenomenon 287, 288
  thromboangiitis obliterans 276, 278
  thrombophlebitis 272
  von Willebrand disease 253
gene, defined 139, 508
gene therapy
  hemophilia 234, 237, 242, 249–52
  sickle cell disease treatment 130
General Accounting Office (GAO) xi, 429n, 449n, 475n, 485n
genetic counseling
  disease carriers 37
  sickle cell disease 131
genetic engineering 242, 479, 491
genetic factors
  hemochromatosis 156
  hemophilia 234, 239–40
  leukemia 171
  sickle cell disease 121, 123, **124**

Information Network, Inc., leukemia
information 169n
infusion therapy
hemophilia 240–41
home-based 241
inheritance *see* heredity
intensification therapy 192
interferon, leukemia treatment 176,
225
interleukin-3 (IL-3) 486
aplastic anemia treatment 45, 47
intraoperative blood collection 493–
94
intrathecal chemotherapy 175–76,
192, 193, 219
iron
absorption 155
Desferal treatment 59–61, 84–87
iron overload 38, **60, 72,** 84–87
Iron Overload Diseases Association,
Inc., contact information 519
"Iron Overload" (Mayo) 526
iron supplements 34
iron-deficiency anemia 34, 54, 110
Ironic Blood (Iron Overload Diseases
Foundation) 525
ischemic lesion, defined 295, 511
isolation
aplastic anemia 43
bone marrow transplants 28
isotrentinoin 403

J

jaundice, sickle cell disease 125
joint problems, hemophilia 233, 244

K

Kaufman, Linda B. 50
Kay, Mark 251
Kessler, David A. 401, 404
kidney disorders
hypertension 329, 331
thalassemia intermedia 93
kissing bug 463
Kogenate 491, 498
Krikker, M. A. 161

L

Landsteiner, Karl 11, 12
Lane, Samuel Armstrong 10
laser therapy
plaques 383, 388–89
sickle cell disease treatment 127
varicose veins 300
LDL cholesterol *see* cholesterol; low-
density lipoprotein (LDL) cholesterol
Lee, Roger 11
Lee-White clotting time 11
Leishmaniasis 446, 473
Lenfant, Claude 249
leukemia 169–227
bone marrow transplants 25, 26, 30
causes 171
clinical trials 528
defined 511
described 169–71
diagnosis 6, 173–74
HTLV 462–63
hydroxyurea 153
information resources 181–82
research 181
symptoms 172–73
treatment 174–81
side effects 178–80
types see also *individual types*
acute lymphocytic leukemia (ALL)
172
acute myeloid leukemia (AML) 172
acute nonlymphocytic leukemia
(ANLL) 172
chronic lymphocytic leukemia
(CLL) 172
chronic myeloid leukemia (CML)
172
hairy cell leukemia 172
leukemia cells 170–71, 172–73
Leukemia Society of America (LSA),
contact information 182, 519
Leukine (sargramostim) 498–99
leukocytes 170
defined 49, 511
described 4
see also white blood cells (WBC)
leukopenia, defined 49, 511

Diabetes Sourcebook, 2nd Edition

Basic Information about Insulin-Dependent Diabetes, Noninsulin-Dependent Diabetes, Gestational Diabetes, and Related Disorders, Including Diabetes Prevalence Data, Management Issues, the Role of Diet and Exercise in Controlling Diabetes, Insulin and Other Diabetes Medicines, and Complications of Diabetes Such as Eye Diseases, Digestive Disorders, Periodontal Disease, Amputation, and End-Stage Renal Disease; Along with Reports on Current Research Initiatives, a Glossary, and Resource Listings for Further Help and Information

Edited by Karen Bellenir. 800 pages. 1998. 0-7808-0224-1. $78.

Diet & Nutrition Sourcebook, 1st Edition

Basic Information about Nutrition, Including the Dietary Guidelines for Americans, the Food Guide Pyramid, and Their Applications in Daily Diet, Nutritional Advice for Specific Age Groups, Current Nutritional Issues and Controversies, the New Food Label and How to Use It to Promote Healthy Eating, and Recent Developments in Nutritional Research

Edited by Dan R. Harris. 662 pages. 1996. 0-7808-0084-2. $78.

"Useful reference as a food and nutrition sourcebook for the general consumer."
— *Booklist Health Sciences Supplement, Oct '97*

"Recommended for public libraries and medical libraries that receive general information requests on nutrition. It is readable and will appeal to those interested in learning more about healthy dietary practices."
— *Medical Reference Services Quarterly, Fall '97*

"An abundance of medical and social statistics is translated into readable information geared toward the general reader."
— *Bookwatch, Mar '97*

"With dozens of questionable diet books on the market, it is so refreshing to find a reliable and factual reference book. Recommended to aspiring professionals, librarians, and others seeking and giving reliable dietary advice. An excellent compilation."
— *Choice, Feb '97*

Diet & Nutrition Sourcebook, 2nd Edition

Basic Information about Nutrition, Including General Nutritional Recommendations, Recommendations for People with Specific Medical Concerns, Dieting for Weight Control, Nutritional Supplements, Food Safety Issues, the Relationship between Nutrition and Disease Development, and Other Nutritional Research Reports; Along with Statistical and Demographic Data, Lifestyle Modification Recommendations, and Sources of Additional Help and Information

Edited by Karen Bellenir. 600 pages. 1998. 0-7808-0228-4. $78.

Ear, Nose & Throat Disorders Sourcebook

Basic Information about Disorders of the Ears, Nose, Sinus Cavities, Pharynx, and Larynx, Including Ear Infections, Tinnitus, Vestibular Disorders, Allergic and Non-Allergic Rhinitis, Sore Throats, Tonsillitis, and Cancers That Affect the Ears, Nose, Sinuses, and Throat, Along with Reports on Current Research Initiatives, a Glossary of Related Medical Terms, and a Directory of Sources for Further Help and Information

Edited by Karen Bellenir and Linda M. Shin. 592 pages. 1998. 0-7808-0206-3. $78.

Endocrine & Metabolic Disorders Sourcebook

Basic Information for the Layperson about Pancreatic and Insulin-Related Disorders Such as Pancreatitis, Diabetes, and Hypoglycemia; Adrenal Gland Disorders Such as Cushing's Syndrome, Addison's Disease, and Congenital Adrenal Hyperplasia; Pituitary Gland Disorders Such as Growth Hormone Deficiency, Acromegaly, and Pituitary Tumors; Thyroid Disorders Such as Hypothyroidism, Graves' Disease, Hashimoto's Disease, and Goiter; Hyperparathyroidism; and Other Diseases and Syndromes of Hormone Imbalance or Metabolic Dysfunction, Along with Reports on Current Research Initiatives

Edited by Linda M. Shin. 632 pages. 1998. 0-7808-0207-1. $78.

Environmentally Induced Disorders Sourcebook

Basic Information about Diseases and Syndromes Linked to Exposure to Pollutants and Other Substances in Outdoor and Indoor Environments Such as Lead, Asbestos, Formaldehyde, Mercury, Emissions, Noise, and More

Edited by Allan R. Cook. 620 pages. 1997. 0-7808-0083-4. $78.

". . . a good survey of numerous environmentally induced physical disorders . . . a useful addition to anyone's library ."
— *Doody's Health Science Book Reviews, Jan '98*

". . . provide[s] introductory information from the best authorities around. Since this volume covers topics that potentially affect everyone, it will surely be one of the most frequently consulted volumes in the *Health Reference Series*."
— *Rettig on Reference, Nov '97*

"Recommended reference source."
— *Booklist, Oct '97*

Fitness & Exercise Sourcebook

Basic Information on Fitness and Exercise, Including Fitness Activities for Specific Age Groups, Exercise for People with Specific Medical Conditions, How to Begin a Fitness Program in Running, Walking, Swimming, Cycling, and Other Athletic Activities, and Recent Research in Fitness and Exercise

Edited by Dan R. Harris. 663 pages. 1996. 0-7808-0186-5. $78.

"A good resource for general readers."
— Choice, Nov '97

"The perennial popularity of the topic . . . make this an appealing selection for public libraries."
— Rettig on Reference, Jun/Jul '97

Food & Animal Borne Diseases Sourcebook

Basic Information about Diseases That Can Be Spread to Humans through the Ingestion of Contaminated Food or Water or by Contact with Infected Animals and Insects, Such as Botulism, E. Coli, Hepatitis A, Trichinosis, Lyme Disease, and Rabies, Along with Information Regarding Prevention and Treatment Methods, and a Special Section for International Travelers Describing Diseases Such as Cholera, Malaria, Travelers' Diarrhea, and Yellow Fever, and Offering Recommendations for Avoiding Illness

Edited by Karen Bellenir and Peter D. Dresser. 535 pages. 1995. 0-7808-0033-8. $78.

"Targeting general readers and providing them with a single, comprehensive source of information on selected topics, this book continues, with the excellent caliber of its predecessors, to catalog topical information on health matters of general interest. Readable and thorough, this valuable resource is highly recommended for all libraries."
— Academic Library Book Review, Summer '96

"A comprehensive collection of authoritative information." *— Emergency Medical Services, Oct '95*

Gastrointestinal Diseases & Disorders Sourcebook

Basic Information about Gastroesophageal Reflux Disease (Heartburn), Ulcers, Diverticulosis, Irritable Bowel Syndrome, Crohn's Disease, Ulcerative Colitis, Diarrhea, Constipation, Lactose Intolerance, Hemorrhoids, Hepatitis, Cirrhosis, and Other Digestive Problems, Featuring Statistics, Descriptions of Symptoms, and Current Treatment Methods of Interest for Persons Living with Upper and Lower Gastrointestinal Maladies

Edited by Linda M. Ross. 413 pages. 1996. 0-7808-0078-8. $78.

". . . very readable form. The successful editorial work that brought this material together into a useful and understandable reference makes accessible to all readers information that can help them more effectively understand and obtain help for digestive tract problems."
— Choice, Feb '97

Genetic Disorders Sourcebook

Basic Information about Heritable Diseases and Disorders Such as Down Syndrome, PKU, Hemophilia, Von Willebrand Disease, Gaucher Disease, Tay-Sachs Disease, and Sickle-Cell Disease, Along with Information about Genetic Screening, Gene Therapy, Home Care, and Including Source Listings for Further Help and Information on More Than 300 Disorders

Edited by Karen Bellenir. 642 pages. 1996. 0-7808-0034-6. $78.

"Provides essential medical information to both the general public and those diagnosed with a serious or fatal genetic disease or disorder." *— Choice, Jan '97*

". . . geared toward the lay public. It would be well placed in all public libraries and in those hospital and medical libraries in which access to genetic references is limited."
— Doody's Health Sciences Book Review, Oct '96

Head Trauma Sourcebook

Basic Information for the Layperson about Open-Head and Closed-Head Injuries, Treatment Advances, Recovery, and Rehabilitation, Along with Reports on Current Research Initiatives

Edited by Karen Bellenir. 414 pages. 1997. 0-7808-0208-X. $78.

Health Insurance Sourcebook

Basic Information about Managed Care Organizations, Traditional Fee-for-Service Insurance, Insurance Portability and Pre-Existing Conditions Clauses, Medicare, Medicaid, Social Security, and Military Health Care, Along with Information about Insurance Fraud

Edited by Wendy Wilcox. 530 pages. 1997. 0-7808-0222-5. $78.

"The layout of the book is particularly helpful as it provides easy access to reference material. A most useful addition to the vast amount of information about health insurance. The use of data from U.S. government agencies is most commendable. Useful in a library or learning center for healthcare professional students."
— Doody's Health Sciences Book Reviews, Nov '97

Immune System Disorders Sourcebook

Basic Information about Lupus, Multiple Sclerosis, Guillain-Barré Syndrome, Chronic Granulomatous Disease, and More, Along with Statistical and Demographic Data and Reports on Current Research Initiatives

Edited by Allan R. Cook. 608 pages. 1997. 0-7808-0209-8. $78.

Kidney & Urinary Tract Diseases & Disorders Sourcebook

Basic Information about Kidney Stones, Urinary Incontinence, Bladder Disease, End Stage Renal Disease, Dialysis, and More, Along with Statistical and Demographic Data and Reports on Current Research Initiatives

Edited by Linda M. Ross. 602 pages. 1997. 0-7808-0079-6. $78.

Learning Disabilities Sourcebook

Basic Information about Disorders Such as Dyslexia, Visual and Auditory Processing Deficits, Attention Deficit/Hyperactivity Disorder, and Autism, Along with Statistical and Demographic Data, Reports on Current Research Initiatives, an Explanation of the Assessment Process, and a Special Section for Adults with Learning Disabilities

Edited by Linda M. Shin. 579 pages. 1998. 0-7808-0210-1. $78.

Men's Health Concerns Sourcebook

Basic Information about Health Issues That Affect Men, Featuring Facts about the Top Causes of Death in Men, Including Heart Disease, Stroke, Cancers, Prostate Disorders, Chronic Obstructive Pulmonary Disease, Pneumonia and Influenza, Human Immunodeficiency Virus and Acquired Immune Deficiency Syndrome, Diabetes Mellitus, Stress, Suicide, Accidents and Homicides; and Facts about Common Concerns for Men, Including Impotence, Contraception, Circumcision, Sleep Disorders, Snoring, Hair Loss, Diet, Nutrition, Exercise, Kidney and Urological Disorders, and Backaches

Edited by Allan R. Cook. 760 pages. 1998. 0-7808-0212-8. $78.

Mental Health Disorders Sourcebook

Basic Information about Schizophrenia, Depression, Bipolar Disorder, Panic Disorder, Obsessive-Compulsive Disorder, Phobias and Other Anxiety Disorders, Paranoia and Other Personality Disorders, Eating Disorders, and Sleep Disorders, Along with Information about Treatment and Therapies

Edited by Karen Bellenir. 548 pages. 1995. 0-7808-0040-0. $78.

"This is an excellent new book . . . written in easy-to-understand language."
— *Booklist Health Science Supplement, Oct '97*

". . . useful for public and academic libraries and consumer health collections."
— *Medical Reference Services Quarterly, Spring '97*

"The great strengths of the book are its readability and its inclusion of places to find more information. Especially recommended." — *RQ, Winter '96*

". . . a good resource for a consumer health library."
— *Bulletin of the MLA, Oct '96*

"The information is data-based and couched in brief, concise language that avoids jargon. . . . a useful reference source." — *Readings, Sept '96*

"The text is well organized and adequately written for its target audience." — *Choice, Jun '96*

". . . provides information on a wide range of mental disorders, presented in nontechnical language."
— *Exceptional Child Education Resources, Spring '96*

"Recommended for public and academic libraries."
— *Reference Book Review, '96*

Ophthalmic Disorders Sourcebook

Basic Information about Glaucoma, Cataracts, Macular Degeneration, Strabismus, Refractive Disorders, and More, Along with Statistical and Demographic Data and Reports on Current Research Initiatives

Edited by Linda M. Ross. 631 pages. 1996. 0-7808-0081-8. $78.

Oral Health Sourcebook

Basic Information about Diseases and Conditions Affecting Oral Health, Including Cavities, Gum Disease, Dry Mouth, Oral Cancers, Fever Blisters, Canker Sores, Oral Thrush, Bad Breath, Temporomandibular Disorders, and other Craniofacial Syndromes, Along with Statistical Data on the Oral Health of Americans, Oral Hygiene, Emergency First Aid, Information on Treatment Procedures and Methods of Replacing Lost Teeth

Edited by Allan R. Cook. 558 pages. 1997. 0-7808-0082-6. $78.

"Recommended reference source." — *Booklist, Dec '97*

Pain Sourcebook

Basic Information about Specific Forms of Acute and Chronic Pain, Including Headaches, Back Pain, Muscular Pain, Neuralgia, Surgical Pain, and Cancer Pain, Along with Pain Relief Options Such as Analgesics, Narcotics, Nerve Blocks, Transcutaneous Nerve Stimulation, and Alternative Forms of Pain Control, Including Biofeedback, Imaging, Behavior Modification, and Relaxation Techniques

Edited by Allan R. Cook. 667 pages. 1997. 0-7808-0213-6. $78.

"The information is basic in terms of scholarship and is appropriate for general readers. Written in journalistic style . . . intended for non-professionals. Quite thorough in its coverage of different pain conditions and summarizes the latest clinical information regarding pain treatment."
— *Choice, Jun '98*

"Recommended reference source."
— *Booklist, Mar '98*

Pregnancy & Birth Sourcebook

Basic Information about Planning for Pregnancy, Maternal Health, Fetal Growth and Development, Labor and Delivery, Postpartum and Perinatal Care, Pregnancy in Mothers with Special Concerns, and Disorders of Pregnancy, Including Genetic Counseling, Nutrition and Exercise, Obstetrical Tests, Pregnancy Discomfort, Multiple Births, Cesarean Sections, Medical Testing of Newborns, Breastfeeding, Gestational Diabetes, and Ectopic Pregnancy

Edited by Heather E. Aldred. 737 pages. 1997. 0-7808-0216-0. $78.

". . . for the layperson. A well-organized handbook. Recommended for college libraries . . . general readers."
— *Choice, Apr '98*

"Recommended reference source."
— *Booklist, Mar '98*

"This resource is recommended for public libraries to have on hand."
— *American Reference Books Annual, '98*

Public Health Sourcebook

Basic Information about Government Health Agencies, Including National Health Statistics and Trends, Healthy People 2000 Program Goals and Objectives, the Centers for Disease Control and Prevention, the Food and Drug Administration, and the National Institutes of Health, Along with Full Contact Information for Each Agency

Edited by Wendy Wilcox. 698 pages. 1998. 0-7808-0220-9. $78.

Rehabilitation Sourcebook

Basic Information for the Layperson about Physical Medicine (Physiatry) and Rehabilitative Therapies, Including Physical, Occupational, Recreational, Speech, and Vocational Therapy; Along with Descriptions of Devices and Equipment Such as Orthotics, Gait Aids, Prostheses, and Adaptive Systems Used during Rehabilitation and for Activities of Daily Living, and Featuring a Glossary and Source Listings for Further Help and Information

Edited by Theresa K. Murray. 600 pages. 1998. 0-7808-0236-5. $78.

Respiratory Diseases & Disorders Sourcebook

Basic Information about Respiratory Diseases and Disorders, Including Asthma, Cystic Fibrosis, Pneumonia, the Common Cold, Influenza, and Others, Featuring Facts about the Respiratory System, Statistical and Demographic Data, Treatments, Self-Help Management Suggestions, and Current Research Initiatives

Edited by Allan R. Cook and Peter D. Dresser. 771 pages. 1995. 0-7808-0037-0. $78.

"Designed for the layperson and for patients and their families coping with respiratory illness. . . . an extensive array of information on diagnosis, treatment, management, and prevention of respiratory illnesses for the general reader."
— *Choice, Jun '96*

"A highly recommended text for all collections. It is a comforting reminder of the power of knowledge that good books carry between their covers."
— *Academic Library Book Review, Spring '96*

"This sourcebook offers a comprehensive collection of authoritative information presented in a nontechnical, humanitarian style for patients, families, and caregivers."
— *Association of Operating Room Nurses, Sept/Oct '95*

Sexually Transmitted Diseases Sourcebook

Basic Information about Herpes, Chlamydia, Gonorrhea, Hepatitis, Nongonoccocal Urethritis, Pelvic Inflammatory Disease, Syphilis, AIDS, and More, Along with Current Data on Treatments and Preventions

Edited by Linda M. Ross. 550 pages. 1997. 0-7808-0217-9. $78.